Autism and Pervasive Developmental Disorders

Second edition

Edited by

Fred R. Volkmar

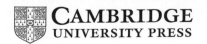
CAMBRIDGE
UNIVERSITY PRESS

CAMBRIDGE UNIVERSITY PRESS

Cambridge, New York, Melbourne, Madrid, Cape Town, Singapore, São Paulo

Cambridge University Press
The Edinburgh Building, Cambridge CB2 8RU, UK

Published in the United States of America by Cambridge University Press, New York

www.cambridge.org
Information on this title: www.cambridge.org/9780521549574

First published 2007

Printed in the United Kingdom at the University Press, Cambridge

A catalog record for this publication is available from the British Library

ISBN-13 978-0-521-54957-4 paperback

Contents

Contributors

Craig A. Erickson
Department of Psychiatry
Indiana University School of Medicine
1111 W. 10th Street
Indianapolis
IN 46202-4800
USA

Deborah Fein
234 Bliss Hall
The College of New Jersey
Ewing
NJ 08629
USA

Eric Fombonne
Department of Psychiatry
Montreal Children's Hospital
4018 Ste. Catherine West
Montreal
QC, H3Z 1P2
Canada

Sandra L. Harris
Graduate School of Applied and Professional
Psychology
P. O. Box 819
Rutgers
The State University of New Jersey
Piscataway
NJ 08855-0819
USA

Patricia Howlin
Department of Psychology
Institute of Psychiatry
Denmark Hill
London SE5 8AF
UK

Marshall B. Jones
Department of Psychiatry
McMaster University
Faculty of Health Sciences
P. O. Box 850
Hamilton L8N 3S5
Canada

Catherine Lord
Departments of Psychology
Psychiatry
and Pediatrics
University of Michigan Autism and
Communicative Disorders Center (UMACC),
Departments of Psychology, Psychiatry, and
Pediatrics
Ann Arbor
Michigan
USA

Christopher J. McDougle
Department of Psychiatry
Indiana University School of Medicine
1111 W. 10th Street
PB A305
Indianapolis
IN 46202-4800
USA

Emily G. W. Nichols
234 Bliss Hall
The College of New Jersey
Ewing
NJ 08629
USA

Sally Ozonoff
MIND Institute and Department of
Psychiatry
University of California – Davis
Sacramento
CA 95817
USA

Rhea Paul
Southern Connecticut State University
P. O. Box 207900
New Haven
CT 06520
USA

David J. Posey
Department of Psychiatry
Indiana University School of Medicine
1111 W. 10th Street
Indianapolis
IN 46202-4800
USA

Fritz Poustka
Department of Child and Adolescent
Psychiatry
J. W. Goethe University
Deutschordenstrasse 50
D-60590 Frankfurt-am-Main
Germany

Margot Prior
School of Behavioural Sciences
University of Melbourne
VIC 3010
Australia

Kimberly A. Stigler
Department of Psychiatry
Indiana University School of Medicine
1111 W. 10th Street
Indianapolis
IN 46202-4800
USA

Peter Szatmari
Offord Centre for Child Studies
McMaster University
Chedoke Site
Patterson Bldg
Hamilton, Ontario
Canada L8N 3Z5

Fred R. Volkmar
Child Study Center
Yale University
P. O. Box 207900
New Haven
CT 06520
USA

Lynn Waterhouse
234 Bliss Hall
The College of New Jersey
Ewing
NJ 08629
USA

Preface to the second edition

Interest in what is now recognized as the pervasive developmental disorders can be traced to the middle of the nineteenth century with the first descriptions of childhood "psychosis" (Volkmar, 1996). This interest stemmed from an increasing awareness of the importance of the factors of both experience and endowment in child development. Early descriptions of childhood "insanity" were followed by descriptions of childhood schizophrenia (DeSanctis, 1906). The latter term became synonymous with all forms of severe mental disorder in children. The particular genius of Leo Kanner was reflected in his description in 1943 of the syndrome of infantile autism, which he initially believed to be quite different from the forms of childhood "psychosis" then recognized. In the subsequent six decades autism has been the focus of considerable interest from clinicians and researchers alike so that, for example, a large body of work both on research and intervention is now available (Volkmar *et al.*, 2005).

Autism has been the focus of a very substantial body of work. While major advances have been made in both treatment (NRC, 2001) and research (Volkmar *et al.*, 2005) precise pathophysiological models have yet to be specified. In an attempt to specify such models essentially all the theories of psychology and neurobiology have been utilized. While specification of such mechanisms remains an important, if as yet unrealized, goal considerable accomplishments have been made.

A substantial body of research has established the validity of autism as a diagnostic concept, e.g. on the basis of its characteristic clinical features and course. The neurobiological basis of the disorder has been established and better and more effective treatment methods have been developed. Recent attention has focused on genetic mechanisms in autism as well as on the spectrum of conditions that share some similarities with autism and which are now included in the category of pervasive developmental disorder. Some of these conditions, such as Asperger's and Rett's syndromes, were proposed after Kanner's classic description of autism whereas others, notably childhood disintegrative disorder, were proposed many years before Kanner's work.

This book reflects the considerable progress that has been made in recent years in our understanding of autism and related conditions. In this second edition the contributors have summarized current knowledge in various areas. The contributors represent various disciplines and provide truly international perspectives on current research in autism and related conditions.

The first chapter provides an overview of current approaches to diagnosis and definition of autism and related conditions. Catherine Lord and I review the development of diagnostic concepts and the rationale for the definitions presently employed in both ICD-10 (1993) and DSM-IV (1994). While these definitions have retained an importantly historical continuity with earlier ones they also reflect advances in knowledge and are based on a large body of empirical data (Volkmar *et al.*, 1994). More importantly the international (ICD-10) and American (DSM-IV) depictions are now conceptually convergent.

Advances in diagnosis have improved methods of case detection and are reflected in the results of more recent epidemiological studies. Such research tells us about the prevalence of these disorders and helps in planning for service delivery. Eric Fombonne provides a helpful summary of present knowledge in this area. As he notes, an even larger group of children has impairments in social interaction, and the characterization of their difficulties remains an important area for future research.

Studies of the cognitive and neurocognitive development of individuals with autism have made it clear that it is necessary to study individuals carefully with different levels of cognitive ability using various approaches. Margot Prior and Sally Ozonoff have summarized the literature on this topic with a particular emphasis on those findings most specific to autism. Their chapter is a masterful summary of a large and diverse literature and outlines areas of work that are of particular interest, e.g. in executive functioning.

Children and adolescents with autism and related conditions exhibit major difficulties in the area of communication. In this second edition we are pleased to have Rhea Paul provide a chapter summarizing what is known both about the fundamental difficulties in this area as well as techniques for intervention. Her chapter addresses an important gap in coverage and will be of great interest to all readers.

The importance of genetic factors in the pathogenesis of autism was relatively underappreciated until quite recently. Somewhat paradoxically the field has gone from a situation in which it was believed that genetic factors had little importance for syndrome pathogenesis to the present situation where it appears that such factors have major importance and where specific genetic mechanisms may indeed be identified in the relatively near future. Peter Szatmari and Marshall Jones' chapter reviews this work and notes the major changes in our understanding of genetic factors in recent years. As he observes, the issue today is not whether autism has a genetic basis but what that basis is.

The relevance of neurobiological factors in the pathogenesis of autism has undergone a similar transformation. At the time of his original description Kanner (1943) minimized the importance of such factors. Now it appears that such factors may be present in 10% or more of cases (Rutter *et al.*, 1994). While the nature of such associations has been debated (Gillberg and Coleman, 1996) these do suggest important areas for research in underlying pathophysiological mechanisms. Fritz Poutska provides a critical summary of this work and notes areas in which knowledge is still lacking.

Given the severity of autism and associated conditions it is probably not surprising that essentially every conceivable intervention has been attempted. Christopher McDougle and colleagues provide a current review of pharmacological treatments. As noted in their chapter recent work suggests important potential benefits of drug treatments in selected cases as one aspect of a total program of intervention.

Over the past 50 years a considerable body of data has established the centrality of intensive, structured, educational intervention as the bedrock of intervention in autism. This work has its origins both in behavioral psychology and special education. As Sandra Harris notes progress continues to be made in behavioral and educational interventions that have improved the outcome of autism and related conditions. Patricia Howlin summarizes these changes in her review of outcome studies. The child with autism or a related condition presents major challenges for parents, siblings, and other family members. However, the improvement in outcome is a major accomplishment of the past 50 years of clinical work and reflects the substantial gains in implementation of remedial programs.

In the final chapter Lynn Waterhouse, Deborah Fein and Emily Nicholas address the nature of the fundamental social disturbance which characterizes autism. The centrality of social deficits in the definition of this, and related conditions, has repeatedly been emphasized in depictions of the disorder beginning with Kanner's initial description. Despite this we continue to have a rather limited understanding of the nature of social deficits in syndrome pathogenesis. The authors provide an interesting synthesis of work in this area.

This book provides a summary of what is known as well as what remains poorly understood. While researchers and clinicians have learned much over the past five decades of work on autism we continue to have little understanding of the nature of the autistic social dysfunction nor, for that matter, of its underlying neurobiological basis. There are, however, reasons to be hopeful. Advances in treatment (both behavioral and pharmacological) have led to improved outcomes. Current work underscores the possibility that at least some form or forms of autism may have a strong genetic component and it is possible that some genetic mechanism may be described in the relatively near future; such a finding will advance research in other areas as well, as we begin to understand pathogenic mechanisms more fully. The chapters in this book are a testament to the advances that have been made as well as to the continuing need for research and treatment of these perplexing conditions.

I am grateful to all the chapter authors for their contributions to this volume. In addition I wish to thank the series editor, Professor Goodyer, as well as Pauline Graham and the staff of Cambridge University Press for their help and support.

REFERENCES

American Psychiatric Association (1980). *Diagnostic and Statistical Manual of Mental Disorders*, 3rd edn (DSM III). Washington, DC: American Psychiatric Association; 3rd edn revised (DSM-III-R), 1987; 4th edn (DSM-IV), 1994.

DeSanctis S. (1906). Sopra alcune varieta della demenzi precoce. *Revista Sperimentale de Feniatria e di Medicina Legale*, **32**, 141–65.

Kanner, L. (1943). Autistic disturbances of affective contact. *Nervous Child*, **2**, 217–50.

Gillberg, C. and Coleman, M. (1996). Autism and medical disorders: a review of the literature. *Developmental Medicine and Child Neurology*, **38**(3), 191–202.

National Research Council (2001). *Educating Children with Autism*. Washington, DC: National Academy of Sciences Press.

Rutter, M., Bailey, A., Bolton, P. and Le Couteur, A. (1994). Autism and known medical conditions: myth and substance. *Journal of Child Psychology and Psychiatry*, **35**(2), 311–22.

Volkmar, F. R. (1996). Childhood and adolescent psychosis: a review of the past 10 years. *Journal of the American Academy of Child and Adolescent Psychiatry*, **35**, 843–51.

Volkmar, F. R., Klin, A., Siegel, B. *et al.* (1994). Field trial for autistic disorder in DSM-IV. *American Journal of Psychiatry*, **151**, 1361–7.

Volkmar, F. R., Klin, A., Paul, R., and Cohen, D. J., eds. (2005). *Handbook of Autism and Pervasive Developmental Disorders*, 3rd edn. New York: John Wiley and Sons.

World Health Organization. (1992). *International Statistical Classification of Diseases and Related Health Problems*, 10th edn (ICD-10). Geneva: World Health Organization.

1

Diagnosis and definition of autism and other pervasive developmental disorders

Fred R. Volkmar
Child Study Center, Yale University

Catherine Lord
Department of Psychology, Psychiatry and Pediatrics, University of Michigan

Introduction

Autism and other pervasive developmental disorders (PDDs) are a phenomenologically related set of neuropsychiatric disorders. These conditions are characterized by patterns of both delay and deviance in multiple areas of development; typically their onset is in the first months of life (APA, 1994; Volkmar & Klin, 2005). Although often associated with some degree of mental retardation, the pattern of developmental and behavioral features differs from that seen in children with mental retardation not associated with PDD in that certain sectors of development, such as social interaction and communication, are most severely affected whereas other areas, such as nonverbal cognitive abilities, may be within normal limits. While the validity of autism has been relatively well established, issues of syndrome boundaries remain the topic of some debate (Bailey *et al.*, 1996). In this chapter, the development of autism as a diagnostic concept, current definitions of the condition and of related diagnostic concepts, and their differentiation from other disorders will be reviewed.

Development of diagnostic concepts

Over the past 150 years, a major point of controversy has been the continuity, or discontinuity, of the severe psychiatric disorders of childhood with the adult psychoses. For example, the great British psychiatrist Maudsley suggested that children, like adults, could exhibit "insanity" (1867). Similarly Kraepelin's

Autism and Pervasive Developmental Disorders, 2nd edn, ed. Fred R. Volkmar.
Published by Cambridge University Press. © Cambridge University Press 2007.

concept of dementia praecox, or what we would now term schizophrenia, was extended to children (dementia praecocissima) (DeSanctis, 1906). While some investigators like Potter (1933) urged the use of more stringent definitions for childhood schizophrenia, there was a general assumption of a fundamental continuity of child and adult "psychosis." The presumption of continuity was based largely on the severity of these conditions with rather little appreciation of the importance of developmental factors in children's understanding of reality. These issues contributed to the confusion and controversy that surrounded Kanner's initial (1943) description of the autistic syndrome.

Kanner's description of autism

Kanner's description of 11 children with "autistic disturbances of affective contact" was atheoretical and quite lucid; present definitions of the autistic syndrome remain profoundly influenced by it. Kanner reported that his patients exhibited a disorder characterized by a profound lack of social engagement starting from, or shortly after, their birth; as they reached toddlerhood they also exhibited a range of communication problems and unusual responses to the inanimate environment. These children might, for example, not be particularly responsive to the comings and goings of their parents but be exquisitely sensitive to a small change in the inanimate environment or routine, such as a kitchen cupboard left open. Three of the 11 children were mute, but the language of those who did speak was remarkable for echolalia, literalness, and pronoun reversal.

Although not cooperative with formal psychometric assessment, these children could sometimes be engaged on certain subtests of cognitive or developmental tests and seemed to do well. Because of this, and because of their usually attractive appearance, Kanner speculated that they probably had good intellectual potential. In his original report, he suggested that the disorder was different from other psychiatric conditions and not associated with specific medical conditions. Kanner also mentioned that in many instances, parents, usually the fathers, were remarkably successful and that interactions with the child often seemed strange or odd; on the other hand, his emphasis on the apparently congenital nature of the problem made it difficult to attribute the disorder exclusively to parent–child disturbance.

In Kanner's view, the essential feature of autism was the children's inability to relate. He put this observation within a developmental context citing the work of Gessel on early social development. The use of Bleuler's (1911/1950) term "autism" for the idiosyncratic, self-centered thinking observed in schizophrenia was intended by Kanner to suggest the notion of the child's living in his or her own world. However, his use of this word and certain aspects of his original report, when interpreted literally, proved to be false leads.

Early studies and false leads for research

Kanner's use of the term "autism" immediately suggested schizophrenia; this was consistent with the very broad and inclusive views of schizophrenia which then were dominant. Many clinicians and researchers did not question longstanding assumptions about severe psychiatric disturbance in children. Unfortunately this meant that there was considerable confusion about autism with some investigators, e.g. Bender (1947), assuming continuity of "psychotic" conditions in younger children with more typical adult forms of schizophrenia. As this has proved not to be the case, it makes it difficult to interpret much of the early work on autism. The issue of continuity of autism and schizophrenia was only resolved in the 1970s as the work of Rutter (1970) and Kolvin (1971) suggested important differences between the conditions, e.g. in course, family history, and clinical features.

As cases of autism were followed for a decade it became apparent that Kanner's original assumption that autism was not associated with any medical condition was also not correct. Many children with autism exhibit signs of overt central nervous system dysfunction including, most strikingly, seizures. As many as 25% of cases developed epilepsy, particularly during adolescence (Volkmar & Nelson, 1990). Other signs of neurological dysfunction were also often observed. Some reports associated autism with diverse medical conditions including chromosomal abnormalities, prenatal infections, various brain abnormalities, and so on. When taken together with the data on neurological dysfunction, these findings seemed to suggest the importance of multiple potential insults which acted through one or more mechanisms to cause autism (Rutter *et al.*, 1994).

Similarly, Kanner's assumption that children with autism had normal intellectual potentials proved mistaken. This notion was based on the accurate observation that "splinter skills" were present in some children with autism and that the occasional individual with autism had truly unusual (and usually very isolated) abilities in one area (Hermelin, 2001). It took over two decades before clinicians and investigators realized that, if *all* aspects of a test of intelligence were administered, many children with autism scored in the mentally retarded range in terms of overall IQ. For many years, low IQ scores were mistakenly attributed to willful noncompliance. In any case, the notion of preserved intellectual skills in individuals with autism, who have otherwise very limited abilities, endures to the present and is the basis for unproven and sometimes fraudulent treatment. Conversely, recent epidemiological studies have indicated that a much higher proportion of children with autism are not mentally retarded than occurred in autism samples 30 to 40 years ago (Fombonne, 2005).

Perhaps, most unfortunately, Kanner's's observation of high levels of parental achievement and unusual parent–child interactions led some clinicians to attribute the source of autism to problems in the parent–child relationship or deficits in child care, e.g. Bettelheim (1967). This view was congruent with the ethos of the time which tended to minimize the importance of biological factors in psychiatric conditions. The ideas seemed superficially consistent with the nature of the disorder, i.e. should it not be the case that a problem characterized by deficits in social interaction is caused by deficiencies in social interaction? However, as controlled studies were conducted, it became clear that the parents of children with autism did not exhibit high degrees of psychopathology (Cox et al., 1975) nor specific deficits in infant caregiving (Cantwell et al., 1978). A growing appreciation of the role of the child in parent–child interactions also suggested that it was just as reasonable to assume that deviance in such interaction might sometimes be a function of a basic disturbance in the child rather than in the parent, i.e. interactions with a child who produces highly deviant social behaviors will differ from interactions with children who do not have this disability. Similarly, the idea that parents of autistic children tended to have much higher levels of occupational and educational achievement proved mistaken. Studies that controlled for possible bias in case detection and referral (Schopler et al., 1980a; Wing, 1980) have suggested that autism is seen in all social classes. It seems likely that the high levels of education in parents of Kanner's original cases resulted from an understandable referral bias, i.e. that the parents who were able to locate Kanner were those who had access to a greater array of resources. It must, however, be noted that good, recent epidemiological data on this issue have been lacking (Rutter, 2005). The lack of studies on potential cultural and ethnic differences is also noteworthy (Brown & Rogers, 2003).

"Nonautistic" pervasive developmental disorders

As noted above, the issue of continuity of adult and child forms of schizophrenia was, until quite recently, a major source of confusion. But over the past century, various diagnostic concepts other than autism have been proposed for patterns of disturbance in children with severe developmental disorders. Three of these conditions are now officially recognized in both DSM-IV and ICD-10.

Childhood disintegrative disorder

Heller (1908, 1930/1969) proposed the term "dementia infantilis," or what now would be termed childhood disintegrative disorder (CDD), to account for children who develop normally for some period prior to profound developmental regression and the development of many "autistic-like" features. This condition (also sometimes referred to as Heller's syndrome or disintegrative psychosis), appears to be very uncommon; over 100 cases have been reported since Heller's original (1908) report (see Volkmar et al., 2005). It is, however, likely that cases have frequently been misdiagnosed (Volkmar & Klin, 2005).

Childhood disintegrative disorder is now included in both DSM-IV and ICD-10 (see Appendix 1.A, pp. 21–25). The condition is difficult to distinguish from autism once it develops. However, the pattern of onset – including a dramatic developmental deterioration and onset of various "autistic-like" behaviors in a previously apparently normal child – is very highly distinctive. The outcome appears to be worse than that in autism (Volkmar, 1992). The presumption in DSM-III and III-R had been that such cases typically resulted from the presence of a significant neuropathological process, e.g. a childhood "dementia"; however, a review of the published cases suggests that this is not the case. There is an increased rate of EEG abnormalities and seizure disorders similar to that in autism, but specific medical conditions that might account for the regression are not usually identified. The relationship, if any, of this condition and "late-onset" or "regressive" autism (see below) merits further study (Siperstein and Volkmar, 2004; Volkmar & Klin, 2005).

Asperger's disorder

In 1944, Hans Asperger, a Viennese medical student unaware of Kanner's earlier report, suggested the concept of autistic psychopathy or what is now usually termed Asperger's disorder. Asperger's description resembled that of Kanner (1943) in some ways, e.g. in the use of the word autism/autistic to describe marked problems in social interaction. However, Asperger suggested that the condition he described was seen only in males, was observed in the face of relatively strong language and cognitive skills, and tended to run in families. Unusual, idiosyncratic interests were common, e.g. affected children would have marked interests in acquiring certain kinds of knowledge. Early research on the condition was largely confined to non-English speaking Europe until Wing's (1981) influential literature review and case series. Subsequent work has yielded somewhat contradictory results (e.g. Pomeroy, 1991; Szatmari et al., 1990; Tantam, 1991); however, this may be a function of the absence, until recently, of generally recognized definitions. While the continuity of Asperger's disorder with autism remains the topic of debate (Klin et al., 1995; Schopler, 1985) the condition has now been included in DSM-IV and ICD-10 (see Appendix 1.A, p. 21).

The overlap of Asperger's disorder with other diagnostic concepts remains an important topic for research (see Klin *et al.*, 2005). One set of issues has to do with the validity of the diagnostic concept as different from "higher functioning autism." Available data on this question remain somewhat contradictory, again reflecting, at least in part, the inconsistencies in approaches to diagnosis (see Klin *et al.*, 2005). Careful reading of the original reports by Kanner (1943) and Asperger (1944; reprinted 1991) as well as a recent review of Asperger's subsequent cases (Hippler & Klicpera, 2003) suggest several possible points of differentiation. Kanner suggested that in autism the condition was congenital; Asperger thought that the syndrome he identified came to attention only after age 3 or 4 years. In Asperger's disorder language skills are usually an area of strength. In contrast, even in higher-functioning individuals with autism, verbal skills tend not to be advanced over nonverbal ones. Several studies have suggested that different IQ profiles characterize the two conditions. Asperger's disorder is associated with higher, often much higher, verbal IQ whereas in autism verbal IQ is either lower or roughly on a par with nonverbal IQ (Klin & Shepard, 1994; Volkmar *et al.*, 1994). Asperger's disorder may also be associated with a characteristic profile on neuropsychological testing referred to as a nonverbal learning disability (Rourke, 1989; Klin & Shepard, 1994). However, the most common finding in comparisons of autism and Asperger's disorder is that whatever feature is used to distinguish the two groups during ascertainment (e.g. severity of autistic characteristics, age of onset, strength of language skills, deficits in visuospatial and motor skills) continues to differentiate them. In the long run, the question will be whether it is scientifically or clinically helpful to classify individuals with these patterns into separate categories of autism and Asperger's disorder or whether it would be better to treat them as part of a greater continuum.

A major series of questions stems from a more complex issue – the broader phenotype of autism (Le Couteur *et al.*, 1996; Pickles *et al.*, 2000). Somewhat paradoxically, the achievement of a consensus on a rigorous definition of autism has led to an awareness of a broader range of difficulties in social interaction, communication, and behavior that affect relatives (see Rutter, 2005 and Chapter 5). As awareness of autism has grown so has awareness of the "broader spectrum" and the large group of individuals with social difficulties. There has been, on the part of the public and media, a tendency to equate such difficulties with "mild" autism and Asperger's disorder; this, and the awareness of the large number of individuals with some social oddity has tended to blur the boundaries between clinical disorders and eccentricity and oddity within the broad range of normal.

It is clear that, compared to work on autism, there has been much less research on the problems of individuals with social difficulties that are more broadly defined. In addition, other diagnostic concepts, derived from diverse disciplines, have been developed; thus, terms like semantic–pragmatic language impairment (Bishop & Norbury, 2002), attention deficit disorder plus PDD (Hellgren *et al.*, 1994), right hemisphere learning problems (Weintraub & Mesulam, 1983), and schizoid disorder (Wolff, 2000) have called attention to specific features that overlap with those of PDDs. The specificity of all of these disorders is unclear. An increased understanding of the relationship of Asperger's disorder to all these conditions and the broader phenotype of autism remains an important area of study.

Rett's disorder

Rett (1966) reported an unusual syndrome, observed only in girls where a very brief period (months) of normal development is followed by decelerated head growth, loss of purposeful hand movements, and the development of severe psychomotor retardation. Characteristic symptoms such as breath-holding spells, air-swallowing, and mid-line hand-wringing or hand-washing stereotypies develop and language skills become severely impaired. By preschool, motor involvement is very significant; an apparent loss of social skills is most evident during this period although social interest will subsequently increase.

Rett's syndrome differs from autism in important ways (van Acker *et al.*, 2005); however, because of the regression, repetitive behaviors, and decrease in social interest, there is the possibility for confusion, particularly during the preschool years. Usually, however, the diagnosis is relatively straightforward (see Hagberg *et al.*, 1983). The condition was included within the PDD group in both ICD-10 and DSM-IV because of the potential for confusion and a concern that it should be listed somewhere in the manuals (Rutter, 1994). Given its distinctive pattern there was also a strong sense that a specific etiology might be found.

The condition is relatively rare, affecting perhaps 1 in 15 000 to 1 in 22 000 females (Fombonne, 2005); the condition almost exclusively occurs in females. A role for genetic factors was suggested by recurrence in family members and in monozygotic twins. The recent identification of methyl CpG binding protein 2 as the cause of a majority of cases of classic Rett's syndrome (Amir *et al.*, 1999) may turn out to provide important clues and promising approaches to genetic studies of other conditions such as CDD (Volkmar *et al.*, 2005).

Pervasive developmental disorder not otherwise specified: atypical autism

The term pervasive developmental disorder not otherwise specified (PDD-NOS) (also referred to as atypical personality development, atypical PDD, or atypical autism) was included in DSM-IV to encompass "subthreshold" cases. It is intended to describe individuals who have a marked impairment of social inter-action and communication difficulties, and/or stereotyped behavior patterns or interests suggestive of a PDD but who do not meet criteria for any of the formally defined disorders in that class. ICD-10 (see Appendix 1.A, pp. 21–24) adopts a somewhat different approach in that the term can be used when a case meets behavioral criteria for autism but fails the onset criteria, or when the onset criteria are met but the behavioral criteria are not, or when individuals appear to have an "autistic-like" illness but meet neither the onset nor behavioral criteria. It seems likely that many possible subtypes are encompassed within this category (Towbin, 2005). Szatmari and colleagues (Mahoney *et al.*, 1998) and other inves-tigators have suggested that this term is used for individuals who meet social and communication criteria for autism but do not have repetitive behaviors or interests. If this distinction is stable across development, it helps increase the homogeneity of a group of individuals with autism spectrum disorder (ASD). Although introduced to encompass "subthreshold' cases in official classifications, the concept also has its origins in earlier notions, e.g. Rank's concept of atypical personality development (Rank, 1949).

The limited available evidence suggest that children with PDD-NOS probably come to professional attention rather later than those with autism. This may reflect the fact that intellectual and language skills tend to be more preserved (Towbin, 2005). Some have argued that PDD-NOS and Asperger's disorder are synonymous terms. As with Asperger's disorder, the validity of PDD-NOS as a separate disorder rather than as a "range" of behaviors will depend on its value in determining etiology or treatment. More research on continuities of all these conditions is needed.

Approaches to the diagnosis of autism

Definitions of autism subsequent to Kanner

The controversy surrounding the nature of autism and the dearth of careful research studies impeded progress for many years. Starting in the 1970s, however, there was a growing appreciation that autism was indeed a distinctive condition, *not* simply the earliest manifestation of childhood schizophrenia. For example, Rutter (1970) also noted the frequency of seizures and the considerable evidence for some degree of neurobiological involvement. In a classic series of clinical studies, Kolvin (1971) demonstrated that autism and childhood schizophrenia differed in clinical features, course, and family history. In addition, there was a growing tendency to de-emphasize the role of theory and establish reliable descriptions of the syndrome in research. As a result of these developments, there were various efforts to develop guidelines for the diagnosis of autism which would facilitate research; this approach paralleled attempts in adult psychiatry to develop precise definitions of syndromes for research purposes, e.g. Spitzer Williams (1988).

Of these early attempts to develop more precise categorical definitions, Rutter's (1978) is undoubtedly the most important. This definition was fundamentally grounded in Kanner's early phenomenological description of the condition, but also recognized the importance of subsequent research. Rutter suggested that there were four features essential for the diagnosis of autism:

(1) an onset prior to 30 months of age;
(2) impaired social development of a distinctive type which did not simply reflect associated mental retardation;
(3) impaired communicative development, which again was distinctive and not simply the result of an overall cognitive delay;
(4) the presence of unusual behaviors subsumed under the concept of "insistence on sameness," i.e. resistance to change, idiosyncratic responses to the environment, and so on.

This definition particularly shaped the first official categorical definition of autism.

The categorical definition of autism

DSM-III

In DSM-III (APA, 1980) autism was accorded diagnostic status for the first time. This inclusion reflected the body of work on autism which had accumulated over the previous decade. In DSM-III, the condition, termed infantile autism, was included in a new class of disorders, the PDDs. Several other conditions, including a separate category for Childhood-onset pervasive developmental disorder, and another category, termed "residual" autism, were also included in this class. Although the term PDD was rather cumbersome, it achieved relatively wide acceptance. The DSM-III definition of infantile autism was much influenced by Rutter's earlier work and emphasized the onset of serious disturbances in social and communicative development and unusual patterns of environmental responsiveness in early childhood. The recognition of autism in DSM-III was a major advance, as was the availability of an officially recognized definition of the condition.

Unfortunately, the other categories proposed and some of the decisions made were less constructive. Partly in response to the early confusion about autism and schizophrenia, the two conditions were made mutually exclusive. While the available data suggested that the two conditions are not, in fact, commonly associated, there is no reason why having autism would necessarily act to *protect* a person from subsequently developing schizophrenia. A few such cases of individuals with autism who then also develop schizophrenia, have, in fact, been observed (Volkmar & Cohen, 1991). Similarly, the term "residual autism" was used in cases where the individual's disorder had once met criteria for infantile autism but no longer did so. In essence, this approach reflected the fact that the criteria proposed for infantile autism emphasized the way the condition presented in early childhood, e.g. with more "pervasive" social deficits. The system did not adequately address the fact that older children and adults continued to exhibit autism which changed somewhat in its expression over the course of development. The term "residual" also had the unfortunate effect of suggesting that somehow children "outgrew" autism; this clearly is *not* usually the case (Howlin, 2005; Rumsey *et al.*, 1985). As a result of these concerns, major changes were made in the definition of autism in DSM-III-R (APA, 1987).

DSM-III-R

In DSM-III-R, the term pervasive developmental disorders was retained to describe the overarching diagnostic class to which autism was assigned. The more problematic diagnostic concepts, e.g. Childhood-onset PDD and residual autism, were eliminated. The DSM-III-R definition was specifically designed to be more developmentally oriented and to be appropriate to the entire range of syndrome expression over both age and developmental level. This was reflected in the new name "autistic disorder" rather than the DSM-III term "infantile autism." DSM-III-R included more criteria and a polythetic definition. Because of various concerns, age of onset was not included as an essential diagnostic feature. Criteria in DSM-III-R were arranged developmentally and grouped in three broad categories relating to social development, communication and play, and restricted activities and interests. This last category reflects an expansion of the earlier concept of "insistence on sameness" included in previous diagnostic schemes. For a diagnosis of autism, an individual was required to exhibit at least 8 of the 16 criteria with at least 2 of the social and 1 from each of the two remaining groups. In DSM-III-R only autism and the "subthreshold" category PDD-NOS were included in the PDD class.

The strong developmental orientation of DSM-III-R was a major improvement. Unfortunately it was quickly apparent that the new scheme had resulted in a significantly broadened diagnostic concept (Volkmar *et al.*, 1988; Factor *et al.*, 1989; Hertzig *et al.*, 1990). This broadening was a source of considerable concern for many reasons. It complicated the task of interpreting research (see Rutter & Schopler, 1992 for a discussion). Differences from the pending revision of the international diagnostic system, the International Classification of Diseases (10th edition; ICD-10) (WHO, 1990), were also marked.

ICD-10

The ICD-10 system provided separate clinical descriptions and research criteria. Major differences in both criteria for autism and disorders from previous diagnostic systems were noteworthy. The draft ICD-10 research definition included age of onset as an essential diagnostic feature and included more detailed and numerous criteria for autism. In addition, other disorders in the PDD class included Rett's syndrome, Asperger's syndrome, childhood disintegrative disorder (Heller's syndrome), and atypical autism as well as the subthreshold PDD-NOS category (Rutter & Schopler, 1992).

DSM-IV

As a result of concerns about the DSM-III-R definition of autism and an awareness of the categories and criteria pending in ICD-10, a large multisite field trial was undertaken for DSM-IV. This field trial (Volkmar et al., 1994) included ratings of nearly 1000 cases by over 100 clinicians of varying backgrounds and experience. Consistent with the previous research, the DSM-III-R system was noted to have a high false-positive rate, particularly in individuals with high levels of mental handicap, regardless of whether DSM-III-R was compared to a clinician's best judgment (clinical diagnosis) or clinician ratings of other diagnostic criteria (e.g. for DSM-III and ICD-10) or to alternative methods of judging the probability of "caseness." While the DSM-III definition (in its "lifetime" sense) had some advantages, it was much less developmentally oriented than DSM-III-R. The ICD-10 system worked reasonably well but tended to err on the side of stringency. The large number and detail of the research criteria were of concern for a system, like DSM-IV, which was meant for both clinical and research use. Together, recent research and data collected in the field trial indicated that reductions in the number and details of the ICD-10 criteria yielded good results even when less experienced clinicians were using the criteria (Lord et al., 1994; Volkmar et al., 1994). Thus a modified version of the original ICD-10 draft criteria for autism was proposed for both the American (DSM-IV) and international (ICD-10) systems. Although primarily focused on the definition of autism, the results of the field trial also provided some support for the inclusion, as in ICD-10, of Rett's disorder, CDD (Heller's syndrome), and Asperger's syndrome in the PDD class in DSM-IV.

The ICD-10 research definitions of autism and other pervasive developmental disorders are provided in Appendix 1.A (p. 21). For a diagnosis of autism, a total of at least six criteria (from impairments in social interaction, communication, and restricted interests and activities) is required, with at least two social impairment criteria present. By definition, the condition must have its onset before age 3 years and not be due to either Rett's disorder or CDD. The choice of 3 years as an arbitrary cut-off point for the onset was consistent with previous research (e.g. Harper & Williams, 1975; Rogers & DiLalla, 1990), and the results of the field trial for autism (Volkmar *et al.*, 1994) suggested that only very rarely does a behavioral syndrome resembling autism have its onset after age 3 years. The convergence of the American and international definitions of autism has enhanced clinical work as well as research (Volkmar & Klin, 2005).

Dimensional approaches to diagnosis

As an alternative, and sometimes as a complement, to categorical "clinical" diagnoses, various diagnostic instruments, rating scales, and diagnostic checklists have been devised relative to autism. These approaches have been concerned with aspects of diagnosis, assessment, and behavioral characterization, and have been used for both research and clinical purposes. In some instances the results of dimensional assessments can be operationalized into categorical diagnoses. For example, the Autism Diagnostic Interview-Revised (ADI-R) (Lord *et al.*, 1994), and the Autism Diagnostic Observation Schedule (ADOS) (Lord *et al.*, 1999) were explicitly designed to generate categorical diagnostic criteria, and are only recently being used as quantitative measures.

Deficits in the three areas that characterize autism are affected by many factors, other than the presence of the disorder. These include chronological age, developmental level, specific language functioning, and comorbidity with other disorders, such as hyperactivity, anxiety, or oppositional behavior (Lord, 1991). The ability to quantify the severity of autism would be helpful both for research and for clinical communication. For example, parents often ask "How severe is my child's autism?" Similarly, many questions in genetic research are dependent on an estimate of the severity of a disorder (Eaves *et al.*, 2000). However, such estimates become very complex because of the developmental nature of autism. For example, restricted and repetitive behaviors are less common in very young (i.e. under age 3) autistic children, probably in part because of their limited independent access to certain events and objects and cognitive level (Lord, 1995). These behaviors appear to increase in frequency from early to late preschool years and then often decrease or change in nature from fascination with particular objects (e.g. balls of string) and repetitive behaviors (e.g. lining them up) to more complicated interests and activities (e.g. an interest in astronomy or Scottish clans) in individuals with sufficient cognitive and language skills. Comparing the severity of these deficits becomes problematic even if a metric of impairment, such as interference in independence or in family life is used, given that families usually adjust to and have different expectations for children who are 2 years of age than those who are 16. Choosing a particular chronological age as a standard, such as the use of the period between 4 and 5 years of age in the ADI-R (Lord *et al.*, 1994), and having different metrics for verbal and nonverbal individuals can minimize this issue to some degree (Pickles *et al.*, 2000), but it still does not control for differences in cognitive functioning. In almost every empirical study of dimensional instruments, severity of quantitative measures is highly correlated with severity of mental handicap (Lord, 1991). Thus it is important for clinicians and researchers to be aware of this relationship in interpreting dimensional scales. This finding also implies that it is very important in interpreting psychometric data from dimensional scales to be certain that autistic and nonautistic groups are equivalent on measures such as cognitive level, language ability, and chronological age before statements about the validity of cut-offs can be made. Finding such groups is not always easy (Lord & Corsello, 2005).

The one clear improvement that multidimensional scales such as the ADI-R and ADOS (Lord *et al.*, 1999) can offer is separate documentation of the presence of abnormalities in each of the areas that define autism: social reciprocity; communication; and restricted, repetitive behaviors. With scales that produce a single score, it is possible that severe deficits in one or two areas (e.g. sensory abnormalities and expressive language) may heighten scores sufficiently to reach a cut-off for autism, even though deficits in other areas are not marked. Having separate scores in the areas that comprise DSM-IV and ICD-10 diagnoses allows confirmation that an individual has the specific pattern of deficits defined as autism.

There are some important issues in the development and use of dimensional assessment instruments and parent interviews. Recently, converging evidence from a number of sources has suggested that many aspects of the social and communication domains overlap, so that having a single domain of social–communication deficits specific to autism may be most appropriate as would be the recognition of language level (Lord *et al.*, 2006). Because the individual with autism may not always be amenable to direct interview, dimensional assessment instruments usually rely either on behavioral observation (in structured or unstructured situations) or parent or caregiver report. Since aspects of syndrome expression change with age, some instruments have focused particularly on the preschool period; when the person being evaluated is older, such an approach entails potential problems with the reliability of parental retrospection. Some behaviors, such as self-injurious behaviors, may be important because of severity but may be low in frequency; this is a problem for instruments which rely exclusively on behavioral observation. Teacher reports bring other questions of reliability particularly when teachers are asked to rate behaviors which they encounter only very rarely. Comparisons to typical peers, if the child is in regular classes, may be different from comparisons to other children with developmental disorders, if the child is in a special class or school (Sigman *et al.*, 1999). Unfortunately aspects of reliability and validity have not always been adequately addressed (Parks, 1983).

Rimland's (1964) diagnostic checklist for the diagnosis of autism is of considerable interest historically. It represents one of the earliest attempts to provide a more truly operational approach to diagnosis. The checklist is completed by parents and contains a set of questions about the development of the child in the first years of life. The total score is used to provide an indication of the likelihood that the person exhibits autism (Rimland, 1964). There has been concern that the questionnaire results in diagnoses that are not equivalent to standard criteria or other measures, but it was an important first step in the creation of standardized instruments in autism (Parks, 1983).

The Childhood Autism Rating Scale (Schopler *et al.*, 1980b) is also based on observation of behavior. A trained rater observes the child during a structured situation or a parent may be interviewed with the scale completed by a teacher or clinician. Various scales are included with scores ranging on a continuum from normal to severely abnormal. It is possible to operationalize the ratings into an estimate of the severity of autism, though this is correlated with intelligence. Reliability and discriminant validity are good, e.g. Teal and Wiebe (1986).

The Aberrant Behavior Checklist (Krug *et al.*, 1979, 1980) is designed for completion by teachers. Dichotomous items are weighted relative to how strongly they predict a diagnosis of autism. The weighted items are then summed across five symptom areas and the probability that the individual exhibits autism can then be estimated. Sums of item weights within area can also be plotted and compared to children of similar chronological age. Volkmar *et al.* (1987) noted that while individual item reliability was not high, the instrument had reasonable sensitivity. However, poor specificity (that is, it accurately identifies autism in the autistic individual but tends to overdiagnose autism in individuals who do not otherwise appear to have autism) is a major limitation. Nevertheless, it may be a useful measure of treatment effects on difficult behavior.

More recently instruments have been developed which have been specifically "keyed" to categorical diagnostic systems. Thus the ADI-R (Rutter *et al.*, 2003) is a semistructured investigator-based interview, applicable for individuals with mental ages from 18 months to adulthood and is specifically linked to ICD-10 and DSM-IV diagnostic criteria. Data on reliability and validity of individual items have been presented and are generally very good to excellent (Rutter *et al.*, 2003). This instrument is particularly useful for research purposes and, as is true for several of the dimensional instruments described here, specific training in its administration and scoring is required. A companion, observational approach, the ADOS has also been developed (Lord, Risi, Lambrecht *et al.*, 2000) and again is explicitly "keyed" to categorical diagnosis. General ratings provided better discrimination between groups of children and adolescents with autism and mild mental retardation than did coding related to specific tasks. The ADOS significantly increases the validity of the ADI-R (see above), and in some cases, when administered by an experienced clinician, may provide as good or better discrimination of autism from other disorders in school-age children. ADOS scores have been shown be to be correlated with extent of activation in particular brain regions on functional magnetic resonance imaging (Schultz *et al.*, 2003), and with independent measures of communication impairment (Joseph *et al.*, 2005).

In addition to rating scales specifically designed for individuals with autism, well-standardized assessments applicable to the general population can be used in the assessment of persons with autism. The social disability associated with autism is highly distinctive (see Chapter 10); there have been some attempts, using the Vineland Adaptive Behavior Scales (VABS) (Sparrow *et al.*, 1984) to provide more dimensional assessments of social dysfunction. Volkmar *et al.* (2003) noted that levels of social skills could be predicted on the basis of a series of regression equations using mental or chronological age as the predictor variable; individuals with autism were much more likely to exhibit lower actual levels of social skill than would otherwise be predicted on the basis of their age or cognitive development. This approach may have particular utility for screening purposes since it relies on a well-standardized, semi-structured interview and is concerned with the acquisition of developmentally expected skills. The development of supplementary norms specific to autism also adds to the usefulness of the VABS in this population (Carter *et al.*, 1998).

Differential diagnosis of autism and related conditions

Autism and related PDDs must be differentiated from other developmental disorders such as mental retardation and language disorders as well as from sensory impairments such as deafness and, less frequently, from other conditions. The use of a developmentally oriented, multiaxial approach is always indicated since behavioral features and diagnostic criteria and guidelines are best interpreted within a developmental context. Assessments of both cognitive (separate verbal and nonverbal) and communicative (separate receptive from expressive) skills are helpful and should be chosen as appropriate to the individual case. Similarly, measures of adaptive skills may provide information, such as about social skills, relevant to diagnosis and help in formulation of remedial programs. Any associated medical conditions should be identified. Additional medical and other investigators should usually be guided by history and examination, e.g. fragile X screening, neurological consultation, and other assessments may be indicated. Audiological evaluation should be obtained if there is concern about the child's ability to hear. Assessment procedures are summarized in Box 1.1.

A careful history from parents significantly facilitates the diagnostic process. In taking a history, it is often helpful to frame questions about specific skills or developmental abilities around certain well-remembered times, e.g. the child's first birthday. The use of videotapes and home movies may also be helpful. The diagnosis of autism is most straightforward in instances where parents report severe problems in social interaction and communication dating from early in the child's life. However, many parents report that socially their autistic children were not obviously unusual until some time in the second year of life (Lord *et al.*, 2004; Luyster *et al.*, 2005). Sometimes parents give clear descriptions of marked changes in children's social behavior sometime in their second year but many report what seems to be a more gradual stagnation of social involvement beyond physical contact (that is, many children continue to enjoy being tickled and roughhoused with, but become less interested in playing peek-a-boo or blowing kisses), once they are walking and more independently mobile.

In addition, about one-quarter of parents report that their autistic children had some words, usually fewer than ten, up to the age of 12 to 18 months, which gradually stopped increasing and then began to disappear after only a few months (Kurita, 1985; Lord *et al.*, 2004). In some cases, these reports may be due to parents' overly optimistic intepretations of their children's early babble, but in many cases it has been possible to verify the presence of a few meaningful words around the first birthday in children who are not speaking at the time of diagnosis at 2 or 3 years (Osterling *et al.*, 2002). As noted above, usually the number of words is very small and they are present for only a period of weeks or months. Often the words are used in appropriate contexts (e.g. saying "buh-buh" for bottle); sometimes they also appear to be intentional and to be part of a general action routine without necessarily being used by the child for communication.

When parents report that a child loses more language than just a few words (including a larger vocabulary or some spontaneous, nonroutinized sentences)

Box 1.1. Evaluation procedures

1. **Historical information**
   - Early development and characteristics of development
   - Age and nature of onset
   - Medical and family history
2. **Psychological/communicative examination**
   - Evaluate social and communicative skills relative to nonverbal intellectual abilities
   - Estimate(s) of intellectual level (particularly nonverbal)
   - Communicative assessment
     receptive and expressive vocabulary
     language skills
     use of nonverbal skills and pragmatic communication
   - Adaptive behavior
3. **Psychiatric examination**
   - Nature of social relatedness
     eye contact, attachment behaviors, interest in peers
     imitation skills, style of interacting
   - Behavioral features
     stereotypy/self-stimulation, resistance to change, unusual interests
     unusual sensitivities to the environment
   - Play skills
     nonfunctional use of play materials
     developmental level of play activities
4. **Medical evaluation**
   - Note associated medical conditions and risk factors including infectious, genetic, pre- and perinatal risk
   - Genetic screen (chromosome analysis for fragile X) and genetic consultation if indicated
   - Hearing test (if indicated)
   - Consultation (neurological, occupational or physical therapy) as indicated by history and current examination
   - Additional evaluations as needed e.g. EEG, CT/MRI scan

or experiences a loss closer to his or her second birthday, then consideration of the diagnosis of CDD should be made. In that condition development up to at least 2 years is supposed to be truly normal. In addition there are cases that are difficult to classify, e.g. a child who appears to have high functioning autism at 2 years of age but loses skills between 2 and 5 years. In Rett's disorder parents report a very early and unusual regression in their daughters, associated with the loss of purposeful hand movements and head-growth deceleration. While there may be some confusion with autism in the preschool years, the usual course of Rett's is quite distinctive (Tsai, 1992). In the syndrome of acquired aphasia with epilepsy (Landau–Kleffner syndrome) language is lost and seizures have their onset but social skills are relatively preserved (Landau, 1992). The study of children who exhibit regression in their early development remains an important topic for research.

It used to be that mental retardation was estimated to be present in about 75% of individuals with autism if the results of formal assessments of nonverbal intelligence were used. If full-scale scores (which include language skills) were employed, the proportion of mental handicap was even higher. However, the frequency of autistic-like symptoms (particularly stereotyped behaviors) increases with more severe retardation and may be the source of some confusion. For a diagnosis of autism to be made in an individual with profound or severe mental retardation, the clinician should be careful to evaluate the presence of social and communicative deficits relative to the person's overall intellectual level. Although these behaviors are highly associated with autism in persons who are not mentally handicapped, they are much more common in individuals with severe to profound mental retardation. The presence of motor mannerisms or stereotyped behaviors only does not establish a diagnosis of autism. In more recent epidemiological studies (Fombonne, 2005), estimates of the proportion of individuals with ASD who have nonverbal mental retardation have decreased to 50% or less. This shift in distribution has been primarily attributed to an increase in the number of children with milder symptoms of autism who are identified early. Many of these children do not have the significant cognitive delays seen in some children with ASD.

In childhood schizophrenia, in most instances, early and subsequent development well into the primary school years is reasonably normal (Werry, 1992). In a smaller group of cases, a longer-standing pattern of neurodevelopmental disability may be present. However, in contrast to autism, marked deficits and deviance in social interaction and communication are not typical. Although differing in some respects from schizophrenia in adults, the main clinical features of schizophrenia in children and adults are quite similar, e.g. delusions, disorganized thinking, hallucinations and so on (Werry, 1992). The onset of schizophrenia in childhood is extremely rare. Very occasionally an individual with autism, particularly during adolescence or young adulthood, may also then develop schizophrenia; in such cases, both diagnoses are made.

The differential diagnosis of Asperger's disorder and higher functioning autism remains an area of controversy. The lack, at least until very recently, of official guidelines for diagnosis has contributed to difficulties in interpreting available research. Some clinicians have used the term Asperger's disorder in ways that are essentially either synonymous with higher functioning autism, with PDD-NOS, or even with reference to adults with autism; none of these uses particularly adds to a classification system. To date, requiring that individuals do not meet criteria for autism if they are to meet criteria for Asperger's Disorder has resulted in very few cases and ongoing confusion. The use of more specific definitions of Asperger's disorder may help to resolve these issues. Consistent with ICD-10 and DSM-IV criteria, cases with Asperger's disorder would be expected to have better language skills than are typically observed in autism. Preliminary work (e.g. Klin *et al.*, 1995) suggests that specifically defined cases of higher-functioning autism and Asperger's disorder differ in important respects. Cases of Asperger's disorder also appear to be at risk for exhibiting a particular profile of learning disability on psychological testing. This profile of "Nonverbal Learning Disability" (Rourke, 1989) includes deficits in tactile perception, psychomotor coordination, and nonverbal problem-solving in the face of well-developed rote verbal and verbal memory skills; problems in social interaction are noted. The neuropsychological pattern associated with this condition differs from that usually seen in autism.

The PDD-NOS category's definition by exclusion is problematic (Towbin, 1994). Essentially this category should be used when an individual fails to meet specific criteria for autism or another explicitly defined PDD but has difficulties of similar quality. Research on this heterogeneous condition has been impeded by the need for a "subthreshold" category and its consequent intrinsic limitations. Attempts to define and validate possible subgroups are needed.

Certain other disorders should also be considered in the differential diagnosis of autism. In attachment disorder, children exhibit deficits in capacities for social interaction which, by definition, arise through markedly deviant caretaking experiences, e.g. institutional rearing or severe neglect. These deficits do, however, typically remit with provision of an appropriately supportive environment. Other features typical of autism are not present. In selective mutism, a child will speak but only in certain situations, e.g. at home. In this condition the characteristic social disturbance observed in autism is not present and the child exhibits a wider range of social communicative functioning than would be expected in autism.

Summary

Considerable progress in the diagnosis and classification of autism has occurred in the six decades that have passed since Kanner's original description of autism. It is clear that autism and related conditions are distinctive and with the publication of DSM-IV and ICD-10 there has been a move towards greater uniformity of diagnosis, a process which has facilitated research and clinical service. The inclusion of "new" disorders within the PDD class has been more controversial. Many of these "new" conditions actually have a rather long history of clinical interest and/or research, sometimes even longer than that for autism. It appears that the inclusion of these conditions has already generated important research contributions, e.g. the discovery of a gene involved in Rett's disorder.

The official recognition of Asperger's disorder has stimulated considerable debate and interest in higher-functioning individuals with social disabilities. There is increasing awareness of the "broader phenotype" of social disability that may be inherited in autism (Rutter, 2005). Issues related to the boundaries and validity of different diagnostic categories of the PDDs, particularly Asperger's disorder and PDD-NOS, remain far from resolved.

For some of the less common conditions, collaborative, multisite projects may be needed if searches for etiological mechanisms are to be successful. Similarly, efforts to understand the broader autism phenotype more fully may require relatively large samples and more attention to different potential pathways into social dysfunction. An understanding of the neural basis of social behavior (Volkmar et al., 2003) may be particularly helpful in this regard.

Although progress has been made, there are many areas that still need much research. Given the body of work (Lord et al., 2001) demonstrating the effectiveness of early intervention in autism, the identification of very young children with autism and related disorders is an important research priority. A decade ago a 4-year-old child with autism was thought of as an example of very early diagnosis, now referrals are made shortly after a child's first birthday (Klin et al., 2004). Longitudinal studies of children referred for possible autism before age 3 years have underscored that while the diagnosis can be made early errors in both directions also occur (Lord & Risi, 2000). Advances have been made in the area of early diagnosis and screening (see Chawarska & Volkmar, 2005; Coonrod & Stone, 2005) but more rigorous and reliable methods – including those which tap specific psychological and neurobiological processes – are needed.

Longitudinal studies are also critically needed. These will address important questions of stability of diagnosis and responses to treatment. It is clear that while many children respond positively to early intervention, some do not, even with good intervention programs. Since most of the available research is cross-sectional in nature, it is difficult for us to understand what factor or factors predict a response to treatment.

Increased knowledge, e.g. the identification of specific genes (see Chapter 5), may require further refinement of diagnosic categories. It is also important to realize that diagnosis involves many purposes including eligibility for services and definition of homogeneous and strictly defined subgroups for research. An understandable and legitimate tension exists among these various purposes (Wing, 2005). It is clear, however, that the development of useful and reliable definitions has significantly advanced research over the past decade.

Acknowledgments

The authors gratefully acknowledge the National Institute of Child Health and Human Development (NICHD) (CPEA program project grant 1PO1HD35482-01). Dr. Volkmar also acknowledges the support of other grants from NICHD (5-P01-HD03008 and R01-HD042127-02) as well as the support of the National Institute of Mental Health (STAART grant U54-MH066494) and of the National Alliance of Autism Research, Cure Autism Now, the Simons Foundation and the Doris Duke Foundation. Dr. Lord also acknowledges the support of the National Institute of Mental Health (R01 MH066496) and the Simons Foundation.

APPENDIX 1.A

ICD-10 definitions of autism and related pervasive developmental disorders

ICD-10 criteria for autism

Childhood autism (F84.0)

A. Abnormal or impaired development is evident before the age of 3 years in at least one of the following areas:
    (1) receptive or expressive language as used in social communication;
    (2) the development of selective social attachments or of reciprocal social interaction;
    (3) functional or symbolic play.
B. A total of at least six symptoms from (1), (2), and (3) must be present, with at least two from (1) and at least one from each of (2) and (3).
    (1) Qualitative impairments in social interaction are manifest in at least two of the following areas:

    (a) failure adequately to use eye-to-eye gaze, facial expression, body pos-
tures, and gestures to regulate social interaction;

    (b) failure to develop (in a manner appropriate to mental age, and despite
ample opportunities) peer relationships that involve a mutual sharing of
interests, activities, and emotions;

    (c) lack of socio-emotional reciprocity as shown by an impaired or deviant
response to other people's emotions; or lack of modulation of behavior
according to social context; or a weak integration of social, emotional,
and communicative behaviors;

    (d) lack of spontaneous seeking to share enjoyment, interests, or achieve-
ments with other people (e.g. a lack of showing, bringing, or pointing
out to other people objects of interest to the individual).

(2) Qualitative abnormalities communication as manifest in at least one of the
following areas:

    (a) delay in or total lack of, development of spoken language that is *not*
accompanied by an attempt to compensate through the use of gestures
or mime as an alternative mode of communication (often preceded by
a lack of communicative babbling);

    (b) relative failure to initiate or sustain conversational interchange (at what-
ever level of language skill is present), in which there is reciprocal responsiveness to the communications of the other person;

    (c) stereotyped and repetitive use of language or idiosyncratic use of words
or phrases;

    (d) lack of varied spontaneous make-believe play or (when young) social
imitative play.

(3) Restricted, repetitive, and stereotyped patterns of behavior, interests, and
activities are manifested in at least one of the following:

    (a) an encompassing preoccupation with one or more stereotyped and
restricted patterns of interest that are abnormal in content or focus;
or one or more interests that are abnormal in their intensity and circumscribed nature though not in their content or focus;

    (b) apparently compulsive adherence to specific, nonfunctional routines or
rituals;

    (c) stereotyped and repetitive motor mannerisms that involve either hand
or finger flapping or twisting or complex whole-body movements;

    (d) preoccupations with part-objects or nonfunctional elements of play
materials (such as their odor, the feel of their surface, or the noise or
vibration they generate).

C.   The clinical picture is not attributable to the other varieties of pervasive developmental disorders; specific development disorder of receptive language (F80.2) with secondary socio-emotional problems' reactive attachment disorder (F94.1) or disinhibited attachment disorder (F94.2); mental retardation (F70–F72) with some associated emotional or behavioral disorders; schizophrenia (F20) of unusually earl onset; and Rett's syndrome (F84.12).

F84.1 Atypical autism

A.   Abnormal or impaired development is evident at or after the age of 3 years (criteria as for autism except for age of manifestation).
B.   There are qualitative abnormalities in reciprocal social interaction or in communication, or restricted, repetitive, and stereotyped patterns of behavior, interests, and activities. (Criteria as for autism except that it is unnecessary to meet the criteria for number of areas of abnormality.)
C.   The disorder does not meet the diagnostic criteria for autism (F84.0).
Autism may be atypical in either age of onset (F84.10) or symptomatology (F84.11); the two types are differentiated with a fifth character for research purposes. Syndromes that are typical in both respects should be coded F84.12.

F84.10 Atypicality in age of onset

A.   The disorder does not meet criterion A for autism (F84.0); that is, abnormal or impaired development is evident only at or after age 3 years.
B.   The disorder meets criteria B and C for autism (F84.0).

F84.11 Atypicality in symptomatology

A.   The disorder meets criterion A for autism (F84.0); that is, abnormal or impaired development is evident before age 3 years.
B.   There are qualitative abnormalities in reciprocal social interactions or in communication, or restricted, repetitive, and stereotyped patterns of behavior, interests, and activities. (Criteria as for autism except that it is unnecessary to meet the criteria for number of areas of abnormality.)
C.   The disorder meets criterion C for autism (F84.0).
D.   The disorder does not fully meet criterion B for autism (F84.0).

F84.12 Atypicality in both age of onset and symptomatology

A.   The disorder does not meet criterion A for autism (F84.0); that is, abnormal or impaired development is evident only at or after age 3 years.

B.   There are qualitative abnormalities in reciprocal social interactions or in commu-
      nication, or restricted, repetitive, and stereotyped patterns of behavior, interests,
      and activities. (Criteria as for autism except that it is unnecessary to meet the
      criteria for number of areas of abnormality.)
C.   The disorder meets criterion C for autism (F84.0).
D.   The disorder does not fully meet criterion B for autism (F84.0).

DSM-IV Criteria for autistic disorder (299.0)

A.   A total of at least six items from (1), (2), and (3), with at least two from (1), and
      one each from (2) and (3):
      (1) Qualitative impairment in social interaction, as manifested by at least two
          of the following:
          (a) marked impairment in the use of multiple nonverbal behaviors such as
               eye-to-eye gaze, facial expression, body postures, and gestures to regulate
               social interaction;
          (b) failure to develop peer relationships appropriate to developmental level;
          (c) markedly impaired expression of pleasure in other people's happiness;
          (d) lack of social or emotional reciprocity.
      (2) Qualitative impairments in communication as manifested by at least one of
          the following:
          (a) delay in or total lack of, the development of spoken language (not
               accompanied by an attemp to compensate through alternative modes of
               communication such as gestures or mime);
          (b) in individuals with adequate speech, marked impairment in the ability
               to initiate or sustain a conversation with others;
          (c) stereotyped and repetitive use of language or idiosyncratic language;
          (d) lack of varied spontaneous make-believe play or social imitative play
               appropriate to developmental level.
      (3) Restricted repetitive and stereotyped patterns of behavior, interests, and
          activities, as manifested by at least one of the following:
          (a) encompassing preoccupation with one or more stereotyped and
               restricted patterns of interest that is abnormal either in intensity or
               focus;
          (b) apparently inflexible adherence to specific, nonfunctional routines or
               rituals;
          (c) stereotyped and repetitive motor mannerisms, e.g. hand or finger flap-
               ping or twisting, or complex whole-body movements;
          (d) persistent preoccupation with parts of objects.

B.   Delays or abnormal functioning in at least one of the following areas, with onset prior to age three: (1) social interaction; (2) language as used in social communication; or (3) symbolic or imaginative play.

C.   Not better accounted for by Rett's disorder or childhood disintegrative disorder.

REFERENCES

American Psychiatric Association (1980). *Diagnostic and Statistical Manual*, 3rd edn. Washington, DC: APA Press.

American Psychiatric Association (1987). *Diagnostic and Statistical Manual*, 3rd revised edn. Washington, DC: APA Press.

American Psychiatric Association (1994). *Diagnostic and Statistical Manual*, 4th edn. Washington, DC: APA Press.

Amir, R. E., Van den Veyver, I. B., Wan, M., Tran, C. Q., Francke, U., & Zoghbi, H. Y. (1999). Rett syndrome is caused by mutations in X-linked MeCP2, encoding methyl-CpG-binding protein 2. *Nature Genetics*, 23, 185–8.

Asperger, H. (1944/1991). Autistic psychopathy in childhood (Uta Frith, trans.). In U. Frith, ed., *Autism and Asperger Syndrome*. Cambridge: Cambridge University Press, pp. 1–36.

Bailey, A., Phillips, W., and Rutter, M. (1996). Autism: towards an integration of clinical, genetic, neuropsychological, and neurobiological perspectives. *Journal of Child Psychology and Psychiatry*, 37(1), 89–126.

Bender, L. (1947). Childhood schizophrenia: clinical study of one hundred schizophrenic children. *American Journal of Orthopsychiatry*, 17, 40–56.

Bettelheim, B. (1967). *The Empty Fortress*. New York: Free Press.

Bishop, D. V. and Norbury, C. F. (2002). Exploring the borderlands of autistic disorder and specific language impairment: a study using standardised diagnostic instruments. *Journal of Child Psychology & Psychiatry & Allied Disciplines*, 43(7), 917–29.

Bleuler, E. (1911/1950). *Dementia Praecox or the Group of Schizophrenia* (J. Zinkin, trans.). New York: International Universities Press (Originally published 1911.) 548 pp.

Brown, J. R. and Rogers, S. J. (2003). Cultural Issues in Autism. In R. L. Hendren, S. Ozonoff and S. Rogers, eds., *Autism Spectrum Disorders*. Washington, DC: American Psychiatric Press, pp. 209–26.

Carter, A. S., Volkmar, F. R., Sparrow, S. S. *et al.* (1998). The Vineland Adaptive Behavior Scales: supplementary norms for individuals with autism. *Journal of Autism and Developmental Disorders*, 28(4), 287–302.

Cantwell, D., Rutter, M., and Baker, L. (1978). Family factors. In M. Rutter and E. Schopler, eds., *Autism: A Reappraisal of Concepts and Treatment*. New York: Plenum, pp. 351–62.

Chawarska, K. and Volkmar, F. (2005). Autism in infancy and early childhood. In F. Volkmar, A. Klin, R. Paul, and D. J. Cohen, eds., *Handbook of Autism and Pervasive Developmental Disorders*, 3rd edn. New York: Wiley.

Cox, A., Rutter, M., Newman, S., and Bartak, L. A. (1975) A comparative study of infantile autism and specific developmental receptive language disorder. I. Parental characteristics. *British Journal of Psychiatry*, **126**, 146–59.

Coonrod, E. E. and Stone, W. L. (2005). Screening for autism in young children. In F. Volkmar, A. Klin, R. Paul, and D. J. Cohen, eds., *Handbook of Autism and Pervasive Developmental Disorders*, 3rd edn. New York: Wiley.

DeSanctis, S. (1906). Sopra alcune varieta della demenza precoce. *Rivista Sperimentale de Feniatria e di Medicina Legale*, **32**, 141–65.

Eaves, L., Rutter, M., Silberg, J. L. *et al.* (2000). Genetic and environmental causes of covariation in interview assessments of disruptive behavior in child and adolescent twins. *Behavior Genetics*, **30**(4), 321–34.

Factor, D. C., Freeman, N. L., and Kardash, A. (1989). A comparison of DSM-III and DSM-III-R criteria for autism. *Journal of Autism and Developmental Disorders*, **19**, 637–40.

Fombonne, E. (2005). Epidemiological studies of Pervasive Developmental Disorders. In F. R. Volkmar, A. Klin, R. Paul & D. J. Cohen, eds. *Handbook of Autism and Pervasive Developmental Disorders*, 3rd edn. Vol. 1. New York: Wiley, pp. 42–69.

Hagberg, B., Aicardi, J., Dias, K., and Ramos, O. (1983). A progressive syndrome of autism, dementia, ataxia, and loss of purposeful hand use in girls: Rett syndrome. Report of 35 cases. *Annals of Neurology*, **14**, 471–9.

Harper, J. and Williams, S. (1975). Age and type of onset as critical variables in early infantile autism. *Journal of Autism and Childhood Schizophrenia*, **5**, 25–35.

Heller, T. (1908). Infantile dementia. *Zeitschrift für die Erforschung und Behandlung des Jugenlichen Schwächsinns*, **2**, 141–65.

Heller, T. (1930). Infantle dementia. *Zeitschrift für Kinderforschung*, **37**, 661–7. Reprinted in J. G. Howells, ed., *Modern Perspectives in International Child Psychiatry*. Edinburgh: Oliver & Boyd, 1969.

Hellgren, L., Gillberg, I. C., Bagenholm, A., and Gillberg, C. (1994). Children with deficits in attention, motor control and perception (DAMP) almost grown up: psychiatric and personality disorders at age 16 years. *Journal of Child Psychology and Psychiatry*, **35**(7), 1255–71.

Hermelin, B. (2001). *Bright Splinters of the Mind*. London: Taylor & Francis.

Hertzig, M., Snow, M., New, E., and Shapiro, T. (1990). DSM-III and DSM-III-R diagnosis of autism and PDD in nursery school children. *Journal of the American Academy of Child Psychiatry*, **29**, 123–6.

Hippler, K. and Klicpera, C. (2003). A retrospective analysis of the clinical case records of "autistic psychopaths" diagnosed by Hans Asperger and his team at the University Children's Hospital, Vienna. *Philosophical Transactions of the Royal Society of London. Series B: Biological Sciences*, **358**(1430), 291–301.

Howlin, P. (2005). Outcomes in autism spectrum disorders. In F. R. Volkmar, A. Klin, R. Paul and D. J. Cohen, eds., *Handbook of Autism and Pervasive Developmental Disorders*, 3rd edn. Vol. 1. New York: Wiley, pp. 201–22.

Joseph, R. M., McGrath, L. M., and Tager-Flusberg, H. (2005). Executive dysfunction and its relation to language ability in verbal school-age children with autism. *Developmental Neuropsychology*, **27**, 361–78.

Kanner, L. (1943). Autistic disturbances of affective contact. *Nervous Child*, **2**, 217–50.

Klin, A. and Shepard, B. A. (1994). Psychological assessment of autistic children. *Child and Adolescent Psychiatry Clinics of North America*, **3**, 131–48.

Klin, A., Volkmar, F. R., Sparrow, S. S., Cicchetti, D.V., and Rourke, B. P. (1995). Validity and neuropsychological characterization of Asperger syndrome convergence with nonverbal learning disabilities syndrome. *Journal of Child Psychology and Psychiatry*, **36**(7), 1127–40.

Klin, A., Chawarska, K., Paul, R. *et al.* (2004). Autism in a 15-month-old child. *American Journal of Psychiatry*, **161**(11), 1981–8.

Klin, A., McPartland, J., and Volkmar, F. R. (2005). Asperger's syndrome. In F. Volkmar, A. Klin, R. Paul, and D. Cohen, eds., *Handbook of Autism and Pervasive Developmental Disorders*, 3rd edn, Vol. 1. New York: Wiley, pp. 88–125.

Kolvin, I. (1971). Studies in childhood psychoses. I. Diagnostic criteria and classification. *British Journal of Psychiatry*, **118**, 381–4.

Krug, D. A., Arick, J. R., and Almond, P. J. (1979). Autism screening instrument for educational planning: background and development. In J. Gilliam, ed., *Autism: Diagnosis, Instruction, Management, and research*. Austin: University of Texas at Austin Press, 1979.

Krug, D. A., Arick, J., and Almond, P. (1980). Behavior checklist for identifying severely handicapped individuals with high levels of autistic behavior. *Journal of Child Psychology and Psychiatry*, **21**, 221–9.

Kurita, H. (1985). Infantile autism with speech loss before the age of 30 months. *Journal of the American Academy of Child and Adolescent Psychiatry*, **24**, 191–6.

Landau, W. M. (1992). Landau–Kleffner syndrome. An eponymic badge of ignorance. *Archives of Neurology*, **49**(4), 353.

Le Couteur, A., Bailey, A., Goode, S. *et al.* (1996). A broader phenotype of autism: the clinical spectrum in twins. *Journal of Child Psychology and Psychiatry*, **37**(7), 785–801.

Lord, C. (1991). Methods and measures of behavior in the diagnosis of autism and related disorders. *Psychiatric Clinics of North America*, **14**(1), 69–80.

Lord, C. (1995). Follow-up of two-year-olds referred for possible autism. *Journal of Child Psychology Psychiatry*, **36**(8), 1365–82.

Lord, C. and Corsello, C. (2005). Diagnostic instruments in autism spectrum disorders. In F. Volkmar, A. Klin, R. Paul and D. J. Cohen, eds., *Handbook of Autism and Pervasive Developmental Disorders*, 3rd edn. Vol. 1. New York: Wiley, pp. 730–71.

Lord, C. and Risi, S. (2000). Diagnosis of autism spectrum disorders in young children. In A. M. Wetherby and B. M. Prizant, eds., *Autism Spectrum Disorders: A Transactional Developmental Perspective Communication and Language Intervention Series. Vol. 9.* pp. 11–30.

Lord, C., Bristol-Power, M., Cafiero, J. M. *et al.* (2001). *Educating Young Children with Autism*. Washington, DC: National Academy Press.

Lord, C., Risi, S., Lambrecht, L. *et al.* (2000). The Autism Diagnostic Observation Schedule-Generic: a standard measure of social and communication deficits associated with the spectrum of autism. *Journal of Autism and Developmental Disorders*, **30**, 205–23.

Lord, C., Rutter, M., and Le Couteur, A. (1994). Autism Diagnostic Interview-Revised: a revised version of a diagnostic interview for caregivers of individuals with possible pervasive developmental disorder. *Journal of Autism and Developmental Disorders*, **24**, 659–85.

Lord, C., Rutter, M., J. DiLavore, P., and Risi, S. (1999). Autism diagnostic observation schedule. Los Angeles, CA: Western Psychological Services.

Lord, C., Risi, S., DiLavore, P., Shulman, C., Thurm, A., and Pickles, A. (2006). Autism from two to nine year of age. *Archives of General Psychiatry*, **63**(6), 694–701.

Lord, C., Shulman, C., and DiLavore, P. (2004). Regression and word loss in autistic spectrum disorders. *Journal of Child Psychology and Psychiatry*, **45**, 936–55.

Luyster, R., Richler, J., Risi, S. *et al.* (2005). Early regression in social communication in autism spectrum disorders: a CPEA Study. *Developmental Neuropsychology*, **27**, 311–36.

Mahoney, W. J., Szatmari, P., MacLean, J. E. *et al.* (1998). Reliability and accuracy of differentiating pervasive developmental disorder subtypes. *Journal of the American Academy of Child and Adolescent Psychiatry*, **37**(3), 278–85.

Maudsley, H. (1867) *The Physiology and Pathology of the Mind*. Macmillan: London.

Osterling, J. A., Dawson, G., and Munson, J. A. (2002). Early recognition of 1-year-old infants with autism spectrum disorder versus mental retardation. *Development and Psychopathology*, **14**(2), 239–51.

Parks, S. L. (1983). The assessment of autistic children: a selective review of available instruments. *Journal of Autism and Developmental Disorders*, **13**, 255–67.

Pickles, A., Starr, E., Kazak, S. *et al.* (2000). Variable expression of the autism broader phenotype: findings from extended pedigrees. *Journal of Child Psychology and Psychiatry and Allied Disciplines*, **41**(4), 491–502.

Pomeroy, J. D. (1991). Autism and Asperger's: same or different? *Journal of the American Academy of Child and Adolescent Psychiatry*, **30**, 152–3.

Potter, H. W. (1933). Schizophrenia in children. *American Journal of Psychiatry*, **89**, 1253–70.

Rank, B. (1949). Adaptation of the psychoanalytic technique for the treatment of young children with atypical development. *American Journal of Orthopsychiatry*, 130–9.

Rett, A. (1966). On an unusual brain atrophy syndrome in hyperammonemia in childhood. *Wien Medizinische Wochenschrift*, **118**, 723–6.

Rimland, B. (1964). *Infantile Autism: The Syndrome and its Implications for a Neural Theory of Behavior*. New York: Appleton-Century-Crofts.

Rogers, S. J. and DiLalla, D. L. (1990). Age of symptom onset in young children with pervasive developmental disorder. *Journal of the American Academy of Child and Adolescent Psychiatry*, **29**, 863–72.

Rourke, B. P. (1989). *Nonverbal Learning Disabilities: The Syndrome and the Model*. New York: Guilford.

Rumsey, J. M., Rapoport, J. L., and Scerry, W. R. (1985). Autistic children as adults: psychiatric, social, and behavioral outcomes. *Journal of the American Academy of Child Psychiatry*, **24**, 465–73.

Rutter, M. (1970). Autistic children: infancy to adulthood. *Seminars in Psychiatry*, **2**, 435–50.

Rutter, M. (1972). Childhood schizophrenia reconsidered. *Journal of Autism and Childhood Schizophrenia*, **2**, 315–38.

Rutter, M. (1978), Diagnosis and definition. In M. Rutter and E. Schopler, eds., *Autism: A Reappraisal of Concepts and Treatment*. New York: Plenum, pp. 139–61.

Rutter, M. (1994). Debate and argument: there are connections between brain and mind and it is important that Rett syndrome be classified somewhere [comment]. *Journal of Child Psychology and Psychiatry*, **35**(2), 379–81.

Rutter, M. (2005). Genetic influences in autism. In F. Volkmar, A. Klin, R. Paul, and D. Cohen, eds., *Handbook of Autism and Pervasive Developmental Disorders*, 3rd edn, Vol. 1. New York: Wiley, pp. 425–52.

Rutter, M. and Schopler, E. (1992). Classification of pervasive developmental disorders: some concepts and practical considerations. *Journal of Autism and Developmental Disorders*, **22**, 459–82.

Rutter, M., Bailey, A., Bolton, P., and Le Couteur, A. (1994) Autism and known medical conditions: myth and substance. *Journal of Child Psychology and Psychiatry*, **35**, 311–22.

Rutter, M., Le Couteur, A., & Lord, C. (2003). ADI-R Autism Diagnostic Interview B Revised. Los Angeles, CA: Western Psychological Services.

Schopler, E. (1985). Convergence of learning disability, higher-level autism, and Asperger's syndrome. *Journal of Autism and Developmental Disorders*, **15**, 359.

Schopler, E., Andrews, C. E., and Strupp, K. (1980a). Do autistic children come from upper middle-class parents? *Journal of Autism and Developmental Disorders*, **10**, 91–103.

Schopler, E., Reichler, R. J., DeVellis, R. F., and Daly, K. (1980b). Toward objective classification of childhood autism: childhood autism rating scale (CARS). *Journal of Autism and Developmental Disorders*, **10**, 91–103.

Schultz, R. T. and Robins, D. L. (2005). Funcitional neuroimaging studies of autism spectrum disorders. In F. Volkmar, A. Klin, R. Paul, and D. J. Cohen, eds., *Handbook of Autism and Pervasive Developmental Disorders*, 3rd edn. Vol. 1. New York: Wiley, pp. 515–33.

Schultz, R. T., Grelotti, D. J., Klin, A. *et al.* (2003). The role of the fusiform face area in social cognition: implications for the pathobiology of autism. *Philosophical Transactions of the Royal Society of London. Series B: Biological Sciences*, **358**(1430), 415–27.

Sigman, M., Ruskin, E., Arbeile, S. *et al.* (1999). *Continuity and Change in the Social Competence of Children with Autism, Down Syndrome, and Developmental Delays*. Monographs of the Society for Research in Child Development, **64**(1), 1–114.

Siperstein, R. & Volkmar, F. (2004). Report: Parental reporting of regression in children with pervasive developmental disorders. *Journal of Autism and Developmental Disorders*, **34**(6), 731–5.

Sparrow, S., Balla, D., and Ciccheti, D. (1984). *Vineland Adaptive Behavior Scales*. Circle Pines, Minnesota: American Guidance Service.

Spitzer, R. and Williams, J. B. W. (1988). Having a dream: a research strategy for DSM-IV. *Archives of General Psychiatry*, **45**, 871–4.

Szatmari, P., Tuff, L., Finlayson, M. A. J., and Bartolucci, G. (1990). Asperger's syndrome and autism: neurocognitive aspects. *Journal of the American Academy of Child and Adolescent Psychiatry*, **29**, 130–6.

Tantam, D. (1991). Asperger syndrome in adulthood. In U. Frith, ed., *Autism and Asperger Syndrome*. Cambridge: Cambridge University Press, pp. 147–83.

Teal, M. B. and Wiebe, M. J. (1986). A validity analysis of selected instruments used to assess autism. *Journal of Autism and Developmental and Disorder*, **16**(4), 485–94.

Towbin, K. E. (1994). Pervasive developmental disorder not otherwise specified: a review and guidelines for clinical care. *Child and Adolescent Psychiatry Clinics of North America*, **3**, 149–60.

Towbin, K. (2005). pervasive developmental disorder Not Otherwise Specified. In F. Volkmar, A. Klin, R. Paul, and D. Cohen, eds, *Handbook of Autism and Pervasive Developmental Disorders*, 3rd edn, Vol. 1. New York: Wiley, pp. 165–200.

Tsai, L. (1992). Is Rett's syndrome a subtype of pervasive developmental disorder. *Journal of Autism and Developmental Disorders*, **22**, 551–62.

Van Acker, R., Loncola, J. A., and van Acker, E. Y. (2005). Rett Syndrome: a pervasive developmental disorder. In F. Volkmar, A. Klin, R. Paul, and D. Cohen, eds., *Handbook of Autism and Pervasive Developmental Disorders*, 3rd edn, Vol. 1. New York: Wiley, pp. 126–64.

Volkmar, F. R. (1992). Childhood disintegrative disorder: issues for DSM-IV. *Journal of Autism and Developmental Disorders*, **22**, 625–42.

Volkmar, F. R. and Cohen, D. J. (1991). Co-morbid association of autism and schizophrenia. *American Journal of Psychiatry*, **148**, 1705–7.

Volkmar, F. R. and Klin, A. (2005). Issues in the classification of autism and related conditions. In F. Volkmar, A. Klin, R. Paul, and D. Cohen, eds, *Handbook of Autism and Pervasive Developmental Disorders*, 3rd edn, Vol. 1. New York: Wiley, pp. 5–41.

Volkmar, F. R. and Nelson, D. S. (1990). Seizure disorders in autism. *Journal of the American Academy of Child and Adolescent Psychiatry*, **29**(1), 127–9.

Volkmar, F. R. and Rutter, M. (1995). Childhood disintegrative disorder: results of the DSM-IV autism field trial. *Journal of the American Academy of Child and Adolescent Psychiatry*, **34**, 1092–5.

Volkmar, F. R., Bregman, J., Cohen, D. J., and Cicchetti, D. V. (1988). DSM-III and DSM-III-R diagnoses of autism. *American Journal of Psychiatry*, **145**(11), 1404–8.

Volkmar, F. R., Cicchetti, D.V., Dykens, E. *et al.* (1987). An evaluation of the Autism Behavior Checklist. *Journal of Autism and Developmental Disorders*, **18**, 81–97.

Volkmar, F., Klin, A., Schultz, R., Chawarska, K., and Jones, W. (2003). The social brain in autism. In M. Brune, H. Ribbert, & W. Schienfenhovel, eds., *The Social Brain: Evolution and Pathology*. New York: Wiley, pp. 167–96.

Volkmar, F. R., Klin, A., Siegel, B. *et al.* (1994). Field trial for autistic disorder in DSM-IV. *American Journal of Psychiatry*, **151**, 1361–7.

Volkmar, F. R., Koenig, K., and State, M. (2005). Childhood disintegrative disorder. In F. Volkmar, A. Klin, R. Paul, and D. J. Cohen, eds., *Handbook of Autism and Pervasive Developmental Disorders*, 3rd edn. Vol. 1. New York: Wiley, pp. 70–8.

Weintraub, S. and Mesulam, M. M. (1983). Developmental learning disabilities of the right hemisphere. Emotional, interpersonal, and cognitive components. *Archives of Neurology*, **11**, 463–8.

Werry, J. (1992). Child and adolescent (early-onset) schizophrenia: a review in light of DSM-III-R.
Journal of Autism and Developmental Disorders, **22**, 601–24.

Wing, L. (1980). Childhood autism and social class: a question of selection? *British Journal of
Psychiatry*, **137**, 410–17.

Wing, L. (1981). Asperger's syndrome: a clinical account. *Psychological Medicine*, **11**, 115–29.

Wing, L. (2005). Problems of categorical classification systems. In F. Volkmar, A. Klin, R. Paul, and
D. J. Cohen, eds., *Handbook of Autism and Pervasive Developmental Disorders*, 3rd edn. Vol. 1.
New York: Wiley, pp. 583–605.

Wolff, S. (2000). Schizoid personality in childhood and Asperger syndrome. In A. Klin and F. R.
Volkmar, eds., *Asperger syndrome*. New York: The Guilford Press, pp. 278–305.

World Health Organization (1990). *International Classification of Diseases, 10th* edn. Diagnostic
Criteria for Research. Geneva: WHO.

2

Epidemiological surveys of pervasive developmental disorders

Eric Fombonne

Department of Psychiatry, McGill University

Introduction

Epidemiological surveys of autism started in the mid 1960s in England (Lotter, 1966, 1967) and have since then been conducted in many countries. Most epidemiological surveys have focused on a categorical–diagnostic approach to autism that has relied over time on different sets of diagnostic criteria; however, all surveys used a definition of autism which comprised severe impairments in communication and language, social interactions, and play and behavior. This chapter is therefore concerned with autism defined as a severe developmental disorder and not with more subtle autistic features or symptoms that occur as part of other, more specific, developmental disorders, as unusual personality traits, or as components of the lesser variant of autism thought to index genetic liability to autism in relatives. With the exception of recent studies, other pervasive developmental disorders (PDDs) falling short of diagnostic criteria for autistic disorder – pervasive developmental disorder not otherwise specified (PDD-NOS), Asperger's syndrome – were generally not included in the case definition used in earlier surveys although several epidemiological investigations yielded useful information on the rates of these particular types of PDD. These data are summarized separately. The aims of this chapter are to provide an up-to-date review of the methodological features and substantive results of published epidemiological surveys. This chapter updates our previous reviews (Fombonne, 1998, 1999, 2003a) with the inclusion of new studies made available since then. Much of this chapter also appeared in the third edition of the *Handbook of Autism and pervasive developmental disorders* (Volkmar, 2005) and tables are reproduced with permission. A key feature of the review was to rely on summary statistics throughout in order to derive quantitative estimates for rates and correlates of autism spectrum disorders. The specific questions addressed in this chapter are:

Autism and Pervasive Developmental Disorders, 2nd edn, ed. Fred R. Volkmar.
Published by Cambridge University Press. © Cambridge University Press 2007.

(1)   What is the range of prevalence estimates for autism and related disorders?
(2)   What proportion of autism cases is attributable to specific associated medical disorders?
(3)   Is the incidence of autism increasing?
(4)   What are the other correlates of autistic-spectrum disorders, particularly with respect to race and ethnicity?
(5)   What is the role, if any, of cluster reports in causal investigations of autism?

The design of epidemiological surveys

Epidemiology is concerned with the study of the repartition of diseases in human populations and of the factors that influence it. There are several measures of disease occurrence used by epidemiologists. Incidence rate refers to the number of new cases (the numerator) of a disease occurring over a specified period in those at risk of developing the disease in the population (the denominator, in x person–years). Cumulative incidence is the proportion of those who were free of the disease at the beginning of the observation period and developed the disease during that period. Measures of incidence are required to estimate properly morbidity due to a disease, its possible changes over time, and the risk factors underlying disease status. Prevalence is a measure used in cross-sectional surveys (there is no passage of time) and reflects the proportion of subjects in a given population who, at that point in time, suffer from the disease. Most epidemiological surveys of autism have not been informative on incidence (with a few recent exceptions) and were of a cross-sectional nature. As a result, prevalence rates have been used to describe autism in populations.

The selection of studies

The studies were identified through systematic searches from the major scientific literature databases (MEDLINE, PSYCINFO) and from prior reviews (Wing, 1993; Fombonne, 1998, 1999, 2003a). Only studies published in the English language were included. Surveys which relied only on a questionnaire-based approach to define caseness were also excluded as the validity of the diagnosis is unsatisfactory in these studies. Overall, 42 studies published between 1966 and 2003 were selected which surveyed PDDs in clearly demarcated, non-overlapping samples. Of these, 36 studies provided information on rates of autistic disorder (Table 2.1), three studies only provided estimates on all PDDs combined, and three studies provided data only on high-functioning PDDs. For several studies, the publication listed in the tables is the most detailed account or the earliest one;

Table 2.1 Prevalence surveys of autistic disorder

No.	Year of publication	Authors	Country	Area	Size of target population	Age	No. of subjects with autism	Diagnostic criteria	% with normal IQ	Gender ratio (M:F)	Prevalence rate/10 000	95% CI
1	1966	Lotter	UK	Middlesex	78 000	8–10	32	Rating scale	15.6	2.6 (23/9)	4.1	2.7; 5.5
2	1970	Brask	Denmark	Aarhus County	46 500	2–14	20	Clinical	–	1.4 (12/7)	4.3	2.4; 6.2
3	1970	Treffert	USA	Wisconsin	899 750	3–12	69	Kanner's	–	3.06 (52/17)	0.7	0.6; 0.9
4	1976	Wing et al.	UK	Camberwell	25 000	5–14	17[a]	24 items rating scale of Lotter	30	16 (16/1)	4.8[b]	2.1; 7.5
5	1982	Hoshino et al.	Japan	Fukushima-Ken	609 848	0–18	142	Kanner's	–	9.9 (129/13)	2.33	1.9; 2.7
6	1983	Bohman et al.	Sweden	County of Västerbotten	69 000	0–20	39	Rutter's	20.5	1.6 (24/15)	5.6	3.9; 7.4
7	1984	McCarthy et al.	Ireland	East	65 000	8–10	28	Kanner's	–	1.33 (16/12)	4.3	2.7; 5.9
8	1986	Steinhausen et al.	Germany	West Berlin	279 616	0–14	52	Rutter's	55.8	2.25 (36/16)	1.9	1.4; 2.4
9	1987	Burd et al.	USA	North Dakota	180 986	2–18	59	DSM-III	–	2.7 (43/16)	3.26	2.4; 4.1
10	1987	Matsuishi et al.	Japan	Kurume City	32 834	4–12	51	DSM-III	–	4.7 (42/9)	15.5	11.3; 19.8
11	1988	Tanoue et al.	Japan	Southern Ibaraki	95 394	7	132	DSM-III	–	4.07 (106/26)	13.8	11.5; 16.2
12	1988	Bryson et al.	Canada	Part of Nova Scotia	20 800	6–14	21	New RDC	23.8	2.5 (15/6)	10.1	5.8; 14.4
13	1989	Sugiyama & Abe	Japan	Nagoya	12 263	3	16	DSM-III	–	–	13.0	6.7; 19.4
14	1989	Cialdella & Mamelle	France	1 district (Rhône)	135 180	3–9	61	DSM-III like	–	2.3	4.5	3.4; 5.6
15	1989	Ritvo et al.	USA	Utah	769 620	3–27	241	DSM-III	34	3.73 (190/51)	2.47	2.1; 2.8
16	1991	Gillberg et al.[d]	Sweden	South-West Gothenburg + Bohuslän County	78 106	4–13	74	DSM-III-R	18	2.7 (54/20)	9.5	7.3; 11.6
17	1992	Fombonne & du Mazaubrun	France	4 regions 14 districts	274 816	9 & 13	154	Clinical ICD-10-like	13.3	2.1 (105/49)	4.9	4.1; 5.7

(cont.)

Table 2.1 (*cont.*)

No.	Year of publication	Authors	Country	Area	Size of target population	Age	No. of subjects with autism	Diagnostic criteria	% with normal IQ	Gender ratio (M:F)	Prevalence rate/10 000	95% CI
18	1992	Wignyosumarto et al.	Indonesia	Yogyakarta (SE of Jakarta)	5 120	4–7	6	CARS	0	2.0 (4/2)	11.7	2.3; 21.1
19	1996	Honda et al.	Japan	Yokohama	8 537	5	18	ICD-10	50.0	2.6 (13.5)	21.08	11.4; 30.8
20	1997	Fombonne et al.	France	3 districts	325 347	8–16	174	Clinical ICD-10-like	12.1	1.81 (112/62)	5.35	4.6; 6.1
21	1997	Webb et al.	UK	South Glamorgan, Wales	73 301	3–15	53	DSM-III-R	–	6.57 (46/7)	7.2	5.3; 9.3
22	1997	Arvidsson et al.	Sweden (west coast)	Mölnlycke	1 941	3–6	9	ICD-10	22.2	3.5 (7/2)	46.4	16.1; 76.6
23	1998	Sponheim & Skjeldal	Norway	Akershus County	65 688	3–14	34	ICD-10	47.1[c]	2.09 (23/11)	5.2	3.4; 6.9
24	1999	Taylor et al.	UK	North Thames	490 000	0–16	427	ICD-10	–	–	8.7	7.9; 9.5
25	1999	Kadesjö et al.	Sweden (central)	Karlstad	826	6.7–7.7	6	DSM-III-R/ICD-10 Gillberg's criteria (Asperger's syndrome)	50.0	5.0 (5/1)	72.6	14.7; 130.6
26	2000	Baird et al.	UK	South-East Thames	16 235		50	ICD-10	60	15.7 (47/3)	30.8	22.9; 40.6
27	2000	Powell et al.	UK	West Midlands	25 377		62	Clinical/ICD10/ DSM-IV	–	–	7.8	5.8; 10.5
28	2000	Kielinen et al.	Finland	North (Oulu and Lapland)	152 732		187	ICD-8/ICD-9/ICD-10	49.8	4.12 (156/50)	12.2	10.5; 14.0
29	2001	Bertrand et al.	USA	Brick Township, New Jersey	8 896		36	DSM-IV	36.7	2.2 (25/11)	40.5	28.0; 56.0

#	Year	Authors	Country	Location	Population	Age	Cases	Criteria				
30	2001	Fombonne et al.	UK	England and Wales	10 438	5–15	27	DSM-IV/ICD-10	55.5	8.0 (24/3)	26.1	16.2; 36.0
31	2001	Magnusson & Saemundsen	Iceland	Whole Island	43 153	5–14	57	Mostly ICD-10	15.8	4.2 (46/11)	13.2	9.8; 16.6
32	2001	Chakrabarti & Fombonne	UK (Midlands)	Staffordshire	15 500	2.5–6.5	26	ICD10/ DSM-IV	29.2	3.3 (20/6)	16.8	10.3; 23.2
33	2001	Davidovitch et al.	Israel	Haifa	26 160	7–11	26	DSM-III-R/DSM-IV	–	4.2 (21/5)	10.0	6.6;14.4
34	2002	Croen et al.	USA	California DDS	4 950 333	5–12	5 038	CDER "full syndrome"	62.8[e]	4.47 (4116/921)	11.0	10.7;11.3
35	2002	Madsen et al.	Denmark	National register	63 859	8	46	ICD-10	–	–	7.2	5.0–10.0
36	2005	Chakrabarti & Fombonne	UK (Midlands)	Staffordshire	10 903	4–7	24	ICD-10/DSM-IV	33.3	3.8 (19/5)	22.0	14.4; 32.2

[a] This number corresponds to the sample described in Wing and Gould (1979);

[b] This rate corresponds to the first published paper on this survey and is based on 12 subjects among children aged 5–14 years;

[c] In this study, mild mental retardation was combined with normal IQ, whereas moderate and severe mental retardation were grouped together;

[d] For the Göteborg surveys by Gillberg et al. (Gillberg, 1984; Steffenburg & Gillberg, 1986; Gillberg et al., 1991), a detailed examination showed that there was overlap between the samples included in the three surveys; consequently only the last survey has been included in this table;

[e] This proportion is likely to be overestimated and to reflect an underreporting of mental retardation in the CDER evaluations;

CARS: Childhood Autism Rating Scale.

CDER: Client Development Evaluation Report.

RDC: Research Diagnosis Criteria.

however, other published articles were used to extract relevant information from the same study, when appropriate.

Survey descriptions

Surveys were conducted in 14 countries and half of the results have been published since 1997. Details on the precise sociodemographic composition and economical activities of the area surveyed in each study were generally lacking; most studies were, however, conducted in predominantly urban or mixed areas, with only 2 (studies 6 and 11) surveys carried out in predominantly rural areas. The proportion of children from immigrant families was generally not available and very low in 5 surveyed populations (studies 11, 12, 19, 23, and 26). Only in studies 4 and 34 there a substantial minority of children with either an immigrant or different ethnic background living in the area. The age range of the population included in the surveys is spread from birth to early adult life, with an overall median age of 8.0. Similarly, in 39 studies, there is huge variation in the size of the population surveyed (range 826–4 590 000), with a median population size of 63 860 subjects (mean 255 000) and about half of the studies relying on targeted populations ranging in size from 15 870 to 166 860.

A few studies have relied on existing administrative databases (i.e. Croen et al., 2002; Gurney et al., 2003) or on national registers (Madsen et al., 2002) for case identification. Most investigations have relied on a two-stage or multi-stage approach to identify cases in underlying populations (Fombonne, 2002a). The first screening stage of these studies often consisted of sending letters or brief screening scales asking schools and health professionals to identify possible cases of autism. Each investigation varied in several key aspects of this screening stage. First, the coverage of the population varied enormously from one study to another. In some (i.e. studies 3, 17, 20, 24, and 33) only cases already known from educational or medical authorities could be identified, whereas in other surveys an extensive coverage of the entire population, including children attending normal schools (studies 1 and 25) or children undergoing systematic developmental checks (studies 13, 19, 22, 32, and 36), was achieved. In addition, the surveyed areas varied in terms of service development as a function of the specific educational or healthcare systems of each country and of the year of investigation. Secondly, the type of information sent out to professionals who were invited to identify children varied from simple letters including a few clinical descriptors of autism-related symptoms or diagnostic checklists rephrased in nontechnical terms, to more systematic screening based on questionnaires or rating scales of known reliability and validity. Thirdly, participation rates in the first screening stages provide another source of variation in the screening efficiency of surveys. Refusal rates were available for 13 studies (studies 1, 5, 6, 9, 12, 14, 19, 20, 23, 25 and 30); the rate of refusal ranged from 0% (study 25) to 35%, with a median value of 14%. Fewer studies could examine the extent to which refusal to participate or uncooperativeness in surveys is associated with the likelihood that the corresponding children have autism. Bryson *et al.* (1988; study 12), however, provided some evidence that those families who refused cooperation in the intensive assessment phase had children with Aberrant Behavior Checklist (ABC) scores similar to other false positives in their study, thereby suggesting that these children were unlikely to have autism. Webb *et al.* (2003) similarly produced data showing an increasing refusal rate in those with fewer ICD-10 PDD symptoms. By contrast, in a Japanese study (Sugiyama and Abe, 1989; study 13) where 17.3% of parents refused further investigations for their 18-month-old children who had failed a developmental check, follow-up data at age 3 suggested that half of these children still displayed developmental problems. Whether or not these problems were connected to autism is unknown, but this study points to the possibility of having higher rates of developmental disorders among nonparticipants to surveys. Similarly, in Lotter's study (1966; study 1), 58 questionnaires covering schools for handicapped children were returned out of the 76 forms sent out, and an independent review of the records showed that 4 of the 18 missing forms corresponded to autistic children. Therefore it is difficult to draw firm conclusions from these different accounts. Although there is no consistent evidence that parental refusal to cooperate is associated with autism in their offspring, it appears that a small proportion of cases may be missed in some surveys as a consequence of non-cooperation at the screening stage. One survey included a weighting procedure to compensate for nonresponse (study 40).

Only two studies (studies 1 and 30) provided an estimate of the reliability of the screening procedure. The sensitivity of the screening methodology is also difficult to gauge in autism surveys. The usual epidemiological approach, which consists of sampling, at random screened negative subjects in order to estimate the proportion of false negatives, has not been used in these surveys for the obvious reason that, due to the very low frequency of the disorder, it would be both imprecise and very costly to undertake such estimations. The consequence of these remarks is that prevalence estimates must be seen as underestimates of "true" prevalence rates because cases are being missed due either to lack of cooperation or to imperfect sensitivity of the screening procedure. The magnitude of this underestimation is unknown in each survey.

Similar considerations about the methodological variability across studies apply to the intensive assessment phases. Participation rates in these second-stage assessments were not always available, either because they had simply not been calculated or because the design and/or method of data collection did not lead easily to their estimation. When available (studies 1, 5, 8, 12, 13, 15, 22, 23, 25, 29, 30, 32, and 36) they were generally high, ranging from 76.1% (study 12) to 98.6% (study 25). The source of information used to determine caseness usually involved a combination of informants and data sources, with a direct assessment of the person with autism in 21 studies.

The assessments were conducted with various diagnostic instruments, ranging from a classical clinical examination to the use of batteries of standardized measures. The Autism Diagnostic Interview (Le Couteur *et al.*, 1989) and/or the Autism Diagnostic Observational Schedule (Lord *et al.*, 2000) were used in the most recent surveys. The precise diagnostic criteria retained to define caseness vary according to the study and, to a large extent, reflect historical changes in classification systems. Thus Kanner's criteria, and Lotter's and Rutter's definitions were used in the first eight surveys (all conducted before 1982), whereas DSM-based definitions took over thereafter as well as ICD-10 since 1990. Some studies have relaxed partially some diagnostic criteria such as the requirement of an age of onset before 30 months (study 6) or that of the absence of schizophrenia-like symptoms (studies 13 and 14). However, most surveys have relied on the clinical judgment of experts to arrive at the final case groupings. It is worth underlining that field trials for recent classifications such as DSM-III-R (Spitzer and Siegel, 1990) or DSM-IV/ICD-10 (Volkmar *et al.*, 1994) have also relied upon the judgment of clinical experts, taken as a gold standard to diagnose autism and calibrate diagnostic algorithms. Therefore the heterogeneity of diagnostic criteria used across surveys is somewhat mitigated by reliance on expert clinical judgment to determine final caseness. It is also difficult to assess the impact of a specific diagnostic scheme or a particular diagnostic criterion on the estimate of prevalence since other powerful method factors confound between-studies comparisons of rates. Surprisingly, few studies have built in a reliability assessment of the diagnostic procedure; reliability during the intensive assessment phase was high in seven surveys (studies 4, 13, 16, 23, 24, 32, and 36) and moderate in one (study 14).

Characteristics of autistic samples

Data on children with autistic disorders were available in 36 surveys (studies 1–36; see Table 2.1). A total number of 7514 subjects were considered to suffer from autism, this number ranging from 6 (studies 18 and 25) to 5038 (study 34) across studies (median 48; mean 209). An assessment of intellectual function was obtained in 21 studies. These assessments were conducted with various tests and instruments; furthermore, results were pooled in broad bands of intellectual level which did not share the same boundaries across studies. As a consequence, differences in rates of cognitive impairment between studies should be interpreted with caution. With these caveats in mind, some general conclusions can nevertheless be reached (see Table 2.1). The median proportion of subjects without intellectual impairment was 29.6% (range 0%–60%) (Study 23, which relied upon different IQ groupings has been excluded). The corresponding figures are 29.3% (range 6.6%–100%) for mild to moderate intellectual impairments, and 38.5% (range 0%–81.3%) for severe to profound levels of mental retardation. Gender repartition among subjects with autism was reported in 32 studies totaling 6963 subjects with autism, and the male:female sex ratio varied from 1.33 (study 7) to 16.0 (study 4), with a mean male:female ratio of 4.3:1. Thus, no epidemiological study ever identified more girls than boys with autism, a finding that parallels the gender differences found in clinically referred samples (Lord *et al.*, 1982). Gender differences were more pronounced when autism was not associated with mental retardation. In 13 studies (865 subjects) where the sex ratio was available within the normal band of intellectual functioning, the median sex ratio was 5.5:1. Conversely, in 12 studies (813 subjects), the median sex ratio was 1.95:1 in the group with autism and moderate to severe mental retardation.

Prevalence estimations for autistic disorder

Prevalence estimates ranged from 0.7 per 10 000 to 72.6 per 10 000 (see Table 2.1). Confidence intervals were computed for each estimate; their width (the difference between the upper and lower limits of the 95% confidence interval, CI) indicates the variation in sample sizes and in the precision achieved in each study (range 0.3–115.9; mean 11.3). Prevalence rates were negatively correlated with sample size (Spearman $r = -0.73$; $p < 0.01$); small-scale studies tended to report higher prevalence rates.

When surveys were combined in two groups according to the median year of publication (1994), the median prevalence rate for 18 surveys published in the period 1966–93 was 4.7 per 10 000, and the median rate for the 18 surveys published in the period 1994–2004 was 12.7 per 10 000. Indeed, the correlation between prevalence rate and year of publication reached statistical significance (Spearman $r = 0.65$; $p < 0.01$), and the results of the 22 surveys with prevalence rates over 7 per 10 000 were all published since 1987. These findings point towards an increase in prevalence estimates in the last 15 to 20 years. In order to derive a best estimate of the current prevalence of autism, it was therefore deemed appropriate to restrict the analysis to 28 surveys published since 1987. The prevalence estimates ranged from 2.5 to 72.6 per 10 000 (average 95% CI width 14.1), with an average rate of 16.2 per 10 000 and a median rate of 11.3 per 10 000. Similar values were obtained when slightly different rules and time cutpoints were used, with median and mean rates fluctuating between 10–13 and 13–18 per 10 000, respectively. From these results, a conservative estimate for the current prevalence of autistic disorder is most consistent with values lying somewhere between 10 per 10 000 and 16 per 10 000. For further calculations, we arbitrarily adopted the midpoint of this interval as the working rate for autism prevalence, i.e. the value of 13 per 10 000.

Associated medical conditions

Rates of medical conditions associated with autism were reported in 15 surveys. These medical conditions were investigated by very different means ranging from questionnaires to full medical work-ups.

Conditions such as congenital rubella and phenylketonuria (PKU) account for almost no cases of autism. Prior studies suggesting an association of congenital rubella (Chess, 1971) and PKU (Knobloch & Pasamanick, 1975; Lowe et al., 1980) with autism were conducted before implementation of systematic prevention measures. Similarly, the estimate of 0% for autism and neurofibromatosis is consistent with the 0.3% rate found in a large series of 341 referred cases (Mouridsen et al., 1992). The rates found for cerebral palsy and Down's syndrome equally suggest no particular association. The recognition that Down's syndrome and autism co-occur in some individuals has been the focus of attention in recent reports (Bregman and Volkmar, 1988; Ghaziuddin et al., 1992; Howlin et al., 1995); the epidemiological findings give further support to the validity of these clinical descriptions (i.e. that the two conditions co-occur in some children), although they do not suggest that the rate of comorbidity is higher than that expected by chance once the effects of mental retardation are taken into account. For fragile X syndrome, the low rate available in epidemiological surveys (0.3%) is most certainly an underestimate due to the fact that fragile X was not recognized until relatively recently. In line with prior reports (Smalley et al., 1992), tuberous sclerosis (TS) has a consistently high frequency among autistic samples (1%). Assuming a population prevalence of 1 per 10 000 for TS (Ahlsen et al., 1994; Hunt & Lindenbaum, 1984; Shepherd et al., 1991), it appears that the rate of TS is about 100 times higher than that expected under the hypothesis of no association.

The overall proportion of cases of autism which could be causally attributed to known medical disorders therefore remains low. From the 16 surveys where rates of 1 in 7 clear-cut medical disorders potentially causally associated with autism (cerebral palsy, fragile X, TS, PKU, neurofibromatosis, congenital rubella, and Down's syndrome) were available, we computed the proportion of subjects with at least one of these recognizable disorders. Because the overlap between these conditions is expected to be low and because the information about multiply handicapped subjects was anyhow not available, this overall rate was obtained by summing directly the rates for each individual condition within each study; the resulting rate of 5.5% might, therefore, be slightly overestimated. The fraction of cases of autism with a known medical condition that was potentially etiologically significant ranged from 0% to 16.7%, with a median and mean values of 5.5% and 5.9%, respectively. Even if some adjustment were made to account for the underestimation of the rate of fragile X in epidemiological surveys of autism, the attributable proportion of cases of autism would not exceed the 10% figure for any medical disorder (excluding epilepsy and sensory impairments). Although this figure does not incorporate other medical events of potential etiological significance – such as encephalitis, congenital anomalies, and other rare medical syndromes – it is similar to that reported in a recent review of the question (Rutter *et al.*, 1994).

Rates of epilepsy are high among autism samples. The proportion suffering from epilepsy also tends to be higher in those studies with higher rates of severe mental retardation (as in studies 16, 17, and 20). Age-specific rates for the prevalence of epilepsy were not available. The samples where high rates of epilepsy were reported tended to have a higher median age, although these rates seemed mostly to apply to school-aged children. Thus, in light of the increased incidence of seizures during adolescence among subjects with autism (Deykin & MacMahon, 1979; Rutter, 1970), the epidemiological rates should be regarded as underestimates of the lifetime risk of epilepsy in autism. These rates are nonetheless high and support the findings of a bimodal peak of incidence of epilepsy in autistic samples, with a first peak of incidence in the first years of life (Volkmar & Nelson, 1990).

Rates of other pervasive developmental disorders

Unspecified PDDs: PDD-NOS

Several studies have provided useful information on rates of syndromes similar to autism but falling short of strict diagnostic criteria for autistic disorder (Table 2.2). Because the screening procedures and subsequent diagnostic assessments differed from one study to another, these groups of disorders are not

Table 2.2 Relative rates of autism and other pervasive developmental disorders (PDDs)

No.	Study	Rates of autism	Prevalence rate of other PDD	Combined rate autism [a] other PDDs	Prevalence rate ratio [b]	Case definition for other PDDs
1.	Lotter, 1966	4.1	3.3	7.8	0.90	Children with some behavior similar to that of autistic children
2.	Brask, 1970	4.3	1.9	6.2	0.44	Children with "other psychoses" or "borderline psychotic"
4.	Wing et al., 1976	4.9	16.3	21.2	3.33	Socially impaired (triad of impairments)
5.	Hoshino et al., 1982	2.33	2.92	5.25	1.25	Autistic mental retardation
9.	Burd et al., 1987	3.26	>7.79[a]	>11.05[a]	2.39	Children referred by professionals with "autistic-like" symptoms, not meeting DSM-III criteria for IA, COPDD, or atypical PDD
14.	Cialdella & Mamelle, 1989	4.5	4.7	9.2	1.04	Children meeting criteria for other forms of "infantile psychosis" than autism or a broadened definition of DSM-III.
17.	Fombonne & du Mazaubrun (1992) [c]	4.6	6.6	11.2	1.43	Children with mixed developmental disorders
20.	Fombonne et al., 1997	5.3	10.94	16.3	2.05	Children with mixed developmental disorders
26.	Baird et al., 2000	30.8	27.1	57.9	0.9	Children with other PDDs
27.	Powell et al., 2000	7.8	13.0	20.8	1.7	Children with other PDDs
29.	Bertrand et al., 2001	40.5	27.0	67.4	0.7	Children with PDD-NOS and Asperger's disorder
32	Chakrabarti & Fombonne, 2001	16.8	36.1	52.9	2.15	Children with PDD-NOS
35.	Madsen et al., 2002	7.2	22.2	29.4	3.08	
36.	Chakrabarti & Fombonne, 2005	22.0	24.8	46.8	1.13	Children with PDD-NOS

[a] Computed by the author;

[b] Other PDD rate divided by autism rate;

[c] These rates are derived from the complete results of the survey of three birth cohorts of French children (Rumeau-Rouquette et al., 1994).

COPDD: Childhood Onset Pervasive Developmental Disorder.

IA: Infantile Autism.

strictly comparable across studies. In addition, as they were not the group on which the attention was focused, details are often lacking on their phenomenological features in the available reports. Different labels (see Table 2.2) have been used to characterize them such as the triad of impairments involving impairments in reciprocal social interaction, communication, and imagination (Wing & Gould, 1979). These groups would be overlapping with current diagnostic labels such as atypical autism and PDD-NOS. Fourteen of the 36 surveys yielded separate estimates of the prevalence of these developmental disorders, with 10 studies showing higher rates for the nonautism disorders than the rates for autism. The ratio of the rate of nonautistic PDD to the rate of autism varied from 0.44 to 3.33 (see Table 2.2) with a mean value of 1.6, which translates into an average prevalence estimate of 20.8 per 10 000. In other words, for every two children with autism assessed in epidemiological surveys, three were found to have severe impairments of a similar nature but falling short of strict diagnostic criteria for autism. This group has been much less studied in previous epidemiological surveys but progressive recognition of its importance and relevance to autism has led to changes in the design of more recent epidemiological surveys (see below) which are now designed to include these less typical children in the case definition adopted in surveys. It should be clear from these figures that they represent a very substantial group of children whose treatment needs are likely to be as important as those of children with autism.

Asperger's syndrome and childhood disintegrative disorder

The reader is referred to recent epidemiological reviews for these two conditions (Fombonne, 2002b; Fombonne & Tidmarsh, 2003).

In brief, epidemiological surveys of Asperger's syndrome are sparse, probably due to the fact that it was acknowledged as a separate diagnostic category only recently in both ICD-10 and DSM-IV. Only two epidemiological surveys have been conducted which specifically investigated its prevalence (Ehlers & Gillberg, 1993; Kadesjö et al., 1999). However, only a handful ($n < 5$) of cases were identified in these surveys, with the resulting estimates of 28 and 48 per 10 000 being extremely imprecise. By contrast, other recent autism surveys have consistently identified smaller numbers of children with Asperger's syndrome than those with autism within the same survey. In seven such surveys (studies 23–27, 32 reviewed in Fombonne & Tidmarsh, 2003; and study 36) the ratio of autism to Asperger's syndrome rates in each survey was above unity, suggesting that the rate was consistently lower than that for autism (Table 2.3). How much lower is difficult to establish from existing data, but a ratio of 5 to 1 would appear an acceptable, albeit conservative, conclusion based on this limited available evidence.

Table 2.3 Asperger's syndrome in recent autism surveys

Study	Size of population	Age group	Informants	Instruments	Diagnostic criteria	Autism n	Autism Rate/10000	AS n	AS Rate/10000	Autism/AS ratio
23. Sponheim & Skjeldal, 1998	65 688	3–14	Parent, child	Parental interview + direct observation, CARS, ABC	ICD-10	32	4.9	2	0.3	16.0
24. Taylor et al., 1999	490 000	0–16	Record	Rating of all data available in child record	ICD-10	427	8.7	71	1.4	6.0
25. Kadesjö et al., 1999	826	6.7–7.7	Child, parent, professional	ADI-R, Griffiths scale or WISC, AS Screening Questionnaire	DSM-III-R/ ICD-10 Gillberg's criteria (AS)	6	72.6	4	48.4	1.5
26. Baird et al., 2000	16 235	7	Parents, child, other data	ADI-R psychometry	ICD-10 DSM-IV	45	27.7	5	3.1	9.0
27. Powell et al., 2000	25 377	1–4.9	Records	ADI-R available data	DSM-III-R, DSM-IV, ICD-10	54	—	16	—	3.4
32. Chakrabarti & Fombonne, 2001	15 500	2.5–6.5	Child, parent, professional	ADI-R, 2 weeks' multidisciplinary assessment, Merrill–Palmer, WPPSI	ICD-10, DSM-IV	26	16.8	13	8.4	2.0
36. Chakrabarti & Fombonne, 2005	10 903	2.5–6.5	Child, parent, professional	ADI-R, 2 weeks' multidisciplinary assessment, Merrill–Palmer, WPPSI	ICD-10, DSM-IV	24	22.0	12	11.0	2.0
Overall	614					123				5.0

ABC: Aberrant Behavior Checklist. CARS: Childhood Autism Rating Scale.
ADI-R: Autism Diagnostic Interview–Revised. WISC: Wechsler Intelligence Scale for Children.

This translates into a rate for Asperger's syndrome which would be 1/5 that of autism. We therefore used, for subsequent calculations, an estimate of 2.6 per 10 000 for Asperger's syndrome. A recent survey of high-functioning PDDs in Welsh mainstream primary schools has yielded a relatively high (uncorrected) prevalence estimate of 14.5 per 10 000. Of the 17 children contributing to this figure, 10 had either Asperger's disorder or high-functioning autism as a primary diagnosis. Assuming that half of these would have Asperger's disorder, we could extrapolate a 4.3 per 10 000 prevalence, a figure that is in line with other studies. However, much caution should be applied to this calculation as it is based on several assumptions that are impossible to verify.

Few surveys have provided data on childhood disintegrative disorder (CDD), also known as Heller's syndrome, disintegrative psychosis (ICD-9) or late-onset autism (see Volkmar, 1992). In addition to the four studies (studies 9, 23, 31, and 32) of our previous review (Fombonne, 2002b), another survey has provided new data on CDD (study 36). Taking the five studies into account (Table 2.4), prevalence estimates ranged from 1.1 to 9.2 per 100 000. The pooled estimate based on seven identified cases and a surveyed population of 358 633 children, was 1.9 per 100 000. The upper-bound limit of the associated CI (4.15 per 100 000) indicates that CDD is a very rare condition, with one case occurring for every 65 cases of autistic disorder. As cases of CDD were both rare and already included in the numerator alongside autism cases in most surveys, we do not provide separate estimates of the numbers of subjects suffering from CDD in subsequent calculations.

Prevalence for combined PDDs

Taking the aforementioned conservative estimates, the prevalence for all PDDs is at least 36.4 per 10 000, i.e. the sum of estimates for autism (13 per 10 000), PDD-NOS (20.8 per 10 000), and AS (2.6 per 10 000). This global estimate is derived from a conservative analysis of existing data.

However, eight recent epidemiological surveys yielded even higher rates in six instances (Table 2.5); the two surveys that did not might have underestimated the rates. In the Danish investigation (study 35), case finding depended upon notification to a National Registry, a method which is usually associated with lower sensitivity for case finding. The Atlanta survey by the Centers for Disease Control (study 38) was based on a very large population (which typically yields lower prevalence; see above) and age-specific rates were in fact in the 40–45 per 10 000 range in some birth cohorts (Fombonne, 2003b). The common design features of the four other epidemiological enquiries (studies 26, 29, 32, and 36) that yielded

Table 2.4 Surveys of childhood disintegrative disorder

Study	Country (region/state)	Size of target population	Age group	Assessment	n	M/F	Prevalence estimate (/100 000)	95% CI[1] (/100 000)
Burd et al., 1987	USA (North Dakota)	180 986	2–18	Structured parental interview and review of all data available: DSM-III criteria	2	2/–	1.11	0.13; 3.4
Sponheim & Skjeldal, 1998	Norway (Akershus County)	65 688	3–14	Parental interview and direct observation (CARS, ABC)	1	?	1.52	0.04; 8.5
Magnusson et Saemundsen, 2001	Iceland (whole island)	85 556	5–14	ADI-R, CARS, and psychological tests: mostly ICD-10	2	2/–	2.34	0.3; 8.4
Chakrabarti & Fombonne, 2001	UK (Staffordshire, Midlands)	15 500	2.5–6.5	ADI-R, two weeks' multidisciplinary assessment, Merrills–Palmer, WPPSI: ICD-10/DSM-IV	1	1/–	6.4	0.16; 35.9
Chakrabarti & Fombonne, 2005	UK (Staffordshire, Midlands)	10 903	2.5–6.5	ADI-R, two weeks' multidisciplinary assessment, Merrill–Palmer, WPPSI: ICD-10/DSM-IV	1	1/–	9.2	0–58.6
Pooled estimates		**358 633**			**7**	**6/–**	**1.9**	**0.87–4.15**

CI: Confidence interval.

Table 2.5 Newer epidemiological surveys of pervasive developmental disorders (PDDs)

No.	Study	Age	Autism			PDD-NOS + AS			All PDDs
			Rate/10 000	M/F ratio	% IQ normal	Rate/10 000	M/F ratio	% IQ normal	Rate/10 000
26	Baird et al., 2000	7	30.8	15.7	60	27.1	4.5	–	57.9
29	Bertrand et al., 2001	3–10	40.5	2.2	37	27.0	3.7	51	67.5
32	Chakrabarti & Fombonne, 2001	4–7	16.8	3.3	29	44.5	4.3	94	61.3
35	Madsen et al., 2002	8	7.7	–	–	22.2	–	–	30.0
36	Chakrabarti & Fombonne, 2005	4–7	22.0	4.0	33.3	35.8	8.7	91.6	58.7
37	Scott et al., 2002	5–11	–	–	–	–	–	–	58.3[a]
38	Yeargin-Allsopp et al., 2003	3–10	–	–	–	–	–	–	34.0
39	Gurney et al., 2003	6–11	–	–	–	–	–	–	52.0

[a] Computed by the author; AS: Asperger's syndrome; PDD-NOS: pervasive developmental disorders not otherwise specified.

higher rates are worthy of mention. First, the case definition chosen for these investigations was that of a PDD as opposed to the narrower approach focusing on autistic disorder typical of previous surveys. Investigators were concerned with any combination of severe developmental abnormalities occurring in one or more of the three symptomatic domains defining PDD and autism. Second, case-finding techniques employed in these surveys were proactive, relying on multiple and repeated screening phases, involving both different informants at each phase and surveying the same cohorts at different ages, which certainly maximized the sensitivity of case identification. Third, assessments were performed with standardized diagnostic measures (i.e. Autism Diagnostic Interview-Revised and Autism Diagnostic Observation Schedule), which closely match the dimensional approach retained for case definition. Finally, these samples comprised young children around their fifth birthdays, thereby optimizing sensitivity of case-finding procedures. Furthermore, the size of targeted populations was reasonably small (between 9000 and 16 000), probably allowing for the most efficient use of research resources. Conducted in different regions and countries by different teams, the convergence of estimates is striking.

Two further results are worth noting. First, in sharp contrast with the prevalence for combined PDDs, the separate estimates for autistic disorder and PDD-NOS vary widely in studies where separate figures were available, as if the reliability of the differentiation between autistic disorder and PDD-NOS was mediocre at that young age, despite the use of up-to-date standardized measures. Second, the rate of mental retardation was, overall, much lower than in previous surveys of autism. While this should not be a surprise for children in the PDD-NOS/Asperger's syndrome groups, this trend was also noticeable within samples diagnosed with autistic disorder. To what extent this trend reflects the previously mentioned differential classification issues between autism and PDD-NOS or a genuine trend over time towards a decreased rate of mental retardation within children with autistic disorder (possibly as a result of earlier diagnosis and intervention) remains to be established.

In conclusion, the convergence of surveys around an estimate of 60 per 10 000 for all PDD combined is striking, especially when coming from studies with improved methods. This estimate now appears to be the best estimate for the prevalence of PDDs currently available.

Time trends

The debate on the hypothesis of a secular increase in rates of autism has been obscured by a lack of clarity in the measures of disease occurrence used by investigators, or rather in their interpretation. In particular, it is crucial to differentiate *prevalence* (the proportion of individuals in a population who suffer from a defined disorder) from *incidence* (the number of new cases occurring in a population over a period of time). Prevalence is useful to estimate needs and plan services but only incidence rates can be used for causal research. Both prevalence and incidence estimates will be inflated when case definition is broadened and case ascertainment is improved. Time trends in rates can therefore only be gauged in investigations that hold these parameters under strict control over time. These methodological requirements must be borne in mind while reviewing the evidence for a secular increase in rates of PDDs.

Five approaches to assess this question have been used in the literature.

1   Referral statistics

Increasing numbers of children referred to specialist services or known to special education registers have been taken as evidence for an increased incidence of autism-spectrum disorders. However, trends over time in referred samples are confounded by many factors such as referral patterns, availability of services, heightened public awareness, decreasing age at diagnosis, and changes over time in diagnostic concepts and practices, to name only a few. Failure to control for these confounding factors was obvious in some recent reports (Fombonne, 2001), such as the widely quoted reports from California educational services (Department of Developmental Services, DDS, 1999, 2003). First, these reports applied to numbers rather than rates, and failure to relate these numbers to meaningful denominators left the interpretation of an upward trend vulnerable to changes in the composition of the underlying population. For example, the population of California was 19 971 000 in 1970 and rose to 35 116 000 as at July 1, 2002, an increase of 75.8%. Thus part of the increase in numbers of subjects identified with autism merely reflects the change in population size, but this has not been taken (or only incompletely) into account in the DDS reports. Second, the focus on the year-to-year changes in absolute numbers of subjects known to California state-funded services detracts from more meaningful comparisons. For example, as at December 2002, the total of subjects with a PDD diagnosis was 17 748 in the 0–19 year age group (including 16 108 autism codes 1 and 2, and 1640 other PDDs; Department of Developmental Services, 2003). The population of 0 to 19-year-olds in California was 10 462 273 in July 2002. If one applies a rather conservative PDD rate of 30 per 10 000, one would expect to have 31 386 subjects within this age group with a PDD living in California. These calculations do not support the "epidemic" interpretation. Rather, they suggest that children identified in the DDS database were only a subset of the population prevalence pool and that the increasing numbers merely reflect an increasing proportion of children accessing services. Third, no attempt was ever made to adjust the trends for changes in diagnostic concepts and definitions. However, major nosographical modifications were introduced during the corresponding years with a general tendency in most classifications to broaden the concept of autism (as embodied in the terms "autism spectrum" or "pervasive developmental disorder"). Fourth, age characteristics of the subjects recorded in official statistics were portrayed in a confusing manner where the preponderance of young subjects was presented as evidence of increasing rates in successive birth cohorts (Fombonne, 2001). The problems associated with disentangling age from period and cohort effects in such observational data are well known in the epidemiological literature and can be handled more effectively as in recent studies (Gurney *et al.*, 2003; Newschaffer *et al.*, 2005). Fifth, the decreasing age at diagnosis leads in itself to increasing numbers of young children being identified in official statistics or referred to already busy specialist services. Earlier identification of children from the prevalence pool may result in increased service activity; however, it does not mean increased incidence.

Another study of this dataset was subsequently launched to demonstrate the validity of the "epidemic" hypothesis (MIND Institute, 2002). The investigation was, however, flawed in its design. The authors relied on DDS data and aimed at ruling out changes in diagnostic practices and immigration into California as factors explaining the increased numbers. While immigration was reasonably ruled out, the study comparing diagnoses of autism and mental retardation over time was impossible to interpret in light of the extremely low ($<20\%$) response rates. Furthermore, a study based only on cases registered for services cannot rule out that the proportion of cases within the general population who registered with services has changed over time. For example, assuming a constant incidence and prevalence at two different time points (i.e. there is no epidemic), the number of cases known to a public agency delivering services could well increase by 200% if the proportion of cases from the community referred to services rises from 25% to 75% in the interval. In order to rule out this (likely, see above) explanation, data over time are needed both on referred subjects and on nonreferred (or referred to other services) subjects. Failure to do that precludes any inference to be drawn from a study of the DDS database to the California population (Fombonne, 2003b). The conclusions of this report were therefore simply unwarranted.

Some United Kingdom (UK) data also suggest that switches in diagnostic practices between autism and specific developmental disorders (including language disorders) could also play a role (Jick & Kaye, 2003) although these findings have not been replicated in the United States (USA) (Newschaffer *et al.*, 2005).

On the whole, evidence from these referral statistics is therefore very weak and certainly does not deserve the media attention that has been orchestrated around it. Accordingly, proper epidemiological surveys are needed in order to assess secular changes in the incidence of a disorder.

2   Comparison of cross-sectional epidemiological surveys

Because of their cross-sectional methodology, most epidemiological investigations of autism have all been concerned with prevalence. As shown earlier, epidemiological surveys of autism each possess unique design features which could account almost entirely for between-studies variations in rates; time trends in rates of autism are therefore difficult to gauge from published prevalence rates. The significant correlation previously mentioned between prevalence rate and year of publication could merely reflect increased efficiency over time in case identification methods used in surveys as well as changes in diagnostic concepts and practices. Thus changes in diagnostic practices were reported in Magnusson and Saemundsen's study (2001) where ICD-9 rates for the oldest cohorts born in the years 1964–83 were lower than the ICD-10 rates of the most recent 1984–92 birth cohorts. Similarly, lower rates in the oldest birth cohorts were thought to reflect changes in diagnostic practices and boundaries in Webb *et al.*'s study (1997). One large survey recently conducted in the UK (study 24) also documented a steep rise in the number of cases diagnosed with autism or atypical autism, and a similar trend for AS. The interpretation of these trends is, however, unclear since there was no control of drift over time in diagnostic practices nor of changes in service development. The impact of changes in diagnostic criteria on rates of autism is best illustrated in the Finnish survey of Kielinen *et al.* (2000) where a threefold increase in the rate of autism (from 2.3 to 7.6 per 10 000) was observed in 15 to 18-year-olds when either Kanner's criteria or ICD-10 spectrum criteria were applied to the same survey data.

The most convincing evidence that method factors could account for most of the variability in published prevalence estimates comes from a direct comparison of eight recent surveys conducted in the UK and the USA (Table 2.6). In each country, four surveys were conducted around the same year and with similar age groups. As there is no reason to expect huge between-area differences in rates, prevalence estimates should therefore be comparable within each country. However, an inspection of estimates obtained in each set of studies (see Table 2.6, right-hand column) shows a sixfold variation in rates for UK surveys, and a 14-fold variation in US rates. In each set of studies, high rates derive from surveys where intensive population-based screening techniques were employed whereas lower rates were obtained from studies relying on administrative methods for

Table 2.6 Study design impact on prevalence

	Location	Size	Age group	Method	PDD rate/ 10 000
UK studies					
Chakrabarti & Fombone, 2001	Stafford shire	15 500	$2^{1}/_{2}$–$6^{1}/_{2}$	Intense screening + assessment	62.6
Baird et al., 2000	South-east Thames	16 235	7	Early screening+follow-up identification	57.9
Fombonne et al., 2001	England and Wales	10 438	5–15	National household survey of psychiatric disorders	26.1
Taylor et al., 1999	North Thames	490 000	0–16	Administrative records	10.1
US studies					
Bertrand et al., 2001	Brick Township, NJ	8 896	3–10	Multiple sources of ascertainment	67
Sturmey & James, 2001	Texas	3 564 577	6–18	Educational services	16
DDS, 1999	California	3 215 000	4–9	Educational services	15
Hillman et al., 2000	Missouri	–	5–9	Educational services	4.8

PDD: pervasive developmental disorders.

case-finding. Since no passage of time was involved, the magnitude of these gradients in rates can only be attributed to differences in case-identification methods across surveys, and the replication of the pattern in two countries provides even more confidence in this interpretation. Thus, following this analysis of recent and contemporaneous studies, it should become obvious that no inference on trends in the incidence of PDDs can be derived from a simple comparison of prevalence rates over time, since studies conducted at different periods are likely to differ even more with respect to their methodology.

The next two approaches are in essence comparable to this one although specific attempts are made to maintain some design features of surveys constant.

3   Repeat surveys in defined geographical areas

Repeated surveys, using the same methodology and conducted in the same geographical area at different points in time, can potentially yield useful information on time trends provided that methods are kept relatively constant. The Göteborg studies (Gillberg, 1984; Gillberg et al., 1991) provided three prevalence estimates which increased over a short period from 4.0 (1980) to 6.6 (1984) and 9.5 per 10 000 (1988). However, comparisons of these rates is not straightforward as different age groups were included in each survey. For example, the rate in the first survey for the youngest age group (which resembles more closely the children included in the two other surveys) was 5.1 per 10 000. Second, the increased prevalence in the second survey was explained by improved detection among the mentally retarded, and that of the third survey by cases born to immigrant parents. That the majority of the latter group was born abroad suggests that migration into the area could be a key explanation. Taken in conjunction with a change in local services and a progressive broadening of the definition of autism over time acknowledged by the authors (Gillberg et al., 1991), these findings do not provide evidence for an increased incidence in the rate of autism.

Two separate surveys conducted on children born in 1992–95 and 1996–98 in Staffordshire, UK (see Table 2.1; studies 32 and 36) were performed with rigorously identical methods for case definition and case identification. The prevalence for combined PDD was comparable and not statistically different in the two surveys (Chakrabarti & Fombonne, 2005), suggesting no upward trend in overall rates of PDD during the studies' time interval.

4   Successive birth cohorts

In large surveys encompassing a wide age range, increasing prevalence rates among the most recent birth cohorts could be interpreted as indicating a secular increase in the incidence of the disorder, provided that alternative explanations can confidently be ruled out. This analysis was used in two French surveys (studies 17 and 20), which derived from large sample sizes. In the first study (study 17), prevalence estimates were available for the two birth cohorts of children born in 1972 and 1976 surveyed in 1985–86. The rates were similar (5.1 and 4.9 per 10 000) and not statistically different (Fombonne & du Mazaubrun, 1992). Furthermore, in a subsequent investigation conducted in 1989–90 in exactly the same areas, the age-specific rate of autism for the 1981 birth cohort was slightly lower (3.1 per 10 000) (Rumeau-Rouquette et al., 1994). In any instance, the findings were not suggestive of increasing rates in the most recent cohorts. Another survey conducted with the same methodology, but in different French regions a few years later (study 20), led to a similar overall prevalence estimate as compared to the first survey (see Table 2.1). The latter survey included consecutive birth cohorts from 1976 to 1985, and, pooling the data of both surveys, age-specific rates showed no upward trend (Fombonne et al., 1997). Some weight should be given to these results as they derive from a total target population of 735 000 children, 389 of whom had autism. However, the most retarded children with autism were reflected in these studies and, as a consequence, any upward trend which would apply specifically to high-functioning subjects might have gone undetected.

A recent analysis of special educational disability from Minnesota showed a 16-fold increase in the number of children identified with a PDD from 1991–92 to 2001–02 (Gurney *et al.*, 2003; study 39). The increase was not specific to autism since during the same period an increase of 50% was observed for all disability categories (except severe mental handicap), especially for the category including attention deficit and hyperactivity disorder. The large sample size allowed the authors to assess age, period, and cohort effects. Prevalence increased regularly in successive birth cohorts; for example, amongst 7-year-olds, the prevalence rose from 18 per 10 000 in those born in 1989, to 29 per 10 000 in those born in 1991 and to 55 per 10 000 in those born in 1993, suggestive of birth cohort effects. Within the same birth cohorts, age effects were also apparent since for children born in 1989 the prevalence rose with age from 13 per 10 000 at age 6, to 21 per 10 000 at age 9, and 33 per 10 000 at age 11. As argued by the authors, this pattern is not consistent with what one would expect from a chronic nonfatal condition diagnosed in the first years of life. Their analysis also showed a marked period effect that identified the early 1990s as the period where rates started to increase in all ages and birth cohorts. Gurney *et al.* (2003) further argued that this phenomenon coincided closely with the inclusion of PDDs in the federal Individual with Disabilities Educational Act funding and reporting mechanism in the USA. A similar interpretation of upward trends had been put forward by Croen *et al.* (2002) in their analysis of the California DDS data and in a nationwide analysis of special education data on US children 6 to 17 years of age (Newschaffer *et al.*, 2005).

5   Incidence studies

Only three studies recently provided incidence estimates (Kaye *et al.*, 2001; Powell *et al.*, 2000; Smeeth *et al.*, 2004). All studies showed an upward trend in incidence over short periods of time. For example, in the largest study of 1410 subjects, there was a 10-fold increase in the rate of first recorded diagnoses of PDDs in United Kingdom general practice medical records from 1988–92 to 2000–01 (Smeeth *et al.*, 2004). The increase was more marked for PDDs other than autism but the increase in autism was also obvious. However, none of these studies' investigations could determine the impact of changes over time in diagnostic criteria, improved awareness, and service availability on the upward trend.

Conclusion on time trends

The available epidemiological evidence does not strongly support the hypothesis that the incidence of autism has increased. As it stands now, the recent upward trend in rates of prevalence cannot be directly attributed to an increase in the incidence of the disorder. There is some evidence that diagnostic substitution and changes in the policies for special education and the increasing availability of services are responsible for the higher prevalence figures. Most of the existing epidemiological data are inadequate to properly test hypotheses on changes in the incidence of autism in human populations. Moreover, due to the low frequency of autism and PDDs, power is seriously limited in most investigations and variations of small magnitude in the incidence of the disorder are very likely to go undetected. Future investigations should aim at setting up surveillance programs which will allow an estimate of the incidence of PDDs (as opposed to autism only) and to monitor its changes over time. It will be crucial to set up parallel investigations in different geographical areas in order to replicate findings across areas as a validating tool. Such programs should focus on age groups where the identification and diagnosis of the range of PDDs is less likely to fluctuate over time. Rapid changes in the age at first diagnosis and concerns about the validity and stability of diagnostic assessments among preschool samples are required to focus on older age groups. On the other hand, changes in the autistic symptomatology in adolescence and difficulties in service delivery to teenagers (and therefore in case identification) suggest that the focus should be on rather younger children. The school age years (7–12) should therefore be selected for efficient monitoring. Mandatory education at that age would facilitate identification, and potential difficulties in diagnosing high-functioning subjects would be minimized at the upper end of this age range. Diagnostic assessments should rely on standardized measures of known reliability and validity. Furthermore, developmental and phenomenological data should be collected at a symptomatic level, and uniformly across the whole spectrum of PDDs, remaining free of particular nosological contingencies. Secondary application of diagnostic algorithms (current and / or future) on datasets containing detailed developmental and symptomatic data will then allow for meaningful comparisons over time to be performed, with diagnostic groupings being held constant. Finally, good psychometric data on cognitive functioning will also be needed to assess trends in various subgroups in the light of the preliminary evidence that patterns of mental retardation in autism may be changing. Obviously, measures of risk factors hypothesized to exert causal influences for this group of disorders should also be incorporated in surveillance programs.

Other correlates

Autism, race, and immigrant status

Some investigators have mentioned the possibility that rates of autism might be higher among immigrants (Gillberg, 1987; Gillberg *et al.*, 1991; Gillberg *et al.*, 1995; Wing, 1980). Five of the 17 children with autism identified in the Camberwell, UK, study were of Caribbean origin (study 4; Wing, 1980) and the estimated rate of autism was 6.3 per 10 000 for this group as compared to 4.4 per 10 000 for the rest of the population (Wing, 1993). However, the wide CIs associated with rates from this study (see Table 2.1) indicate no statistically significant difference. In addition, this area of London had received a large proportion of immigrants from the Caribbean region in the 1960s and, under circumstances where migration flux in and out of an area is happening, estimation of population rates should be viewed with much caution. Yet, Afro-Caribbean children referred from the same area were recently found to have higher rates of autism than referred controls (Goodman & Richards, 1995); however, the sample was again very small ($n = 18$) and differential referral patterns to a tertiary center also providing services for the local area could not be ruled out. It is worth noting that only one child with autism was born from British-born Afro-Caribbean parents in a recent UK survey (study 21; Webb *et al.*, 1997), providing little support to this particular hypothesis. Similarly, the findings from the Göteborg studies paralleled an increased migration flux in the early 1980s in this area (Gillberg, 1987); they, too, were based on relatively small numbers (19 children from immigrant parents). In the same geographical area, Arvidsson *et al.* (1997; study 22) had five children out of nine in their sample with either both parents ($n = 2$) or one parent ($n = 3$) having immigrated to Sweden; however, there were no systematic comparisons with rates of immigrants in the population. It is worth noting that a positive family history for developmental disorders was reported in three such cases and a chromosomal abnormality in one further case. In the Icelandic survey (study 31), 2.5% of the autism parents were from non-European origin compared to a 0.5% corresponding rate in the whole population, but it was unclear if this represented a significant difference. In study 23, the proportion of children with autism and a non-European origin was marginally but not significantly raised as compared to the population rate of immigrants (8% vs. 2.3%) but this was based on a very small sample (two children of non-European origin). A UK survey found comparables rates in areas contrasting for their ethnic composition (Powell *et al.*, 2000). In the Utah survey, where a clear breakdown by race was achieved (Ritvo *et al.*, 1989; study 15; see Table 2.1), the autism parents showed no deviation from the racial distribution of this state. The proportion of nonwhites in this study and state was, however, noticeably low, providing little power to detect departures from the null hypothesis. Unfortunately, other studies have not systematically reported the proportion of immigrant or ethnic groups in the areas surveyed. However, in four studies where the proportions of immigrant groups were low (studies 11, 12, 19, and 21), rates of autism were in the upper range of rates. Conversely, in other populations where immigrants contributed substantially to the denominators (studies 14, 17, and 20), rates were in the rather low band. The analysis of a large sample ($n = 4356$) of Californian PDD children showed a lower risk of autism in children of Mexico-born mothers and a similar risk for children of mothers born outside the USA as compared to California-born mothers (Croen *et al.*, 2002). In this study, the risk of PDD was raised in African-American mothers with an adjusted rate ratio of 1.6 (95% CI 1.5–1.8); by contrast, the prevalence was similar in white, black, and other races in the population-based survey of Atlanta (Yeargin-Allsopp *et al.*, 2003) where case ascertainment is likely to be more complete than in the previous study.

Taken altogether, the combined results of these reports should be interpreted in the specific methodological context of these investigations. Most studies had low numbers of identified cases, and especially small numbers of autistic children born from immigrant parents, and many authors in these studies relied upon broadened definitions of autism. Statistical testing was not rigorously conducted and doubts could be raised in several studies about the appropriateness of the comparison data that were used. Thus the overall proportion of immigrants in the population may be an inappropriate figure with which to compare observed rates of children from immigrant parents amongst autistic series; fertility rates of immigrant families are likely to be different from those in the host populations and call for strictly age-adjusted comparisons of individuals at risk for the disorder. The proportion of immigrants in the entire population might seriously underestimate that for younger age groups, and, in turn, this could have given rise to false-positive results. In addition, studies sampling children through services or clinical sources may be biased as ethnicity and race are likely to affect differentially access to these settings. Studies were generally poor in their definition of immigrant status, with some unclear amalgamation of information on country of origin, citizenship, immigrant status, race, and ethnicity. Finally, it is unclear what common mechanism could explain the putative association between immigrant status and autism since the origins of the immigrant parents (especially in study 16; Gillberg & Gillberg, 1996) were very diverse and, in fact, represented all continents. With this heterogeneity in mind, what common biological features might be shared by these immigrant families and what would be a plausible mechanism explaining the putative association between autism and immigrant status? The possibility of an increased vulnerability to intrauterine infections in nonimmunized immigrant mothers was raised but not supported in a detailed analysis of 15 autistic children from immigrant parents (Gillberg & Gillberg, 1996). These authors instead posited that parents, and in particular fathers, affected with autistic traits would be inclined to travel abroad in order to find female partners more naïve to their social difficulties. This speculation was based, however, on three observations only, and assessment of the autistic traits in two parents was clearly not independently obtained.

The hypothesis of an association between immigrant status or race and autism, therefore, remains largely unsupported by the empirical results. Most of the claims about these possible correlates of autism derived from *post hoc* observations of very small samples and were not subjected to rigorous statistical testing. Large studies have generally failed to detect such associations.

Autism and social class

Twelve studies provided information on the social class of the families of autistic children. Of these, four studies (1, 2, 3, and 5) suggested an association between autism and social class or parental education. The year of data collection for these four investigations was before 1980 (see Table 2.1) and all studies conducted thereafter provided no evidence for the association. Thus the epidemiological results suggest that the earlier findings were probably due to artifacts in the availability of services and in the case-finding methods, as already shown in other samples (Schopler *et al.*, 1979; Wing, 1980).

Cluster reports

Occasional reports of space or time clustering of cases of autism have raised concerns in the general public. In fact, only one such report has been published in the professional literature (Baron-Cohen *et al.*, 1999) which described seven children with either autism or PDD-NOS living within a few streets of each other in a small town in the British Midlands. The cluster was first identified by a parent and the subsequent analysis was uninformed with proper statistical procedures and inconclusive as to whether or not this cluster could have occurred by chance only. The comparison of the incidence or prevalence rate within the cluster to that of the general population (as performed by Baron-Cohen *et al.*, 1999) is an inappropriate technique to assess cluster alarms since, by definition, a pre-selection bias occurs in the delineation of the cluster boundaries (Kulldorf, 1999). Thus finding an increased incidence or prevalence rate ratio in a cluster does not prove anything; this erroneous approach has been referred to in the literature as the Texan sharpshooter effect, referring to the gunman who shot first and then painted a target around the bullet hole. On the other hand, a negative finding would certainly suggest a random phenomenon.

When cluster alarms are associated to a possible causal mechanism, it is recommended to perform focused tests of clustering at other suspected sources of risk exposure. For example, the cluster alarms for childhood leukemia occurring near a nuclear plant in England were followed by investigations of disease incidence at other nuclear plants, which proved to be negative (Hoffmann & Schlattmann, 1999). However, the potential source of the cluster alarm is not always identified and, in these instances, it is suggested that the incidence of future cases is monitored in the area of first alarm. Chen *et al.* (1993) have outlined post-alarm monitoring techniques, which allow the confirmation or rejection of alarms, based on the observation of the time intervals preceding each of the first five cases diagnosed subsequent to the alarm. The approach is a confirmatory technique, which ignores the cluster alarm data and thus avoids the aforementioned pre-selection bias. Other techniques, such as space-time scan statistics (Kulldorf, 1999), exist which can confirm or reject a cluster alarm by extending the investigation to a larger area while avoiding selection biases, adjusting for population density, confounding variables and multiple testing, and allowing for the precise location of clusters.

Cluster alarms are likely to represent random occurrences in most instances, as illustrated by several recent investigations of cluster alarms for other rare disorders of childhood. Cluster alarms in autism have not been investigated with scientific rigor whereas research strategies and ad hoc statistical procedures exist for that purpose. The approach to such cluster alarms should be to confirm the alarm in the first place, using the available techniques to assess the significance of clusters and to exclude random noise in spatial and time distribution of the disorder. It is only when an alarm has been confirmed that more complex epidemiological investigations should be set up to investigate risk factors and causal mechanisms.

Conclusion

Epidemiological surveys of autism and PDDs have now been carried out in several countries. Methodological differences in case definition and case-finding procedures make between-survey comparisons difficult to perform. Nevertheless, in spite of these differences, some common characteristics of autism and

PDDs in population surveys have emerged with some consistency. Autism is associated with mental retardation in about 70% of the cases and is overrepresented among males (with a male:female ratio of 4.3:1). Autism is found in association with some rare and genetically determined medical conditions, such as tuberous sclerosis. Overall, the median value of about 5.5% for combined rate of medical disorders in autism derived from this review is consistent with the 5% (Tuchman *et al.*, 1991) to 10% (Rutter *et al.*, 1994) figures available from other investigations. A majority of surveys has ruled out social class as a risk factor for autism, a result once supported by studies of clinical, i.e. less representative, samples. The putative association of autism with immigrant status or race is, so far, not borne out by epidemiological surveys. The conclusion of a lack of variation in the incidence of autism according to race or ethnicity is reached, however, from a weak empirical base and future studies might address this issue more efficiently. In fact epidemiological surveys of autism and PDDs have generally been lacking sophistication in their investigation of most other risk factors.

The same considerations apply to the issue of secular changes in the incidence of autism. The little evidence that exists does not support this hypothesis, but the power to detect time trends is seriously limited in existing datasets. The debate has been largely confounded by a confusion between prevalence and incidence. While it appears that prevalence estimates have gone up over time, this increase most likely represents changes in the concepts, definitions, service availability, and awareness of autistic-spectrum disorders in both the lay and professional public. To assess whether or not the incidence has increased, method factors which account for an important proportion of the variability in rates must be tightly controlled. Nevertheless, the current prevalence estimates carry straightforward implications for current and future needs in services and early educational intervention programs.

REFERENCES

Ahlsen, G., Gillberg, C., Lindblom, R., and Gillberg, C. (1994). Tuberous sclerosis in Western Sweden: a population study of cases with early childhood onset. *Archives of Neurology*, **51**, 76–81.

Arvidsson, T., Danielsson, B., Forsberg, P. *et al.* (1997). Autism in 3–6-year-old children in a suburb of Göteborg, Sweden. *Autism*, **2**, 163–73.

Baird, G., Charman, T., Baron-Cohen, S. *et al.* (2000). A screening instrument for autism at 18 months of age: a 6-year follow-up study. *Journal of the American Academy of Child and Adolescent Psychiatry*, **39**, 694–702.

Baron-Cohen, S., Saunders, K., and Chakrabarti, S. (1999). Does autism cluster geographically? A research note. *Autism*, **3**, 39–43.

Bertrand, J., Mars, A., Boyle, C. et al. (2001). Prevalence of autism in a United States population: the Brick Township, New Jersey, investigation. *Pediatrics*, **108**, 1155–61.

Bohman, M., Bohman, I. L., Björck, P. O., and Sjöholm, E. (1983). Childhood psychosis in a northern Swedish county: some preliminary findings from an epidemiological survey. In M. H. Schmidt and H. Remschmidt, eds., *Epidemiological Approaches in Child Psychiatry*. New York: Georg Thieme Verlag, pp. 164–73.

Brask, B. H. (1970). A prevalence investigation of childhood psychoses. In *Nordic Symposium on the Care of Psychotic Children*. Oslo, Norway: Barnepsychiatrist Forening, Universitetsforlagets Trykningssentral, pp. 45–143.

Bregman, J. D. and Volkmar, F. R. (1988). Autistic social dysfunction and Down's syndrome. *Journal of the American Academy of Child and Adolescent Psychiatry*, **27**, 440–1.

Bryson, S. E., Clark, B. S., and Smith, I. M. (1988). First report of a Canadian epidemiological study of autistic syndromes. *Journal of Child Psychology and Psychiatry*, **4**, 433–45.

Burd, L., Fisher, W., and Kerbeshan, J. (1987). A prevalence study of pervasive developmental disorders in North Dakota. *Journal of the American Academy of Child and Adolescent Psychiatry*, **26**(5), 700–3.

Chakrabarti, S. and Fombonne, E. (2001). Pervasive developmental disorders in preschool children. *Journal of the American Medical Association*, **285**(24), 3093–9.

Chakrabarti, S. and Fombonne, E. (2005). Pervasive developmental disorders in preschool children: confirmation of high prevalence. *American Journal of Psychiatry*, **162**, 1133–41.

Chen, R., Connelly, R., and Mantel, N. (1993). Analysing post-alarm data in a monitoring system in order to accept or reject the alarm. *Statistics in Medicine*, **12**, 1807–12.

Chess, S. (1971). Autism in children with congenital rubella. *Journal of Autism and Childhood Schizophrenia*, **1**, 33–47.

Cialdella, P. and Mamelle, N. (1989). An epidemiological study of infantile autism in a French department. *Journal of Child Psychology and Psychiatry*, **30**(1), 165–75.

Croen, L. A., Grether, J. K., Hoogstrate, J., and Selvin, S. (2002). The changing prevalence of autism in California. *Journal of Autism and Developmental Disorders*, **32**(3), 207–15.

Davidovitch, M., Holtzman, G., and Tirosh, E. (2001). Autism in the Haifa area: an epidemiological perspective. *Israeli Medical Association Journal*, **3**, 188–9.

Department of Developmental Services (1999). Changes in the population of persons with autism and pervasive developmental disorders in California's Developmental Services System: 1987 through 1998; http://www.dds.ca.gov, accessed July 16, 2004.

Department of Developmental Services (2003). Autism spectrum disorders: changes in the California caseload. An update 1999 through 2002; http://www.dds.ca.gov/Autism/pdf/AutismReport2003.pdf, accessed August 22, 2006.

Deykin, E. Y. and MacMahon, B. (1979). The incidence of seizures among children with autistic symptoms. *American Journal of Psychiatry*, **136**(10), 1310–12.

Ehlers, S. and Gillberg, C. (1993). The epidemiology of Asperger syndrome: a total population study. *Journal of Child Psychology and Psychiatry*, **34**, 1327–50.

Fombonne, E. (1998). Epidemiological surveys of infantile autism. In F. Volkmar, eds., *Autism and Pervasive Developmental Disorders*. Cambridge: Cambridge University Press, pp. 32–62.

Fombonne, E. (1999). The epidemiology of autism: a review. *Psychological Medicine*, **29**, 769–86.

Fombonne, E. (2001). Is there an epidemic of autism? *Pediatrics*, **107**, 411–13.

Fombonne, E. (2002a). Case identification in an epidemiological context. In M. Rutter and E. Taylor, eds., *Child and Adolescent Psychiatry*. Oxford: Blackwell, pp. 52–69.

Fombonne, E. (2002b). Prevalence of childhood disintegrative disorder (CDD). *Autism*, **6**(2), 147–55.

Fombonne, E. (2003a). Epidemiological surveys of autism and other pervasive developmental disorders: an update. *Journal of Autism and Developmental Disorders*, **33**(4), 365–82.

Fombonne, E. (2003b). The prevalence of autism. *Journal of the American Medical Association*, **289**(1), 1–3.

Fombonne, E. and du Mazaubrun, C. (1992). Prevalence of infantile autism in 4 French regions. *Social Psychiatry and Psychiatric Epidemiology*, **27**, 203–10.

Fombonne, E. and Tidmarsh, L. (2003). Epidemiological data on Asperger disorder. *Child and Adolescent Psychiatric Clinics of North America*, **12**, 15–21.

Fombonne, E., du Mazaubrun, C., Cans, C., and Grandjean, H. (1997). Autism and associated medical disorders in a large French epidemiological sample. *Journal of the American Academy of Child and Adolescent Psychiatry*, **36**(11), 1561–6.

Fombonne, E., Simmons, H., Ford, T., Meltzer, H., and Goodman, R. (2001). Prevalence of pervasive developmental disorders in the British nationwide survey of child mental health. *Journal of the American Academy of Child and Adolescent Psychiatry*, **40**(7), 820–7.

Ghaziuddin, M., Tsai, L., and Ghaziuddin, N. (1992). Autism in Down's syndrome: presentation and diagnosis. *Journal of Intellectual Disability Research*, **36**, 449–56.

Gillberg, C. (1984). Infantile autism and other childhood psychoses in a Swedish region: epidemiological aspects. *Journal of Child Psychology and Psychiatry*, **25**, 35–43.

Gillberg, C. (1987). Infantile autism in children of immigrant parents. A population-based study from Göteborg, Sweden. *British Journal of Psychiatry*, **150**, 856–8.

Gillberg, I. C. and Gillberg, C. (1996). Autism in immigrants: a population-based study from Swedish rural and urban areas. *Journal of Intellectual Disability Research*, **40**, 24–31.

Gillberg, C., Steffenburg, S., and Schaumann, H. (1991). Is autism more common now than ten years ago? *British Journal of Psychiatry*, **158**, 403–9.

Gillberg, C., Schaumann, H., and Gillberg, I. C. (1995). Autism in immigrants: children born in Sweden to mothers born in Uganda. *Journal of Intellectual Disability Research*, **39**, 141–4.

Goodman, R. and Richards, H. (1995). Child and adolescent psychiatric presentations of second-generation Afro-Caribbeans in Britain. *British Journal of Psychiatry*, **167**, 362–9.

Gurney, J. G., Fritz, M. S., Ness, K. K. *et al.* (2003). Analysis of prevalence trends of autism spectrum disorder in Minnesota [comment]. *Archives of Pediatrics and Adolescent Medicine*, **157**(7), 622–7.

Hillman, R., Kanafani, N., Takahashi, T., and Miles, J. (2000). Prevalence of autism in Missouri: changing trends and the effect of a comprehensive state autism project. *Missouri Medicine*, **97**, 159–63.

Hoffmann, W. and Schlattmann, P. (1999). An analysis of the geographical distribution of leukemia incidence in the vicinity of a suspected point source: a case study. In A. B. Lawson, A. Biggeri, D. Böhning, E. Lesaffre, J.-F. Viel, and R. Bertollini, eds., *Disease Mapping and Risk Assessment for Public Health*. Chichester, UK: Wiley, pp. 396–409.

Honda, H., Shimizu, Y., Misumi, K., Niimi, M., and Ohashi, Y. (1996). Cumulative incidence and prevalence of childhood autism in children in Japan. *British Journal of Psychiatry*, **169**, 228–35.

Hoshino, Y., Yashima, Y., Ishige, K. *et al.* (1982). The epidemiological study of autism in Fukushi-maken. *Folia Psychiatrica et Neurologica Japonica*, **36**, 115–24.

Howlin, P., Wing, L., and Gould, J. (1995). The recognition of autism in children with Down syndrome: implications for intervention and some speculations about pathology. *Developmental Medicine and Child Neurology*, **37**, 406–14.

Hunt, A. and Lindenbaum, R. H. (1984). Tuberous sclerosis: a new estimate of prevalence within the Oxford region. *Journal of Medical Genetics*, **21**, 272–7.

Jick, H. and Kaye, J. A. (2003). Epidemiology and possible causes of autism. *Pharmacotherapy*, **23**(12), 1524.

Kadesjö, B., Gillberg, C., and Hagberg, B. (1999). Autism and Asperger syndrome in seven-year-old children: a total population study. *Journal of Autism and Developmental Disorders*, **29**(4), 327–31.

Kaye, J. A., Melero-Montes, M., and Jick, H. (2001). Mumps, measles, and rubella vaccine and the incidence of autism recorded by general practitioners: a time trend analysis. *British Medical Journal*, **322**, 460–3.

Kielinen, M., Linna, S. L., and Moilanen, I. (2000). Autism in Northern Finland. *European Child and Adolescent Psychiatry*, **9**, 162–7.

Knobloch, H. and Pasamanick, B. (1975). Some etiologic and prognostic factors in early infantile autism and psychosis. *Pediatrics*, **55**, 182–91.

Kulldorff, M. (1999). Statistical evaluation of disease cluster alarms. In A. B. Lawson, A. Biggeri, D. Böhning, E. Lesaffre, J.-F. Viel, and R. Bertollini, eds., *Disease Mapping and Risk Assessment for Public Health*. Chichester, UK: Wiley, pp. 143–9.

Le Couteur, A., Rutter, M., Lord, C. *et al.* (1989). Autism diagnostic interview: a standardized investigator-based instrument. *Journal of Autism and Developmental Disorders*, **19**, 363–87.

Lord, C., Schopler, E., and Revecki, D. (1982). Sex differences in autism. *Journal of Autism and Developmental Disorders*, **12**, 317–30.

Lord, C., Risi, S., Lembrecht, L. *et al.* (2000). The Autism Diagnostic Observation Schedule-Generic: a standard measure of social and communication deficits associated with the spectrum of autism. *Journal of Autism and Developmental Disorders*, **30**, 205–23.

Lotter, V. (1966). Epidemiology of autistic conditions in young children. I. Prevalence. *Social Psychiatry*, **1**, 124–37.

Lotter, V. (1967). Epidemiology of autistic conditions in young children. II. Some characteristics of the parents and children. *Social Psychiatry*, **1**(4), 163–73.

Lowe, T. L., Tanaka, K., Seashore, M. R., Young, J. G., and Cohen, D. J. (1980). Detection of phenylketonuria in autistic and psychiatric children. *Journal of the American Medical Association*, **243**, 126–8.

Madsen, K. M., Hviid, A., Vestergaard, M. *et al.* (2002). A population-based study of measles, mumps, and rubella vaccination and autism. *New England Journal of Medicine*, **347**(19), 1477–82.

Magnusson, P. and Saemundsen, E. (2001). Prevalence of autism in Iceland. *Journal of Autism and Developmental Disorders*, **31**, 153–63.

Matsuishi, T., Shiotsuki, M., Yoshimura, K. *et al.* (1987). High prevalence of infantile autism in Kurume City, Japan. *Journal of Child Neurology*, **2**, 268–71.

McCarthy, P., Fitzgerald, M., and Smith, M. A. (1984). Prevalence of childhood autism in Ireland. *Irish Medical Journal*, **77**(5), 129–30.

MIND Institute (2002). *Report to the Legislature on the Principal Findings from the Epidemiology of Autism in California: A Comprehensive Pilot Study*. Davis: University of California.

Mouridsen, S. E., Bachmann-Andersen, L., Sörensen, S. A., Rich, B., and Isager, T. (1992). Neurofibromatosis in infantile autism and other types of childhood psychoses. *Acta Paedopsychiatrica*, **55**, 15–18.

Newschaffer, C. J., Falb, M. D., and Gurney, J. G. (2005). National autism prevalence trends from United States special education data. *Pediatrics*, **115**(3), 277–82.

Powell, J., Edwards, A., Edwards, M. *et al.* (2000). Changes in the incidence of childhood autism and other autistic spectrum disorders in preschool children from two areas of the West Midlands, UK. *Developmental Medicine and Child Neurology*, **42**, 624–8.

Ritvo, E. R., Freeman, B. J., Pingree, C. *et al.* (1989). The UCLA–University of Utah epidemiologic survey of autism: prevalence. *American Journal of Psychiatry*, **146**(2), 194–9.

Rumeau-Rouquette, C., du Mazaubrun, C., Verrier, A. *et al.* (1994). *Prévalence des Handicaps: Évolution dans Trois Générations d'Enfants 1972, 1976, 1981*. Paris: Editions INSERM.

Rutter, M. (1970). Autistic children: infancy to adulthood. *Seminars in Psychiatry*, **2**, 435–50.

Rutter, M., Bailey, A., Bolton, P., and Le Couteur, A. (1994). Autism and known medical conditions: myth and substance. *Journal of Child Psychology and Psychiatry*, **35**, 311–22.

Schopler, E., Andrews, C. E., and Strupp, K. (1979). Do autistic children come from upper middle-class parents? *Journal of Autism and Developmental Disorders*, **9**(2), 139–51.

Scott, F. J., Baron-Cohen, S., Bolton, P., and Brayne, C. (2002). Brief report: prevalence of autism spectrum conditions in children aged 5–11 years in Cambridgeshire, UK. *Autism*, **6**(3), 231–7.

Shepherd, C. W., Beard, C. M., Gomez, M. R., Kurland, L. T., and Whisnant, J. P. (1991). Tuberous sclerosis complex in Olmsted County, Minnesota, 1950–1989. *Archives of Neurology*, **48**, 400–1.

Smalley, S. L., Tanguay, P. E., Smith, M., and Gutierrez, G. (1992). Autism and tuberous sclerosis. *Journal of Autism and Developmental Disorders*, **22**, 339–55.

Smeeth, L., Cook, C., Fombonne, E. *et al.* (2004). Rate of first recorded diagnosis of autism and other pervasive developmental disorders in United Kingdom general practice, 1988 to 2001. *BMC Medicine*, **2**, 39.

Spitzer, R. L. and Siegel, B. (1990). The DSM-III-R field trial of pervasive developmental disorders. *Journal of the American Academy of Child and Adolescent Psychiatry*, **6**, 855–86.

Sponheim, E. and Skjeldal, O. (1998). Autism and related disorders: epidemiological findings in a Norwegian study using ICD-10 diagnostic criteria. *Journal of Autism and Developmental Disorders*, **28**, 217–22.

Steffenburg, S. and Gillberg, C. (1986). Autism and autisticlike conditions in Swedish rural and urban areas: a population study. *British Journal of Psychiatry*, **149**, 81.

Steinhausen H.-C., Göbel, D., Breinlinger, M., and Wohlloben, B. (1986). A community survey of infantile autism. *Journal of the American Academy of Child Psychiatry*, **25**(2), 186–9.

Sturmey, P. and James, V. (2001). Administrative prevalence of autism in the Texas school system. *Journal of the American Academy of Child Psychiatry*, **40**(6), 621.

Sugiyama, T. and Abe, T. (1989). The prevalence of autism in Nagoya, Japan: a total population study. *Journal of Autism and Developmental Disorders*, **19**(1), 87–96.

Tanoue, Y., Oda, S., Asano, F., and Kawashima, K. (1988). Epidemiology of infantile autism in Southern Ibaraki, Japan: differences in prevalence in birth cohorts. *Journal of Autism and Developmental Disorders*, **18**, 155–66.

Taylor, B., Miller, E., Farrington, C. P. *et al.* (1999). Autism and measles, mumps, and rubella vaccine: no epidemiological evidence for a causal association. *Lancet*, **353**, 2026–9.

Treffert, D. A. (1970). Epidemiology of infantile autism. *Archives of General Psychiatry*, **22**, 431–8.

Tuchman, R. F., Rapin, I., and Shinnar, S. (1991). Autistic and dysphasic children. II. Epilepsy. *Pediatrics*, **88**, 1219–25.

Volkmar, F. R. (1992). Childhood disintegrative disorder: issues for DSM-IV. *Journal of Autism and Developmental Disorders*, **22**, 625–42.

Volkmar, F. R., ed. (2005). *Handbook of Autism and Pervasive Developmental Disorders*, 3rd edn. New York: Wiley.

Volkmar, F. R. and Nelson, D. S. (1990). Seizure disorders in autism. *Journal of the American Academy of Child and Adolescent Psychiatry*, **1**, 127–9.

Volkmar, F. R., Klin, A., Siegel, B. *et al.* (1994). Field trial for autistic disorder in DSM-IV. *American Journal of Psychiatry*, **151**(9), 1361–7.

Webb, E., Lobo, S., Hervas, A., Scourfield, J., and Fraser, W. I. (1997). The changing prevalence of autistic disorder in a Welsh health district. *Developmental Medicine and Child Neurology*, **39**, 150–2.

Webb, E., Morey, J., Thompsen, W. *et al.* (2003). Prevalence of autistic spectrum disorder in children attending mainstream schools in a Welsh education authority. *Developmental Medicine and Child Neurology*, **45**(6), 377–84.

Wignyosumarto, S., Mukhlas, M., and Shirataki, S. (1992). Epidemiological and clinical study of autistic children in Yogyakarta, Indonesia. *Kobe Journal of Medical Sciences*, **38**(1), 1–19.

Wing, L. (1980). Childhood autism and social class: a question of selection? *British Journal of Psychiatry*, **137**, 410–17.

Wing, L. (1993). The definition and prevalence of autism: a review. *European Child and Adolescent Psychiatry*, **2**, 61–74.

Wing, L. and Gould, J. (1979). Severe impairments of social interactions and associated abnormalities in children: epidemiology and classification. *Journal of Autism and Developmental Disorders*, **9**(1), 11–29.

Wing, L., Yeates, S. R., Brierly, L. M., and Gould, J. (1976). The prevalence of early childhood autism: comparison of administrative and epidemiological studies. *Psychological Medicine*, **6**, 89–100.

Yeargin-Allsopp, M., Rice, C., Karapurkar, T. *et al.* (2003). Prevalence of autism in a US metropolitan area. *Journal of the American Medical Association*, **289**(1), 49–55.

3

Psychological factors in autism

Margot Prior
School of Behavioural Sciences, Melbourne University

Sally Ozonoff
MIND Institute and Department of Psychiatry, University of California

Introduction

Reviewing psychological factors in autism presents a major challenge, given the vast amount of research that has accumulated over the past 50 years. In that time we have moved from largely speculative notions of what underlies the puzzling set of symptoms that children with autism present to us (Kanner, 1943) to a comprehensive knowledge of their strengths and weaknesses in a broad range of psychological domains. Our understanding of psychological factors has informed increasingly well-designed and productive approaches to the education and treatment of children with autism, so that theory and practice can build on each other in a synergistic way. This review of psychological aspects of autism is divided into sections covering the major domains of perception, cognition, affect, language, social behaviors, and neuropsychological factors.

One important issue that needs to be kept in mind concerns the powerful and pervasive influence of level of functioning on the symptoms, behaviors, and capabilities of children with autism. Low- and high-functioning children with autism are both similar in their core deficits, and very different in their adaptive level, and this makes some of our conclusions about psychological factors rather qualified. While the central social and communicative deficits may be common, there are clear differences in levels and profiles of abilities across the range of severity of autistic conditions; these differences affect adaptive behavior as well as intervention opportunities and outcome in later life. Since the first edition of this book there has been a surge of publications focusing on children at the upper end of what is currently termed a "spectrum of autistic disorders," that is those children with high-functioning autism and Asperger's syndrome. These recent developments have served to highlight even further the differences

Autism and Pervasive Developmental Disorders, 2nd edn, ed. Fred R. Volkmar.
Published by Cambridge University Press. © Cambridge University Press 2007.

between children functioning at different levels, perhaps most notably in the picture presented by children with Asperger's syndrome.

Children with Asperger's syndrome or high-functioning autism share key symptom criteria for autism, but they are generally at the upper end of the spectrum in terms of their cognitive and language capacities and they are also less severely socially impaired. So far, the data indicate that the similarities between high-functioning autism and Asperger's syndrome may well outweigh any differences, and hence it is debatable whether they require separate diagnostic categories on the basis of current research data (Mayes & Calhoun, 2003a). There is currently a very active area of research which focuses on putative distinguishing features of autism and Asperger's syndrome or, alternatively, seeks evidence which supports the validity of a "spectrum of severity" heuristic (Gillberg & Gillberg, 1989; Ozonoff *et al.*, 1991; Szatmari *et al.*, 1989, 1995). Recent papers by Mayes *et al.* (2001), Miller and Ozonoff (1997), Tager-Flusberg (2003) and numerous others lead to the conclusion that there are no clear, reliable, or valid clinical or empirical ways of separating Asperger's syndrome from high-functioning autism; rather Asperger's syndrome should be considered as part of the spectrum (Frith, 1991).

A variety of standard neuropsychological tests are now available which are suitable for assessing the cognitive capacities of high-functioning individuals with autism spectrum disorders (ASDs). One of the challenges in continuing research on psychological factors of autism is to develop experimental designs and measures which will expand further investigation of the problems for the lower-functioning children, who are in the majority but who are unable to participate in the more sophisticated tests. Nevertheless, the creativity and ingenuity shown by researchers in autism, in designing ways of exploring key psychological factors in a seriously handicapped population, is a feature of this field.

Sensorimotor and perceptual development

Many early studies of children with autism investigated their sensory and perceptual abilities. As this disorder is of very early onset, it seems reasonable to suggest that perceptual development at its most basic level is disturbed in some way. Overall, both earlier and recent studies converge towards the conclusion that basic sensory and perceptual abilities are not fundamentally abnormal. Nevertheless, children with autism are well known for their deviant response patterns to various kinds of sensory stimuli, and both under- and overresponsiveness are seen, not only to differing degrees within the autistic population, but even within the one child. Disturbed perception of auditory stimulation, including voice perception, has been particularly noted (Dawson *et al.*, 1998; Klin, 1991; Prior, 1979).

Many low-functioning children show sensory anomalies similar to those seen in sensorily handicapped children, such as peculiar and perseverative gazing at lights or moving fans; running water or sand through their hands repetitively; peering closely and persistently at objects; and flicking fingers in front of the eyes. A study of young low-functioning children with autism based on observations via home movies reported by Losche (1990) suggested that sensory motor development was normal at least during the infancy period, but that with increasing age children with autism showed increasing delays and even regressions in their development, with aimless and stereotyped behavior particularly being a feature.

Testing young children with autism using Piagetian scales of sensorimotor development indicates that they develop normal object permanence, but show notable deficits in vocal and gestural imitation (Sigman & Ungerer, 1984). These deficits appear to diminish with age and with verbal skill development (Morgan *et al.*, 1989). Children with autism often develop adequate rote learning ability (figurative schemas of representation according to Piagetian theory), at least commensurate with their mental age level (Green *et al.*, 1995), but do not develop operative representation, or the ability to form and manipulate symbolic material, and do not develop conceptual structures. Hence, for a high proportion of children with autism, there is a low ceiling on their sensorimotor and cognitive development.

The acquisition of imitation and language skills is associated with more sophisticated levels of Piagetian-type skills such as means-end reasoning (Abrahamsen & Mitchell, 1990). Lack of imitation skills is a notable feature of autism and is a distinguishing diagnostic characteristic. Deficiencies are apparent from the first year of life (Prior *et al.*, 1975) when the normally expected simple imitative games do not appear. Difficulties in using gestures and in imitating communicative and social behaviors are persistent and pervasive (Wing, 1976, 1981), except perhaps in the very highest functioning children. Ohta (1987), Sigman and Ungerer (1984), and Hertzig *et al.* (1989) have all reported autism-specific imitation deficits in comparative studies covering motor, vocal, sensorimotor, symbolic, and affective behaviors across a range of ages. Recent research has questioned whether the deficits are due to conceptual and symbolic impairments, or perhaps to more basic problems with organizing, coordinating, and integrating body movements (Rogers & Williams, 2006). Smith and Bryson (1994) in reviewing imitation and action in autism have suggested that difficulties with motor imitation are characteristic of children with other developmental disorders, especially those involving language impairments; hence at least some of the difficulties may be nonspecific. The relations are complex as these impairments seem to be present even when other areas of cognitive and language functioning are relatively preserved (Green *et al.*, 2002; Manjiviona & Prior, 1995), and some groups with similar levels of language impairment and mental retardation, such as children with Down's syndrome, nevertheless show good imitation skills (Prior, 1977).

The other salient line of argument is that children with autism have representational deficits, and hence imitation and action deficits may be the product of lack of social cognitive abilities, which are necessary for the understanding of why and how imitation works in the social and communicative domain. The "chicken and egg" problem here is one that requires prospective studies of very young children with autism, in which stages of development of various skills, and the sequence of their emergence, can be minutely tracked.

Most researchers would agree with Shapiro and Hertzig (1991) that it is "integrative deficits" that are central to any sensory and perceptual dysfunction, i.e. the child with autism is unable to coordinate and integrate varying kinds of sensory input to form a coherent functional picture of the world. This applies across all modalities and may be fundamental to all of the other deficits. Temple Grandin, an adult with autism, in reflecting on her early life has described her experience as "sensory jumbling" (Grandin, 1995), an expression that seems to describe well the problems for children with autism. However, paradoxically it is also often observed that children with autism can show extraordinary sensitivity to miniscule changes to particular patterns which are associated with their obsessive behavior, for example, in arrangements of objects or minor flaws in well-known visual stimuli. This "enhanced" perception usually involves low-level processing of particular features and is commonly domain-specific rather than generalized.

Mottron and Burack (2001) have drawn attention to the fact that savants with autism can show greatly enhanced perceptual abilities in their specific skills such as pitch perception and drawing. Plaisted and colleagues (1998) gave adults with autism novel discrimination problems presented in a computerized task. The task had multiple conditions, starting with simple discrimination training, then learning key experimental stimuli (beachball circles in different positions), then training in stimulus discrimination, and lastly to the critical tests of discrimination between stimuli similar to those they had learned previously and completely novel stimuli. The participants appeared better able than nonautistic individuals both at the end of the pre-exposure phase and in the novel discrimination condition, suggesting that they were better at processing unique features, while poorer at processing common features (see the later discussion on central coherence theory with reference to this point). Generally, the picture with regard to perceptual development in autism is not a clear or straightforward one, with anomalies and idiosyncrasies within this population across developmental periods, which require further research.

Motor development

Evidence that children with autism show neurodevelopmental and motor abnormalities has gathered steadily over the years. Early descriptions of these children suggested that they were graceful and skillful and had few signs of motor impairment. This was part of the puzzle relating to the origins of the disorder. Later systematic studies of motor performance in low-functioning cases, including those of DeMyer *et al.* (1972) and Jones and Prior (1985), uncovered clear signs of delayed or abnormal motor and sensorimotor development, however. Wing (1976) had also described clumsiness and difficulties in planning and executing organized motor programs such as riding a tricycle or managing more than one motor task at a time. Bennetto (1999), in reporting on the nature of motor imitation problems in children with high-functioning autism, noted basic motor functioning problems or dyspraxias which were significant handicaps to imitation (see also Rogers *et al.*, 1996). Problems in producing gesture, either by imitation or spontaneously, may underlie the well-known failure of children with autism to use gesture to communicate like normal children. Motor dyspraxias and neurodevelopmental signs such as choreiform movements, balance problems, gait abnormalities, and impaired body imitation abilities are confirmed as significant characteristics of autism (Damasio & Maurer, 1978; Goldstein *et al.*, 2001a; Manjiviona & Prior, 1995).

Further, motor milestones are reported to be slow in a substantial proportion of cases (DeMyer *et al.*, 1981), although it is unknown whether clearly neurologically handicapped children with autism are different in other significant ways from those without measurable signs on these indices. There is increasing evidence that a significant proportion of children appear to have central nervous system (CNS) dysfunction along with their autism. For example, Noterdaeme *et al.* (2002) compared children with autism with those who had language disorder and with controls on a neurological examination. They found motor problems across balance, coordination, fine, gross and oromotor functions. Recent moves toward the use of more standardized tests of motor impairment have allowed improved assessment of motor development (Smith, 2000). Using standardized tests of motor impairment and including children with Asperger's syndrome and higher-functioning autism as subjects (Ghaziuddin *et al.*, 1994; Goldstein *et al.*, 2001b; Manjiviona & Prior, 1995), it has been shown that both groups show signs of neuromotor clumsiness across a range of motor systems. These findings have been of particular interest given the belief that clumsiness is a marked feature of Asperger's syndrome rather than autism, and that it might be a diagnostically differentiating sign. It appears that this belief is questionable (Prior, 2003). Mayes and Calhoun (2003a, 2003b) studied ability profiles in a substantial sample of children aged 3 to 15 years and found that the majority of children with IQs both above and below 80 had a reported history of normal motor development. Most children who achieved early motor milestones on time functioned in the normal IQ range in the school-age years. However, their graphomotor scores, as ascertained from testing with standard visuomotor tests, remained an area of weakness in ability profiles from early to later ages. In the academic domain, although the higher IQ group had normal range scores in numeracy and literacy, their written expression was a notable weakness. Ongoing problems with written work in the school curriculum, which of course requires fine motor skills and effort, were also documented by Manjiviona (2003) supporting the longer-term significance of such deficits, even in higher-functioning cases.

A recent review of motor functioning in autism and Asperger's syndrome (Smith, 2000) pointed to many anomalies and inconsistencies in the literature on this topic, and the need to evaluate the evidence in the context of the literature regarding executive functioning problems (see below). It should be noted, though, that psychomotor slowness, poor coordination, and neurological signs are frequent in a range of nonautistic developmental disorders (Green *et al.*, 2002), hence their presence in autism signals impairments in neuromotor development as part of the biological basis for the disorder, rather than distinctive features of ASD.

Attention

Many investigations have documented attentional abnormalities in individuals with autism, but the deficits in this area appear rather different from those in other disorders. It has been noted in case studies and in the clinical literature for many years that individuals with autism appear to have "overfocused" attention, responding only to a subset of environmental cues during learning situations, e.g. Lovaas *et al.* (1979). Several experimental paradigms have been used to explore this clinical observation; for a review see Allen and Courchesne (2001). Deficits relative to controls have been found in the shifting of attention between sensory modalities. In one study, average IQ adults with autism performed as well as typical controls on a task that required no shifting of attention, but performance was over six standard deviations (SDs) below that of controls when rapid alternation of attention between auditory and visual channels was required

(Courchesne *et al.*, 1994). Several studies using the visuospatial orienting task of Posner (1980) have documented that people with autism take longer to disengage and move attention than controls matched on ability (Casey *et al.*, 1993; Townsend *et al.*, 1999; Wainwright-Sharp & Bryson, 1993). New studies have also pointed to deficits in the size of the attentional spotlight, suggesting that the attention of people with autism is too narrow and takes longer than controls to spread to peripheral spatial locations (Mann & Walker, 2003; Townsend & Courchesne, 1994; Townsend *et al.*, 1996). These difficulties may underlie the executive dysfunction and weak central coherence processes discussed below.

In contrast, a number of studies have suggested that the ability to *sustain* attention is a relatively spared function in autism, with normal performance on continuous performance tests found in several investigations (Buchsbaum *et al.*, 1992; Casey *et al.*, 1993; Garretson *et al.*, 1990). Individuals with autism have been shown to perform similarly to controls on tests of selective attention as well, although they may use different neural networks to accomplish the task than the controls do (Allen & Courchesne, 2003). A few studies have administered a battery of attention tests and confirmed both strengths in sustained and focused attention, and weaknesses in disengaging and shifting attention (Goldstein *et al.*, 2001; Noterdaeme *et al.*, 2001). This profile of attentional strengths and weaknesses distinguishes children with autism from those with attention deficit hyperactivity disorder (ADHD). While children with ADHD have little difficulty disengaging and shifting attention (Swanson *et al.*, 1991), they demonstrate severe impairment in sustaining attention and controling impulses. More work comparing children with autism to other clinical groups is needed because attention deficits are such a ubiquitous phenomenon in a range of psychiatric disorders. As many less able children with autism are unable to participate in the common experimental tasks used to assess attention, there is a great challenge in finding ways to assess their problems objectively.

Abnormal attentional processes in autism are highly likely to be associated with difficulties in understanding the meaning of environmental stimuli, leading to poor choices of what to attend to in the absence of clear directives, and strong tendencies to overfocus in an attempt to achieve some measure of control over overwhelming input. This in turn restricts adaptive learning and perpetuates the difficulties.

General intellectual function

It has long been stated that the majority of children with autism function intellectually in the mentally handicapped range (e.g. IQ < 70). In an initial and influential study, DeMyer *et al.* (1974) reported that close to half their sample functioned in the severe–profound range of mental retardation (IQ < 35); one-quarter demonstrated abilities in the moderately handicapped range (IQ 35–50); a fifth functioned in the mildly retarded range (IQ 50–70); and only 6% obtained IQ scores in the nonretarded range (IQ > 70). More recent estimates suggested that approximately a quarter of children with autism function intellectually in the borderline range or above and do not demonstrate comorbid mental retardation (Freeman et al., 1985; Lord & Schopler, 1988). The low representation of higher-functioning cases in early samples is likely because there was not nearly as great a recognition of mild forms of autism as there is today. A recent epidemiological study of a preschool-aged sample found that 31% with autism and 94% with other ASDs (such as Asperger's syndrome and pervasive developmental disorder not otherwise specified) demonstrated IQ scores above the mentally handicapped range (Chakrabarti & Fombonne, 2001), suggesting that the higher-functioning forms of autism, with IQ > 70, may in fact be the more common form. In general, girls with autism obtain lower scores on intellectual tests and represent a smaller proportion of high-functioning cases than boys (Konstantareas et al., 1989; Lord & Schopler, 1985).

Children with autism demonstrate a wide scatter of skills on intellectual testing. They perform least well on intellectual tasks that require language, abstract reasoning, integration, and sequencing (Green et al., 1995; Lincoln et al., 1995). They tend to perform better on intellectual tasks that require visual–spatial processing, attention to detail, and rote memory abilities (Green et al., 1995; Lincoln et al., 1995). This general pattern of strengths and weaknesses contributes to a characteristic profile on intellectual testing. On standard intelligence tests such as the Wechsler scales, most studies report higher Performance than Verbal IQ (for a review see Lincoln et al., 1995). Intersubtest variability is the norm. Reflecting the strengths in visual–spatial processing and rote memory often seen in autism, scores on the Block Design, Object Assembly, and Digit Span subtests are often the highest in a profile (Asarnow et al., 1987; Dennis et al., 1999; Freeman et al., 1985; Goldstein et al., 2001b; Happe, 1994a; Lincoln et al., 1988; Shah & Frith, 1983, 1993). In contrast, the Comprehension subtest is often the lowest verbal score (Asarnow et al., 1987; Dennis et al., 1999; Freeman et al., 1985; Goldstein et al., 2001b; Lincoln et al., 1988), reflecting deficits in conceptual reasoning, social judgment, and perhaps the ability to reason about others' minds (Happe, 1994a, 1994b). Scores on the Picture Arrangement and Coding subtests are often the lowest in the Performance scale profile (Freeman et al., 1985; Lincoln et al., 1988), probably associated with the sequential and analytical difficulties of autism. These patterns appear to be independent of IQ level and severity of autistic symptomatology (Fein et al., 1985; Freeman et al., 1985; Lincoln et al., 1988) and differentiate individuals with ASDs from those with learning disabilities (Goldstein *et al.*, 2001b). Similar patterns are also obtained on other intelligence tests. For example, on the Kaufman Assessment Battery for Children, higher scores are obtained on both the Triangles subtest, a measure analogous to the Wechsler Block Design task, and Number Recall, similar to Digit Span (Allen *et al.*, 1991). Similarly, profile patterns on the Stanford–Binet Intelligence Scales demonstrate highest performance on the Pattern Analysis subtest, a measure of visuospatial function, and lowest performance on the Absurdities subtest, a measure of verbal conceptual reasoning and social judgment (Carpentieri & Morgan, 1994; Harris *et al.*, 1990).

These intellectual profiles have been suggested to be so consistent and universal in children with autism that they can be used for diagnostic purposes. Lincoln *et al.* (1988: pp. 521–2) wrote, " . . . the pattern of subtest scaled scores should not provide the exclusive criteria to make the diagnosis of autism. It does appear, however, that the pattern of subtest scaled scores is robust enough to support history and other test results in developing a diagnosis in nonretarded children, adolescents, and adults suspected of having a disorder of autism." However, in a large (*n* = 81) sample of high-functioning adults (Full Scale IQ > 70) meeting research criteria for autism, only 20% had a significantly higher Performance than Verbal IQ and almost as many (16%) showed the opposite pattern (Siegel *et al.*, 1996). Block Design was the highest subtest for only 22% and Comprehension was the lowest for 33% of this sample. Similarly, in a group of 47 children with ASDs, all but 5 of whom met research criteria for autism, 62% demonstrated verbal–nonverbal intelligence discrepancies, which occurred equally in both directions (Tager-Flusberg & Joseph, 2003). So while there appear to be profiles that are common within the autism spectrum, they should never be used for diagnostic purposes.

There has been some suggestion that the cognitive profile of individuals with Asperger's syndrome may differ from that of autism. In his initial description of the syndrome, Asperger (1944) stated that the children he was studying were extremely clumsy and demonstrated delays in both gross and fine motor development. Motor deficits have been shown to correlate with poor visuospatial skills (Henderson *et al.*, 1994), stimulating recent exploration of visuospatial functions in individuals with Asperger's syndrome. One study found that Verbal IQ was significantly higher than Performance IQ in a sample with Asperger's syndrome (Klin *et al.*, 1995), a pattern opposite to many findings in autism. Additionally, subjects with Asperger's syndrome in this study showed deficits on tests of fine and gross motor ability, visuomotor integration, visuospatial perception, visual memory, and nonverbal concept formation. Conversely, subjects with high-functioning autism of similar overall IQ performed well on these tests, but demonstrated deficits on measures of auditory perception, verbal memory, articulation, vocabulary, and verbal output (Klin *et al.*, 1995). However, several research teams have failed to replicate these findings (Ghaziuddin *et al.*, 1994; Manjiviona & Prior, 1995; Mayes & Calhoun, 2003a; Miller & Ozonoff, 2000; Szatmari *et al.*, 1995) so we reiterate our warning that IQ or cognitive profiles should not be used for differential diagnosis purposes.

The IQ scores of individuals with autism are relatively stable across time and development. Correlations of IQ scores in preschool and school age are generally statistically significant and similar to values seen in nonhandicapped children (Lord & Schopler, 1988). Scores are more stable and predictive the older the age at initial assessment (Lord & Schopler, 1989). Scores can and do change, however, with a proportion of children changing IQ grouping levels as they age (Freeman *et al.*, 1991; Lord & Schopler, 1989; Mayes & Calhoun, 2003a), and in response to early intervention (Rogers, 1998). Thus, narrow categorization of intellectual level based on early IQ scores may not be appropriate. However, IQ scores remain one of the best predictors of later outcome, with both early studies (Lotter, 1974; Rutter, 1984) and more recent investigations conducted during the era of widespread early intensive intervention (Freeman *et al.*, 1999; Harris & Handleman, 2000; Stevens *et al.*, 2000) upholding the finding that intelligence during preschool is significantly positively correlated with functional level later in life.

Academic functioning

The performance profile seen on measures of academic function is consistent with that obtained on intellectual tests. Academic skills requiring primarily rote, mechanical, or procedural abilities are generally intact, while those relying upon more abstract, conceptual, or interpretive abilities are typically deficient. For example, in the reading domain, Minshew and colleagues (1994) found that individuals with high-functioning autism performed as well as or better than normal controls matched on age and IQ on tests of single-word oral reading, non-word reading, and spelling. These measures all require phonological decoding skills and thus indicate preserved or even advanced knowledge of grapheme–phoneme correspondence rules in autism. In contrast, subjects with autism performed less well than controls on two measures of reading comprehension. This pattern, in its most extreme form, is called hyperlexia. This term is used to describe individuals with word recognition skills that are significantly better than predicted by intellectual or educational level. Excellent decoding skills are typically accompanied by relatively poor comprehension abilities (Silberberg & Silberberg, 1967). Hyperlexia has been documented in individuals with autism by a number of researchers (Burd et al., 1987; Nation et al., 2006; Tirosh & Canby, 1993; Welsh et al., 1987).

The pattern is quite different from that typically obtained by reading disabled individuals (Pennington, 1991; Vellutino, 1979). In two studies directly comparing the reading profiles of autism and dyslexia, subjects with dyslexia demonstrated deficits on phonological processing measures but strengths in comprehension and interpretation, while subjects with autism displayed the opposite pattern (Frith & Snowling, 1983; Rumsey & Hamburger, 1990). While there does appear to be a characteristic pattern of academic strengths and weaknesses, variability is very common and cautions against diagnosis-specific conclusions (Manjiviona, 2003).

There has been less empirical work examining mathematical and other academic abilities in autism. Rumsey and Hamburger (1990) found that adult males with high-functioning autism performed as well as matched normal controls and better than dyslexic individuals on a test of arithmetical calculation. Similarly, Minshew and colleagues (1994) found that high-functioning individuals with autism performed as well as controls on math computation tasks. Interestingly, in this study subjects with autism showed no deficits in applied aspects of math, thus failing to demonstrate the same discrepancy between mechanical and conceptual abilities apparent in the reading realm. This finding requires independent replication by other research teams, but may suggest that math is a relatively spared academic ability in high-functioning cases of autism.

Investigators have also examined age differences in performance on academic tests. Goldstein et al. (1994) compared children with autism to adolescents/adults with autism of similar IQ level. They found that both age groups performed better on measures of phonological decoding and math than on measures of reading comprehension and abstract, complex reasoning. In comparison with matched normal controls, some interesting differences as a function of age emerged. Younger subjects with autism performed as well as controls on most tests, but older individuals with autism performed significantly less well than matched controls on many of the same measures. These findings may reflect the kinds of skills emphasized in the educational system across the course of development. School-work in the early years emphasizes mastery of rote, mechanical procedures (such as letter–sound correspondences), and multiplication tables. Later educational curricula, on the other hand, highlight comprehension, conceptualization, and analysis skills. Therefore, as Goldstein *et al.* (1994) suggest, individuals with high-functioning autism may perform as well as peers until grade levels in which abstractive, interpretive skills are emphasized, at which point they fall behind (Prior, 2003).

Predictors of school achievement in people with autism have also been studied. Venter *et al.* (1992) found that performance on academic tests in adolescence was significantly predicted by early nonverbal IQ and functional speech before the age of 5 years, while the severity of repetitive, stereotyped behavior in preschool was negatively correlated with later academic achievement. Similar findings regarding the validity of IQ, as well as severity of autism, in predicting academic achievement were reported by Eaves and Ho (1997).

These studies suggest that high-functioning individuals with autism perform capably in a number of academic domains, at least relative to others of similar intellectual and mental age level. Deficits are not universal and tend to cluster in areas requiring conceptual and abstract reasoning. This mirrors the characteristic profile obtained on measures of intellectual function (Lincoln *et al.*, 1995). However, academic variability is common and academic profiles should not be used diagnostically, just as intellectual profiles should not.

Idiot savant or splinter abilities

Early studies of autism and its particular characteristics highlighted cases where there were "islets of ability" or splinter skills in a background of general intellectual disability. This was likened to examples of *idiot savant* abilities documented in the mental retardation literature for some time. Rimland (1978) suggested that these cases should be called "autistic savants." He reported that about 10% of people with autism showed some high-level special ability or in some cases more than one savant ability. The particular association between savant abilities and autism is demonstrated by the fact that the estimate of such cases in the mentally retarded population is about 1 in 2000 (Hill, 1977, cited in Pring *et al.*, 1995). Their special talents are notable for the fact that they are of little help in other cognitive and social domains of their lives.

The kinds of talents described in autistic savants include mathematics, especially "lightning calculation," music, art, mechanical ability, calendrical calculation, memory, and geographical knowledge (maps, routes, etc.). The most common in this list according to Rimland's (1978) study are musical, memory, artistic, mathematical, geographical, and pseudoverbal abilities (remembering, spelling, and pronouncing, but not understanding words). (The latter is probably what is currently called "hyperlexia" although the term is often used in the context of normal intellectual ability.) Most of these cases showed their gifts by the age of 4 years, and had reached their peak by 10 according to parental reports. The autistic savants are usually functioning in the intellectually disabled range and are unable to describe or explain their abilities (but for counterexamples on this last point, see Pring *et al.*, 1995). Rimland, in seeking theoretical and biological explanations for this phenomenon, stressed the ability of these individuals to concentrate intensely on their interests, to fixate on details, and to demonstrate abnormal memory processes.

The research group of Hermelin, O'Connor, and colleagues in the United Kingdom (UK) has provided sophisticated analyses of some autistic savant talents using experimental methods to try to identify the processes involved and their relations to facets of intelligence. They report that preoccupations or obsessions and repetitive behavioral tendencies are closely associated with *idiot savant* abilities (Hermelin & O'Connor, 1991). Their experiments indicate that autistic savants do use cognitive strategies such as following simple rules to help them in recall and to calculate dates, for example; furthermore, they are able to abstract, a capacity which is usually extremely limited in the general autistic population (O'Connor, 1989). A study of calendrical calculators (O'Connor & Hermelin, 1984) suggested that their exceptional ability was not based just on rote memory for dates and days, but involved "rule-governed calculations and strategies," and that speed of access to the correct calendar information was influenced by the distance of the date to be recalled from the present. Musical savants have illustrated a cognitive style of focusing on parts rather than wholes in playing heard music from memory. They were very accurate and were able to preserve the structure of the music, reminiscent of the facility with calendrical rules demonstrated in calendrical calculators.

In seeking explanations for exceptional artistic ability, Pring *et al.* (1995) emphasized the fact that a substantial proportion of those with autism show notable superiority with block design tasks by comparison with other subtests of intelligence, which suggests that they have a special ability to segment a holistic stimulus into its component parts (see "Central coherence" from p. 106). This, they argue, can be especially significant in drawing and painting, and is an ability that appears to be independent of general intelligence in artistically talented people. A parallel argument can be made with regard to musical ability and the particular facility with pitch discrimination (i.e. subcomponents of music) within a musical "gestalt," which has been described (Hermelin, 2001). Such dissociations may also be important in, for example, geographical abilities, where individuals can remember with absolute fidelity the details of particular streets, places, maps, and routes no matter how unusual or obscure they might be. Hermelin's group has linked such abilities to Frith's (1989) "central coherence" theory in which the core deficit in autism is seen as a failure to derive coherence (meaningful wholes) from the information they may apprehend, leaving them prone to "modular" (noncoherent) abilities (see further discussion on this in the final section of the chapter).

In a recent monograph providing an overview of many studies of autistic savant abilities, Hermelin (2001) draws out valuable insights from in-depth examination of the abilities of particular cases, carried out by the UK group. Their series of elegant, well-controlled, and systematic investigations have immensely enhanced our understanding of these extraordinary modular abilities of artists, musicians, and mathematicians with autism. Hermelin concludes that IQ does have some influence on abilities, at least in some domains of savant abilities, and further, that the capacity to make use of repetitive rules, predictability, and intense focus on particular "parts" rather than "wholes" of information (for example, in calculating dates or remembering information such as detailed bus routes), fits with many core behavioral and cognitive characteristics of autism. She notes that with all her cases it is the *engagement* in the activity that counts, rather than any finished product or its affective or esthetic value. Some of Hermelin's accounts also illustrate that creativity and the ability to generate new forms and ideas, as in music, are not absent in the pattern of savant abilities. This is contrary to the results obtained from extensive psychological and executive functioning testing, and from social cognition experiments, which highlight impairment in such capacities, and suggests that in specific highly valued contexts these abilities may be elicited.

Although there is minimal substantive evidence on differential outcome for autistic savants, Rimland (1978) has claimed that many of those who "recover" to some extent from their autism lose their exceptional abilities. A common feature of Asperger's syndrome and high-functioning autism is an intense preoccupation with special interests. Since by definition this is present in a context of normal or near-normal overall intellectual ability it does not have the status of a savant ability. However, like savants, such children are extraordinarily knowledgeable (and pedantic) about favorite topics (such as computers, trains, timetables, sports, astronomy, anatomy, geography, etc.), often in a nonfunctional way. Such individuals are rarely able to reflect upon and describe how they have acquired this knowledge. While specialized and detailed knowledge may enhance employment opportunities in some cases (Howlin, 2003), for most it lacks adaptive value.

Memory

The memory of people with autism has been extensively studied. Some investigators have suggested that autism is a primary disorder of memory, likening
it to an amnesic syndrome (Bachevalier, 1994; Boucher & Warrington, 1976;
DeLong, 1992; Hetzler & Griffin, 1981). This theory was first put forth by
Boucher and Warrington (1976) who outlined the behavioral similarities between
children with autism and animals with hippocampal and other medial temporal
lesions. The amnesic analogy has received some support from anatomical data
(Aylward *et al.*, 1999; Bauman & Kemper, 1985, 1988; Saitoh *et al.*, 2001; Salmond
et al., 2003; White & Rosenbloom, 1992) and renewed interest due to the current
popularity of an "amygdala" theory of autism (Baron-Cohen *et al.*, 2000). The
pattern of functioning on memory tests has also been proposed to be similar in
patients with autism and amnesia (Bachevalier, 1994; Boucher & Warrington,
1976; DeLong, 1992). Amnesic subjects typically demonstrate three patterns that
have been hypothesized to also exist in autism:

(1)   intact short-term, rote, and recognition memory abilities;
(2)   reduced primacy but normal recency effects;
(3)   better performance under cued than free recall conditions.

A number of experimental investigations have been carried out to explore the
validity of this analogy and are reviewed below.

Short-term, rote, and recognition memory

In the opening paragraphs of his seminal paper describing the syndrome of
autism, Kanner (1943) commented upon the extraordinary memories of the
children he was describing, particularly their ability to recite long lists of items
or facts. Many have suggested that the echolalic tendencies of children with
autism indicate an above-average auditory rote memory (Hermelin & Frith,
1971; Hermelin & O'Connor, 1970). Early experimental studies confirmed the
observations that short-term and rote memorial processes were largely intact in
autism. In a series of studies, Hermelin and Frith (1971) demonstrated that the
short-term auditory memory of children with autism was as good as that of normal and mentally handicapped individuals of similar mental age. Subjects with
autism were as able to repeat back strings of words as the other groups, although
there were some qualitative differences in how they did this (see below). Prior and
Chen (1976) demonstrated that once subjects with autism, mental retardation,
or typical development matched on mental age were equated for pre-existing
list learning and acquisition differences, the three groups were equally capable
of recalling both single items and lists in a visual memory task. They concluded

that differences in performance on memory tasks between samples with and without autism may be a function of learning and acquisition deficiencies rather than primary memory difficulties.

Several studies have documented normal recognition memory in autism, in higher functioning, older participants (Bennetto *et al.*, 1996; Beversdorf *et al.*, 2000), school-aged lower-functioning children (Barth *et al.*, 1995), and preschool-aged children (Dawson *et al.*, 2001).

However, the rote memory of people with autism appears to diverge from that of amnesia in the ability to learn paired associate lists. Boucher and Warrington (1976) found that children with autism were able to learn lists of word pairs as easily as typical children and better than controls with mental retardation but of higher verbal ability. Similar results on a paired associate learning task have been reported more recently by Minshew and Goldstein (2001) in high-functioning adolescents and adults with autism. This is in contrast to adults with amnesia, who typically demonstrate extraordinary difficulty on this type of learning task (Boucher & Warrington, 1976), thus weakening the strongest version of the autism–amnesia analogy.

Primary versus recency effects

O'Connor and Hermelin (1967) were the first to note that primacy effects in list learning tended to be weaker than recency effects in autism; these results were replicated by Boucher (1981). This pattern is also characteristic of adults with amnesia (Baddeley & Warrington, 1970). Hermelin and Frith (1971) attempted, unsuccessfully, to attenuate strong recency effects by composing sentences in which the beginning part of the word string was made up of meaningful sentence fragments, while the latter part was composed of random verbal material. The children with autism continued to demonstrate strong recency and weak primacy effects even under these conditions. Deficient primacy but intact recency memory has been replicated more recently by Renner *et al.* (2000). As recency effects rely more purely on rote auditory mechanisms, while recall of the first part of a list requires further processing and encoding of the material, less developed primacy effects in autism may be secondary to organizational and encoding impairments rather than to memory deficits per se, an issue to which we return below.

Free versus cued recall

Another suggested point of similarity between autism and amnesia is the finding that cued recall is significantly better than free recall for both groups (Boucher & Warrington, 1976). Some studies have demonstrated that providing semantic or phonological cues improves recall (Mottron *et al.*, 2001; Tager-Flusberg, 1991).

Others, however, have found mild impairments relative to controls in both free and cued recall conditions, suggesting a general recall inefficiency in autism that is not specific to the method of testing retention (Minshew & Goldstein, 1993).

Other patterns: the role of organization and meaning

It has been suggested that individuals with autism encounter difficulty remembering material that requires further encoding, organization, or use of meaning to facilitate recall (DeLong, 1992; Minshew & Goldstein, 1993, 2001). In a pioneering series of experiments, Hermelin, O'Connor, and colleagues found that the advantage in remembering meaningful over random material typically seen in normally developing individuals is not apparent in autism, i.e. individuals with autism do not appear to use the syntactic and semantic cues that aid others in recalling material. For example, two studies demonstrated that children with autism were just as capable of recalling random verbal material, e.g. unconnected words, as they were of remembering meaningful sentences (Hermelin & Frith, 1971; Hermelin & O'Connor, 1967). In contrast, matched mentally handicapped children demonstrated a significant advantage in remembering words in the context of a meaningful sentence. Similarly, early studies demonstrated that children with autism did not semantically cluster or "chunk" related items when recalling word lists (Hermelin & Frith, 1971; O'Connor & Hermelin, 1967).

Later experiments clarified, however, that children with autism are not incapable of using semantic cues in recall, perhaps just less efficient in doing so, or less likely to use this strategy spontaneously. Fyffe and Prior (1978) failed to replicate earlier results, finding that children with autism recalled sentences significantly better than random word lists. Relative to controls, however, recall of sentences was deficient, while recall of random material was adequate. Thus, while the group with autism did appear to make use of meaning in recall, their advantage was not as great as in the mentally handicapped or typically developing control groups. Tager-Flusberg (1991) replicated this pattern, finding that recall of related and unrelated word lists was equivalent within the group with autism; however, their memory for meaningful material was less efficient than that of controls. Thus the ability of people with autism to use meaning, structure, and semantic cues in recall may be poorer than that of matched controls, but is by no means absent.

Working memory

Deficits in working memory have also been found in autism. Working memory is defined as the ability to maintain information in an activated, online state to guide cognitive processing (Baddeley, 1986). Typical working memory tasks require subjects to simultaneously hold information online, process it, and store results for later recall, thus requiring a significant amount of organization and processing of the material to be remembered. An initial study found that subjects with autism were significantly impaired relative to controls on working memory tasks, but not on measures of short- and long-term recognition memory, cued recall, or new learning ability (Bennetto *et al.*, 1996). Later studies have not confirmed this finding, however. In an investigation by Russell and colleagues, a group with both autism and mental retardation did not differ from matched controls on three measures of verbal working memory (Russell *et al.*, 1996). No group differences were found in a higher-functioning sample, relative to matched comparison groups with Tourette's syndrome and typical development, on three tasks of working memory in another study (Ozonoff & Strayer, 2001). One hypothesis of the latter study was that performance would be more impaired on tasks of verbal working memory than on measures of nonverbal working memory. This prediction was not borne out and the group with autism performed as well as both comparison groups on all tasks, despite having a nonsignificant but still substantial IQ disadvantage of approximately two-thirds of an SD. Thus, at present, it is not clear whether working memory is a specific difficulty for people with autism and more research is needed.

The evidence reviewed here suggests that autism is not a primary disorder of memory. Rather, difficulty appears to occur at the stage of encoding and organizing material. It is the overlay or additional requirement of higher-order processing that makes certain memory tasks difficult for people with autism. As summarized by DeLong (1992), the deficit does not appear to be an acquisition, storage, or retention impairment, but an interaction with the kind of information being processed and the operations being performed on the information. As with attention, intellectual, and academic functions, memory deficits appear to be selective, rather than widespread and all-encompassing. Concrete, rote, and mechanical memory processes are spared – in some studies, even enhanced (Toichi & Kamio, 2002); once abstraction, organization, and use of meaning are required, however, performance declines (Minshew & Goldstein, 2001, Williams *et al.*, 2006).

Social development and behavior

Impairments in perceiving and processing social and emotional cues in people and in the environment from the beginning of life seem to be at the heart of the disorder (Rutter, 1983). On the basis of a large epidemiological study of children with autism and developmental disorders, Wing and Gould (1979) proposed that the deficits of children with autism were encompassed by a "triad of impairments" in imagination, communication, and socialization. This conceptualization is immediately appealing because it captures the core features across all levels of functioning and it provides direction for exploring why these features might co-occur, and clues about the basis of the autistic disorder. In the remainder of this chapter, social behavior, communicative/language capacities, and theoretical approaches to bringing together research in these domains are the focus.

Social impairments are apparent very early in life in the majority of cases. As infants, individuals with autism are reported as not cuddly but rather stiff and resistant to contact, or else passive and floppy. They do not mold their bodies in anticipation of being picked up. Some appear placid and undemanding of human attention and are described as exceptionally "good" babies; others are difficult to manage, their needs are hard to identify and to satisfy, and they are difficult to comfort.

Their self-isolation and lack of communication is sometimes interpreted as a sign of deafness even though they may show an unpredictable or idiosyncratic reaction to particular sounds. While earlier researchers (e.g. DeMyer, 1976) suggested that severely handicapped young children with autism do not discriminate between people, more recent research (e.g. Dissanayake & Crossley, 1996; Walters et al., 1990) has shown that children with autism do show responsiveness and attachment to familiar carers, at least at a level consistent with their mental age. A number of studies during the last decade have reported evidence of attachment to carers in young children with autism that is not too dissimilar from that seen in nonautistic groups (Rogers et al., 1991; Sigman et al., 1986). This has represented a breakthrough in understanding, since for decades it had been widely believed that a central and causal mechanism in autism was a complete lack of bonding and attachment. This work suggests that their nonresponsiveness is not always "pervasive." Attachment behavior can be seen across the spectrum in various forms but may be more likely to be observable in higher-functioning children.

Nevertheless it is true that children with autism seek help and comfort less often than do normal and intellectually disabled children; they show less mutual eye contact, reduced attention to people and events, and more avoidant behavior. Contact is most frequently "on their terms" (Wing, 1976).

Aloofness, indifference, passivity, distractibility, and noncompliance, along with lack of cooperation and engagement in the activities of others, are characteristic of these children although this may vary on a continuum from almost totally withdrawn to occasional or "active but odd" contact based entirely on their own interests and needs (Wing & Gould, 1979). The severity of social deficits is related to IQ and language capacities, with the lowest-functioning children the most difficult to engage. Children and adolescents with Asperger's syndrome may be aware of their social deficiencies; they often desire and seek interaction (Attwood, 1998; Howlin, 2003; Shaked & Yirmiya, 2003), but are unable to develop the reciprocity, creativity, fluency, and "naturalness" that are characteristic in the social interactions of most normally developing children. This impairment, which in later life is associated with difficulties in developing intimate relationships, can be a great source of frustration and distress to them (Prior, 2003).

In the search for the antecedents of these deficits, a number of researchers have examined "joint attention" and social behavior in children with autism in both laboratory and naturalistic settings. Joint attention refers to the child's propensity, normally present from around 12 months of age, to show by pointing, bringing, or otherwise indicating an object or event they wish to share with a partner. It also encompasses eye contact with the partner related to interest in the object, so-called "referential looking." It is a key component of normal social development and one which is notably absent in most children with autism. This deficit is believed to offer a key to the understanding of their deviance in social development because of its high salience in the normal developmental pathway to social and communicative competence. It is argued that joint-attention skills underlie the development of all social and communication skills, and hence this deficit represents a fundamental neurobiological underpinning of autism (Wetherby et al., 2000).

Mundy and Sigman (1989a) have summarized a number of studies confirming the universality of joint-attention deficits in young children with autism, and have drawn on this work in developing a theory that incorporates the cognitive and affective impairments central to autism (on this topic see debate among Baron-Cohen, 1989a; Mundy & Sigman, 1989a, 1989b; Sigman, 1998). Baron-Cohen (1989b) has shown that deficits in pointing are in the shared interest aspect (protodeclarative), rather than representing an inability to indicate the presence of an object or request it (protoimperative pointing). Joint-attention behavior can be increased when adult carers provide structure and modeling for such interaction, although it is rarely spontaneously shown (Kasari et al., 1993).

Although a lack of joint-attention behaviors is evident even when controlling for IQ (Mundy et al., 1990), like other deficit behaviors it is less marked in higher-functioning children. Joint-attention skills are also associated with the development of language skills (Mundy et al., 1987), with correlations around 0.5 and 0.6 being reported by Mundy et al. (1990) in a longitudinal study of 4 to 5-year-olds, based on observations of social and play interactions in the laboratory, and assessment with the Reynell Developmental Language Scales. Mundy and Sigman (1989a) assert that "a disturbance of nonverbal joint attention behaviors is a fundamental characteristic of young children with autism" and that this "may be regarded as an important manifestation of early aspects of autistic developmental process." They question whether social skill deficits are better explained via a model that emphasizes cognitive impairments (Baron-Cohen, 1988) or one that emphasizes deficits in the development of affect in interaction with carers (Hobson, 1989; Kanner, 1943). They argue that problems in gestural joint attention skills reflect deficits in *both* affective processes and social/cognitive factors (see also Leekam & Ramsden, 2006).

While there is little disagreement that joint-attention deficits are one of the keys to autism and that they are related to the expression of other core social impairments, the precise nature of their influence on the developmental pathways in autism remains the subject of debate (Baron-Cohen, 1989a; Charman, 2003; Harris, 1989; Mundy & Sigman, 1989a, 1989b). In a recent review and research report, Charman (2003) summarized the evidence that joint attention plays a pivotal role in ASD. Joint-attention behaviors are the most discriminating early symptoms of the disorder; they are associated with later language and social development as well as with symptomatic improvement, as shown in longitudinal studies of early development; and intervention focused upon improving nonverbal social/communicative skills can progress the development of language and social skills. Further longitudinal studies, which can map the timing and emergence of joint attention skills within the context of cognitive and affective development in other domains, will be helpful in understanding the temporal and causal role of these impairments in the development of the disorder. This could provide important information to guide continuing efforts to design adaptive avenues for treating children with autism, e.g. Whalen and Schriebman (2003).

While rarely demonstrating joint interest and reciprocal activities, some children will enlist partners for repetitive games, preoccupations, or obsessions. This may be seen in verbal routines which the child will not permit to vary, and which do not take into account the other person's independent or contributory role. Some will make pseudosocial approaches to complete strangers that are inappropriate and deviant. For example, older children have been known to try to stroke the hair or the breasts of complete strangers.

The hallmark of the condition, at every age and stage, and every level of functioning, is lack of reciprocal social interaction. Even high-functioning individuals with Asperger's syndrome who are actively seeking to make contact with others suffer from lack of insight into the thoughts, feelings, plans, and wishes of others.

Try as they might, they cannot master the skills necessary for true reciprocity of social communication and they have great difficulty forming peer relationships. Empathy remains a mystery even to those who appear to have made a good adjustment (Sigman *et al.*, 1992; Wing, 1981). Individuals with high-functioning autism and Asperger's syndrome are egocentric in their communications and are prone to engage in lengthy, one-sided monologues about their own specific preoccupations or interests. Nevertheless, higher-functioning individuals with autism and Asperger's syndrome sometimes do have a particular "friend," usually a child with similar social problems or obsessive interests.

Apart from the absence of appropriate social skills there is also the presence of much unacceptable deviant and socially embarrassing behavior. These behaviors include stereotypies such as rocking, head banging, self-stimulatory, and self-injurious behavior such as hand-biting and head-punching, screaming, and temper tantrums often in highly public places such as supermarkets; aggressive and hyperactive behavior; purloining desired objects or those that are part of an obsession (e.g. taking certain flowers or leaves from people's gardens); and socially embarrassing eating, toileting, and sometimes verbal behaviors. There are some famous examples in the literature of even high-functioning individuals making comments that might be true but which would rarely be uttered by a nonhandicapped person. These kinds of deviant behaviors contribute to the fact that so many of these children are extraordinarily difficult to manage and to socialize. It is such behaviors that are likely to have some children excluded from normal educational and social environments and make it more likely that they will be kept in segregated and more restrictive settings.

Comparative studies of children with autism and other handicaps as well as normal groups using standardized tests such as the Vineland Adaptive Behaviour Scales show severe handicaps in social and communicative domains, with scores well below expectation taking into account their mental age levels (Boelte & Poustka, 2002). For example, dysfunctional social behaviors found in a study of this genre by Rodrigue *et al.* (1991) were pervasive, especially in the use of play and leisure times, in interpersonal relating and in coping skills. Their subjects with autism also showed behaviors not apparent in normal children at any age. Naturalistic observational studies of social behavior (Buitelaar *et al.*, 1991) confirm deficits in reciprocal social and communicative skills across varying levels of severity of autism. Peer interaction is significantly impaired and most commonly almost completely absent, even in children who relate reasonably well to adults. Attempts to train peer interaction skills have had limited success and there are persistent and seemingly intransigent difficulties in spontaneous initiation of interactions (Walters *et al.*, 1990). It is claimed that social functioning improves after about the age of five years although normalcy, even in high-functioning cases, is very rarely achieved (Volkmar *et al.*, 1997). Social development in the adolescent and adult phases of development has received little study, but it is common for young people to experience continued isolation and preoccupation with their own interests, and to have difficulty sustaining relationships in any reciprocal way even when they want to.

Emotion and face perception

Experimental research on the emotion perception abilities of individuals with autism was originally stimulated by Hobson's account of early affective development (Hobson, 1986a, 1989). Hobson highlighted the inborn capacity of normal infants and children to recognize the salience of social and affective cues, make "emotional touch" with others, and affectively experience close personal relationships. He hypothesized that this inborn mechanism does not develop properly in children with autism, accounting for many of their aberrant social behaviors. In addition, his theory predicted that children with autism should have particular difficulties with experimental tasks that require recognition of emotional states in other people.

Using a crossmodal paradigm in which subjects had to match affective and non-affective auditory and visual stimuli, Hobson (1986a, 1986b) found that the group with autism committed significantly more errors than controls matched on non-verbal IQ when matching affective material, but performed as well as controls on nonaffective crossmodal matching. Weeks and Hobson (1987) demonstrated that children with autism preferred to sort faces by nonemotional attributes, such as hairstyles and accessories, than by emotional expressions. When required to sort faces by emotion, performance was significantly impaired relative to controls.

Other researchers, using different but related paradigms, have replicated the finding that individuals with autism are selectively impaired on affect matching tasks, relative both to performance of comparison subjects matched on nonverbal IQ and to their own performance on nonaffective control tasks (Bormann-Kirschkel *et al.*, 1995; MacDonald *et al.*, 1989). Young children with autism pay little attention to the emotional displays of others, tending to ignore them or to engage in alternate activities, relative to both normally developing and mentally retarded controls (Sigman *et al.*, 1992). Two studies have found that individuals with autism are impaired in recognizing the meanings of emotion-related nouns and adjectives, relative to concrete, nonemotional terms (Hobson & Lee, 1989; van Lancker *et al.*, 1991).

However, two methodological issues have been raised concerning these studies by both Hobson himself (1991) and others (Braverman *et al.*, 1989; Ozonoff *et al.*, 1990). First, in many studies the affective and nonaffective comparison tasks were not of equal difficulty, with the latter typically being easier for all groups. Thus, the finding that group differences exist on emotion recognition tasks, but not on nonaffective control tasks, does not necessarily indicate a specific deficit in emotion perception. Second, and even more importantly, the role of verbal ability in emotion perception was not adequately controlled in early studies. If some verbal mediation is required to process affective information, then failure to match on verbal ability may account for group differences, rather than a primary deficit in emotion perception being responsible. Most studies reviewed above matched control samples on nonverbal IQ alone.

Both of these issues were addressed in three subsequent investigations by Hobson *et al.* (1988a, 1988b, 1989a), who found that when individuals with autism were matched with control subjects on the basis of verbal ability, group differences were no longer apparent on emotion sorting, matching, and naming tasks. The finding that group differences in emotion perception tasks are dependent on the nature of the control group used and disappear when matching on the basis of verbal ability has been replicated by many independent research teams (Braverman *et al.*, 1989; Buitelaar *et al.*, 1999a, 1999b; Davies *et al.*, 1994; Gepner *et al.*, 2001; Loveland *et al.*, 1997; Ozonoff *et al.*, 1990; Prior *et al.*, 1990; Serra *et al.*, 1995). Language ability and verbal IQ can account for large amounts of variance in emotion perception scores, with intercorrelations in the 0.60–0.70 range (Fein *et al.*, 1992). Capps *et al.* (1992) found deficits in recognizing only more complex emotions, such as pride and embarrassment. Since these emotions require some social referencing and social comparison, it has been suggested that deficits on such tasks may be more reflective of theory of mind difficulties than emotion perception impairments (Baron-Cohen, 1991a). Similarly, Adolphs *et al.* (2001) found no group differences in recognition of simple emotions, but impairment when making social judgments, such as trustworthiness or approachability, from faces. Grossman *et al.* (2000) found deficits in emotion recognition only when faces were paired with mismatching verbal descriptions. Celani *et al.* (1999) found deficits in matching emotional expressions only when the target pictures were presented very briefly (for 750 ms) and were not visible when the sample choices were provided, eliminating the possibility of matching based on perceptual strategies alone.

These results suggest that there are a number of moderating variables that account for variance in emotion perception abilities in autism. Group differences between samples with and without autism may be secondary to linguistic, cognitive, pragmatic, or theory of mind deficits of autism, rather than reflecting a specific emotion-processing impairment. Finally, research has demonstrated that emotion perception deficits are not specific to people with autism, having also been documented in individuals with mental retardation (Hobson *et al.*, 1989b), learning disabilities (Holder & Kirkpatrick, 1991) and schizophrenia (Novic *et al.*, 1984; Walker *et al.*, 1984).

Several studies have also explored potential differences in more basic processes involved in understanding faces. As with emotion perception, results have been somewhat mixed, with some studies finding that identity matching and basic facial perception appear to be normal (Adolphs *et al.*, 2001; Bar-Haim *et al.*, 2006; Ozonoff *et al.*, 1990; Volkmar *et al.*, 1989), while other studies find deficits in these abilities (Boucher *et al.*, 1998; Klin *et al.*, 1999).

New techniques that have only recently become available suggest that the mechanisms underlying face-processing, regardless of accuracy, may be different in people with and without autism. Recent eye-tracking and behavioral studies have demonstrated that individuals with autism use an atypical and disorganized approach to viewing faces, including an unusual focus on nonfeature areas of the face, such as the mouth (Dalton *et al.*, 2005; Joseph & Tanaka, 2003; Klin *et al.*, 2002; Pelphrey *et al.*, 2002), instead of the normal focus on the eyes (Emery, 2000). Dawson *et al.* (2002) used event-related potentials (ERPs) to study response to familiar faces (i.e. their mothers') and unfamiliar faces in young children with autism and matched controls. Only those with autism failed to show a difference in ERP response to the familiar versus unfamiliar face, although they did show the expected response to familiar versus unfamiliar objects. Baron-Cohen and colleagues (1999) used fMRI to examine brain function while participants looked at pictures of eyes and made judgments about what emotion the eyes conveyed. They found that typical adults relied heavily on both the amygdala and the frontal lobes to perform this task. In contrast, adults with either high-functioning autism or Asperger's syndrome used the frontal lobes much less than the normal adults and did not activate the amygdala at all when looking at the pictures of eyes. Instead they used the superior temporal gyrus, which is not typically active during this task in people without autism (Baron-Cohen *et al.*, 1999). Another important study, by Schultz *et al.* (2000), found that people with autism and Asperger's syndrome use the inferior temporal gyrus, the part of the brain that normally makes sense of objects, when they look at faces and do not activate typical face-processing structures, such as the fusiform gyrus. These studies suggest that even when people with autism can figure out what someone's eyes or face conveys, they do so in a different, possibly less efficient, manner.

Language

In most children with autism, impairment in language and communication is apparent by the second year of life (Lord & Paul, 1997), and this impairment is almost always the presenting complaint of parents of preschool children subsequently diagnosed with autism (Howlin & Rutter, 1987; Rapin, 1996). The qualitative impairment in communication that affects both verbal and nonverbal skills (APA, 1994; Wing, 1996) varies from failure to develop language at all, to a range of language abnormalities, including echolalia, odd intonation patterns, confusions with pronoun distinctions, and poor comprehension (Bishop & Rosenbloom, 1987; Lord & Paul, 1997; Tager-Flusberg, 2001a). Around half of the population of children with autism do not develop communicative language. A number of these mute children may use grunting, pointing, or instrumental touching or pulling in order to communicate needs, and a minority may have a few words used for similar purposes. Use of gesture to communicate is notably restricted. It is rare for children with autism to gain language if they have not done so by the age of about 6 years. Prognosis for children who have developed some language before 2 years of age appears to be enhanced (Rogers & DiLalla, 1990) but for nonspeaking children it is universally poor. Even for speaking children, the communicative functions of language are impaired or limited in significant ways. The intention to communicate may be said to underlie both language and social behavior and it is this which often appears abnormal in children with autism. An alternative view for which there is some support is that many of these children wish to communicate but lack the capacity or "wiring" to do so effectively, i.e. this is a fundamental, biologically based, cognitive impairment. Most children, though, will have at least some form of needs-driven communication such as nonverbal requesting, pointing, or taking a carer's hand and leading them to a desired object or outcome.

For those who do speak, various characteristic abnormalities have been noted over the years in the language of children with autism. These have included concreteness, literalness, pronomial reversal, deviant or monotonous prosodic features, metaphorical language, inability to initiate or sustain a conversation, ritualistic and inflexible language, and an insensitivity to the listener's response to a conversation (Tager-Flusberg, 1981, 1982). Such deficits, however, exist on a continuum across the population of children with autism and there are marked individual differences (Wetherby, 1986).

The language abnormalities appear to be present early in life as noted in a lack of (or abnormal) babbling, lack of the normal preference for human speech (Klin, 1991), signs of incomprehension of the language environment, failure to

imitate sounds and speech, delay in first words and phrase speech, and sometimes regressions after initial speech development. Also noted are echolalia,
both immediate and delayed, and repeating of rhymes or jingles with no apparent communicative function, often as the only form of speech. Communication
difficulties in children with autism can be compounded by their neuromotor
problems, including dyspraxias, which may handicap their efforts to communicate both verbally and by sign or gesture (Wetherby et al., 2000). Charman et al.
(2003) assessed the development of language in very young children with autism
using the parent-reported MacArthur Communicative Development Inventory.
Considerable variability was found, in the context of significant delay compared
to normal language acquisition timetables, with both comprehension and use
of referential gestures notably impaired. Nevertheless the overall patterns followed the language developmental pathways seen in typically developing young
children.

Perhaps the most universal language deficit in autism is that associated with
pragmatics, i.e. language used to communicate socially (Tager-Flusberg & Anderson, 1991). This transcends the individual differences in level of language and
speech competence, as it is seen in every person with autism to some degree.
Even very high-functioning cases show these pragmatic problems in adapting
their discourse to the listener's response, in turn-taking, in perceiving what the
listener might be wanting or thinking, and in imagining where to go next in the
conversation. Some individuals are able to articulate that they experience such
communication problems, they wish to overcome it, but are unable to adapt their
conversation and thinking no matter how well motivated (see the collection of
personal accounts in Schopler & Mesibov, 1992). They also have difficulty understanding and responding to complex questions and processing higher order,
contextually relevant language. Baron-Cohen et al. (1999), for example, tested
whether children with Asperger's syndrome or high-functioning autism could
recognize a faux pas (inappropriate comment for the context) by presenting them
with stories and asking whether someone has said something they should not
have said. Even though the subjects with ASD clearly understood the stories,
they were much poorer than nonautistic controls in recognizing faux pas.

Tager-Flusberg and colleagues, in a series of studies (e.g. Tager-Flusberg,
1989, 2001b), have explored the acquisition of language in children with autism
over time and compared them with children with typical development and
Down's syndrome. While children with autism are similar to matched comparison groups in the early stages of their language development, especially
with their mothers and in familiar settings, as they grow older they become
increasingly divergent. They become more prone to use routines, recoding, and

simple responses, rather than developing more sophisticated discourse as do normal children, and they appear unaware that conversation provides an opportunity for giving new knowledge or for sharing experience. Their vocabularies can also be limited or stereotyped (Tager-Flusberg, 1981), and prosody is frequently deviant, even in high-functioning cases. Some children may whisper, speak in a flat monotonous tone, or speak too loudly.

A naturalistic observational study of communication in the school setting and including children with autism across a wide range of cognitive abilities (Stone & Caro-Martinez, 1990) showed that the most common form of communication was instrumental, in the form of "motoric acts," i.e. touching another person to gain their attention or to obtain a desired end. The most common recipient was the teacher, although speaking children were also likely to target communication at peers or observers. The speaking group also used more gestures, made comments, and gave information, even though overall any spontaneous communication was rare.

Volden and Lord (1991) have analyzed the indiosyncratic language and neologisms sometimes reported as a feature of autism, and compared their utterances with those of mentally retarded and normal children matched by chronological age. Most of their high-functioning sample with autism produced unusual words, phrases, or neologisms, and these were also seen, albeit to a lesser extent, in mentally handicapped children. The children with autism more often used peculiar forms of speech that were neither semantically nor phonologically similar to the appropriate English word, by comparison with control groups. The linguistic idiosyncrasies were seen as part of a broader language impairment in autism that is not simply a function of developmental delay.

Most recent work confirms that children with autism are consistent with their mental age level in the mechanics or formal aspects of language, such as order of acquisition of speech sounds, measures of syntax and language content, and length and complexity of utterances (Green *et al.*, 1995); it is the semantic and pragmatic, or socially relevant aspects, which they cannot master. Abstract words, i.e. those with no concrete referents, are rarely understood or used; hence "thinking," "feeling," "wanting," kinds of messages in normal social communicative behavior leave all but the highest-functioning cases at a loss. Even high-functioning children with autism are impaired in social discourse, and particularly those with a diagnosis of Asperger's syndrome are known for their tendency towards formal pedantic styles of speech which take little account of the listener's feelings or interests. Capps *et al.* (1998) compared the conversational capacities of relatively high-functioning children with autism (mean IQ 75) to those of children with developmental delay matched on language

age and mental age, via engagement in an informal semistructured conversation. Although children with autism at this level of functioning were willing to engage in conversation, they more often gave no response, were more likely to repeat questions and previous comments, and less often offered new relevant information. Their attempts were marked by disjointedness, lack of reciprocity in responding to questions or comments from conversational partners, fewer personal experience stories, and bizarre language or noncontextual utterances (e.g. sabre-tooth tigers can't fly). However, they did show as much appropriate affect, smiling, and gesture as the developmentally delayed group. Of interest was the finding that the groups were extremely similar in their theory of mind scores in this study, and did not differ in their use of mental state, emotion, or desire terms during conversation.

Impaired comprehension and a lack of focus on the meaning aspects of language have led to the linking of autism to the language disorder known as "semantic–pragmatic disorder" (Bishop, 1989), described as "a set of behaviors that are loosely associated, which shade into autism at one extreme and normality at the other" (Brook & Bowler, 1992: p. 62). Primary characteristics of this communication disorder encompass the use of language, which may be fluent and complex but which is inappropriate or out of tune with the social context. Comprehension is impaired. The semantic pragmatic language impairments shared with high-functioning autism (and Asperger's syndrome) include comprehension deficits, literal interpretations of messages, perseveration, deficits in turn-taking, and problems with maintaining conversational topics (Tager-Flusberg, 2003). The two diagnostic groups also share deficits in symbolic play and joint referencing behavior. Comparisons of social impairments between autism and semantic pragmatic language disorder underline the heterogeneity and variation in levels especially within the latter condition. But as Bishop (1989) has noted, children with autism can have other kinds of language disorders, and children with semantic–pragmatic disorder are often not autistic and their communication difficulties are less extensive than those common in autism.

Attempts to train children with autism in the use of speech and in sign language have proliferated in recent years, with ongoing development of useful strategies and programs (see Quill, 1995). There are, however, serious limitations to progress in that even when children learn words or signs, they are limited in their ability to use such skills to generate spontaneous "new" utterances and tend to remain at a relatively echolalic level (Harris, 1975). At least with higher-functioning children there has been documented success in improving communication and language competence especially through intensive home-based training programs based on behavioral principles (Howlin, 1989; Lovaas,

1987). The communication of children with severe autism often remains quite limited despite the best efforts of parents and teachers. Alternative communication strategies, such as the Picture Exchange Communication System (Bondy & Frost, 1994), have been adopted in interventions catering to severely impaired young children. Knowledge of the long-term effects of such alternative communication systems await systematic evaluations.

Theory of mind

The last part of this chapter provides a brief discussion of recent theorizing and empirical work focused on key underlying deficits in autism including theory of mind, executive functioning, and central coherence, three aspects of the disorder which have been linked heuristically at behavioral and neuropsychological levels. The theory of mind hypothesis, which became prominent in autism research in the 1980s and 1990s, brought together what was known about the social, cognitive, and communication problems of children with autism across the developmental period, with the intention of providing an integrated and comprehensive explanation of the psychological characteristics of the disorder (Frith, 1989). Beginning with the experimental studies of Baron-Cohen, Frith and colleagues in the UK (for a summary, see Happe & Frith, 1995), this hypothesis has had considerable influence over autism research in recent years. Early studies demonstrated that children with autism have specific difficulties in understanding states of mind such as false belief, ignorance, and second-order belief (i.e. beliefs about beliefs) in other people; in the concept of pretence, and in comprehension of emotional reactions based on beliefs (Baron-Cohen, 1991a, 1991b). In essence, the theory of mind explanation of such deficits argues that children with autism are unable to perceive and comprehend the thoughts and feelings of others, i.e. to know that other people have "minds." They suffer from "mind blindness" (Happe & Frith, 1995). They do not apprehend the fact that individuals have beliefs, thoughts, feelings, plans, and intentions, i.e. mental states that influence their actions; nor are they able to comprehend that the thoughts, feelings, and actions of other people need to be taken into account in social transactions as guides to reciprocal behaviors. Their inability to "read" or predict the behavior of others is shown in their characteristic social deficits and reflects the absence of such knowledge. Their difficulties in understanding pretence, states of ignorance, states of knowledge, and emotions that are based on beliefs means that they are unable to provide "mentalistic" explanations for behavior, and they cannot predict others' behavior (Tager-Flusberg & Sullivan, 1994). Their spontaneous language rarely includes terms or comments which refer to mental states such as belief, although some individuals may refer to more primitive mentalistic concepts such as desire, emotion, and perception (Tager-Flusberg, 1992). More sophisticated apperception involving mind-reading, such as cheating, lying, deceiving, and understanding jokes, are a mystery to them by this theory.

A variety of experimental tasks and procedures have been used to assess mentalizing ability in children with autism, usually involving comparisons with other groups of similar levels of language and cognitive capacities. Probably the most common tasks are enacted scenarios involving dolls or people, whose knowledge or belief states must be intuited, in order that predictions about their behavior can be accurately made. For example, children may be asked what another person would think if they were presented with a tube of Smarties (correct answer: there are Smarties in there). While another character, either real or puppet like, is demonstrably absent, the child is shown that there are really pencils in the box. They are then asked what the absent character believes are the contents of the box. Normal children above the age of four years will correctly answer "Smarties." Children with autism are more likely to answer "pencils," thus demonstrating an inability to imagine what the other character will believe on the basis of access to new information. Many other creative ways of assessing this ability at varying levels of sophistication and abstraction have been reported in the literature (Baron-Cohen, 1991b; Bowler, 1992; Happe, 1994c; Leekam & Prior, 1994), and naturalistic studies have also illustrated the mentalizing deficits in autism.

The earliest signs of this key deficit, which according to theorists arises from a missing or dysfunctional "module" in the brain, can be observed in the lack of joint attention skills, communicative gestures and sharing of objects of interest and information with others (Baron-Cohen, 1991b). These behaviors are said to be developmental precursors to mentalizing ability. There is ongoing debate, however, concerning the direction of relations between these impairments, i.e. what is precursor to what? Higher-functioning children with autism, particularly those with good verbal skills, are notably less handicapped in theory of mind abilities, hence it seems that higher levels of social and communicative capacities allow the development of mentalizing ability (Hale & Tager-Flusberg, 2005). This has been cogently argued in recent reviews of this field (e.g. Garfield et al., 2001). It has also been noted that mentalizing deficits may not always be absent in people with autism, even though they are inevitably delayed in their development (Baron-Cohen, 1989c; Happe, 1995).

Klin et al. (1992) have claimed that the social impairments characteristic of autism emerge in the earliest developmental stages, *before* the emergence of precursors to theory of mind capacities, an argument that was also put forth in 1989 by Mundy and Sigman. It is also possible, as Leekam (1993) and others have suggested, that communicative ability and mental state knowledge develop independently, albeit in parallel, rather than being causally related.

Since not all children with autism lack a theory of mind, the early claims to have discovered the "core" and universal explanation for autism are hard to sustain. Findings that children diagnosed with Asperger's syndrome as well as a substantial proportion of more verbally capable individuals with autism are often able to solve the theory of mind tasks conventionally used in this genre of research (Bowler, 1992; Eisenmajer & Prior, 1991; Ozonoff *et al.*, 1991a) have led the proponents of the theory to suggest that such cases may "hack out" or "compute" solutions, using compensatory cognitive mechanisms which, however, do not constitute evidence for a "true" theory of mind (Happe & Frith, 1995). Whether this is true remains a question for exploration, but in any case, however successful the theory might be in explaining the social, language, and imaginative impairments of children with autism, it may not satisfactorily encompass other key deficits such as the lack of spontaneous activity and impairment in language; the repetitive and ritualistic behaviors including obsessions and preoccupations, islets of ability, lack of generalization skills, resistance to learning, and stereotypic behavior.

In recent years there has been increasing debate and re-evaluation of the theory, especially in terms of claims regarding its modularity or componential quality in brain development and dysfunction (Garfield *et al.*, 2001; Tager-Flusberg, 2001b). As noted above, many features of autism cannot be explained by theory of mind, and recent genetic advances make it clear that a number of interacting genes may be needed for the development of the disorder. Hence a single specific modular deficit hypothesis seems naïve. Moreover, the range of social–cognitive and communicative impairments with their diverse levels and balances in individual presentations seen in autism mean that reductionist models are unsatisfactory to explain the spectrum of abilities and deficits seen across this population of children.

Children and adolescents with high-functioning autism and Asperger's syndrome have shown that they have some theory of mind abilities in a number of studies (e.g. Capps *et al.* 1998; Dahlgren & Trillingsgaard, 1996; Leekam & Prior, 1994; Ozonoff *et al.*, 1991b). Methods of testing for this ability make a notable difference to performance since several studies have shown that children with autism do show understanding of false photographs in tasks which are similar in almost every other way to the procedures used in traditional false-belief investigations (Leekam & Perner, 1991; Peterson & Siegal, 1998). Nevertheless, despite their quite well-developed language and cognitive abilities they appear to develop such ability relatively late in development, and solving of more complex theory of mind problems may still elude them. Happe (1995) reviewed this field, based on a combination of published studies from 1985 to 1993, and combined results from her own experimental samples from many studies; she claimed that children with autism need a much higher verbal mental age level in order to pass false-belief tasks compared with nonautistic children. She also reported that only 25% of children from these aggregated studies passed theory of mind tasks.

While "theory of mind" research has made a major contribution in bringing together much of what is known about autistic behaviors, there are some findings that challenge the boundaries, if not the essence, of this theory. Not every child with autism lacks a theory of mind; despite the fact that their core social and communicative deficiencies are clearly apparent, mentalizing capacity is clearly associated with language ability (Eisenmajer & Prior, 1991; Ozonoff et al., 1991a; Tager-Flusberg, 1993). Nor are theory of mind deficits specific to autism. For example, a meta-analysis comparing theory of mind in autism, mental retardation, and normal development (Yirmiya et al., 1998) confirmed theory of mind impairment in individuals with mental retardation as well as those with autism. Other linguistically handicapped children, including deaf individuals (Peterson & Siegal, 1995), may show theory of mind handicaps, but not the other social and pragmatic impairments. Moreover, it is likely that "mentalizing" problems are simply one aspect of a more pervasive collection of cognitive impairments and in that sense the theory does not have comprehensibility. Garfield et al. (2001) have summarized a range of arguments and empirical work that shows that theory of mind is very much interwoven with linguistic and social skill development, and is acquired through the experience of social interaction and conversation.

Although explanations in terms of an autism-specific metarepresentational deficit were originally the primary explanatory focus (e.g. Leslie, 1987), a variety of alternative interpretations for the responses of children with autism on theory of mind tasks have been explored. Success with theory of mind tasks involves a range of cognitive and language abilities, including working memory and inhibition of prepotent responses (Bailey et al., 1996). Finding any kind of biological substrate for such a range of psychological processes remains a great challenge.

Recent research has drawn connections between the kinds of behaviors adduced to indicate theory of mind deficits and those that are believed to indicate problems with executive functions. In the next section, some of this recent experimental and theoretical work is reviewed.

Executive function

Investigation of executive functions has been an active area of research in autism. Executive functions are goal-directed, future-oriented cognitive abilities thought to be mediated by the frontal cortex (Duncan, 1986), including planning, inhibition, flexibility, organization, and self-monitoring. The first empirical investigation of the executive functions (EFs) of people with autism was done by Rumsey (1985) who administered the Wisconsin Card Sorting Test (WCST), a measure of cognitive flexibility, to adult men with high-functioning autism. Relative to a sample of typical adults matched on age, adults with autism demonstrated significant perseveration, sorting by previously correct rules despite feedback that their strategies were incorrect. In a later study, Rumsey and Hamburger (1990) demonstrated that this perseveration was not a general consequence of learning or developmental disorders as impairment was specific to people with autism and was not apparent in matched controls with severe dyslexia.

Prior and Hoffmann (1990) were the first research team to administer the WCST to a pediatric sample with autism. Like adults with autism, the children in this study made significantly more perseverative errors than matched controls. Several research groups have found that executive deficits are apparent in autism even relative to controls with other neurodevelopmental disorders (Ozonoff et al., 1991b; Szatmari et al., 1990). In one study, performance on the Tower of Hanoi (a test of planning) correctly predicted diagnosis in 80% of subjects, while other neuropsychological variables (e.g. theory of mind, memory, emotion perception, spatial abilities) predicted group membership at no better than chance levels. Following the sample longitudinally, Ozonoff and McEvoy (1994) found that deficits on the Tower of Hanoi and WCST were stable over a 2.5-year period. Not only did EF abilities not improve during the follow-up interval, they showed a tendency to decline relative to controls over time. Shu et al. (2001) reported significant deficits on WCST performance in a sample of 26 Taiwanese children with autism, relative to matched controls. Since these children were raised in a completely different culture and environment than the Western children who participate in most EF studies, the authors suggested that executive dysfunction may be a core impairment in autism.

In a review of the EF literature, Pennington and Ozonoff (1996) reported that 13 out of the 14 studies existing at the time of publication demonstrated impaired performance on at least one EF task in autism, including 25 of the 32 executive tasks used across those empirical studies. The magnitude of group differences tended to be quite large, with an average effect size (Cohen's d) across all studies of 0.98, marked by especially large effect sizes for the Tower of Hanoi ($d = 2.07$) and the WCST ($d = 1.04$).

Two research groups have tested age-related EF development in very young children with autism. McEvoy *et al.* (1993) studied preschool children with autism (mean age 5 years) and matched developmentally delayed and typically developing control groups. In the spatial reversal task, an object was hidden in one of two identical wells outside the subject's vision. The side of hiding remained the same until the subject successfully located the object on four consecutive trials, after which the side of hiding was changed to the other well. Thus successful search behavior required flexibility and set-shifting. Significant group differences were found, with the children with autism making more perseverative errors than children in either the mentally or chronologically age-matched groups. However, no group differences were evident on three other EF measures. It was suggested that these tasks may have been less developmentally appropriate for the sample.

However, in another investigation by the same research team (Griffith *et al.*, 1999), studying even younger preschool children with autism (mean age 4 years), there were no differences in performance on any of eight executive tasks (including the spatial reversal task), compared to a developmentally delayed group matched on chronological age and both verbal and nonverbal mental age. Similarly, in a larger study of even younger children with autism (mean age 3 years), Dawson *et al.* (2002) reported no significant differences on six EF tasks (again including spatial reversal), relative to developmentally delayed and typically developing control groups matched on mental age. This work raises the possibility that differential EF deficits emerge with age and are not present (at least relative to other samples with delayed development) early in the preschool range. Since EFs are just beginning to develop during the early preschool period in all children, a relative lack of variance across groups may explain this apparent developmental discontinuity. Differences in the way EF is measured at different ages may also contribute to this finding. The executive tests that have been administered to very young children with autism do not require the same use of arbitrary rules that those given to older individuals do. If arbitrary rule use is central to the EF performance deficits of autism (Biro & Russell, 2001), then the discontinuity between earlier and later development may be due simply to measurement differences. Further work, particularly longitudinal research, is needed to examine when during development specific executive difficulties emerge and what their developmental precursors may be.

Executive function is a multidimensional construct. The category includes a number of skills (flexibility, planning, inhibition, organization, self-monitoring, goal-setting) that appear to be, to some extent, dissociable. The tasks used in initial studies of EF in autism were relatively imprecise, typically measuring several executive operations, with no method to examine variance in individual skills. A recent research trend has been the use of computerized experimental paradigms designed to examine specific aspects of EF and more precisely identify the nature of the EF impairments underlying autism. Ozonoff and colleagues, in a series of papers, have suggested that flexibility is a more dysfunctional component of EF than inhibition. In a computerized Go–NoGo task designed to isolate and separately examine flexibility and inhibition operations in subjects with high-functioning autism (Ozonoff et al., 1994), they found that the group with autism was not impaired relative to controls when inhibiting responses, but was very deficient at shifting set. In contrast, matched comparison subjects with Tourette's syndrome experienced no difficulty in either the inhibition or flexibility conditions. Two additional aspects of inhibitory function, the ability to inhibit voluntary motor responses and the ability to inhibit processing of distractor stimuli during a cognitive task, were found to be unimpaired in subjects with autism in a later study (Ozonoff & Strayer, 1997), a finding that was recently replicated by an independent research team (Brian et al., 2003).

A newly developed EF battery, the Cambridge Neuropsychological Test Automated Battery (CANTAB), has been used in several recent studies (Hughes et al., 1994; Ozonoff et al., 2004; Turner, 1997). Relative to matched controls with mental retardation, individuals with autism plus mental retardation demonstrated intact performance on tasks measuring discrimination learning and inhibitory control, but impairments in shifting from one sorting strategy to another (Hughes et al., 1994). Turner (1997) replicated this shifting deficit in individuals with autism and mental retardation, but not in participants with autism of normal IQ, although small sample size and low power may have contributed to this result. In the most recent study, CANTAB was administered to 79 participants with autism and 70 well-matched typical controls recruited from seven universities who are part of the Collaborative Programs of Excellence in Autism network (Ozonoff et al., 2004). Normal inhibition but significant group differences in shifting relative to controls were found in both lower- and higher-IQ individuals with autism across the age range of 6 to 47 years. In aggregate, these results suggest that inhibition may be a spared component of EF in autism, standing in contrast to the impairments in flexibility found in other studies.

Another recent research trend has been to study the relationships between EF and other cognitive and social–cognitive processes, e.g. Landa and Goldberg (2005). The explanatory power of executive dysfunction to autism would be greatest if individual differences in EF predicted variations in other impairments or in symptoms of autism. The first work in this area was actually done within a study designed to examine theory of mind and strategic deception abilities (Russell *et al.*, 1991). Children with autism were taught to play a game in which they competed with an experimenter for a piece of candy. The candy was placed in one of two boxes with windows that revealed the contents of the box to subjects, but not to the experimenter. The objective of the task was to "fool" the experimenter into looking for the candy in the empty box. It was explained that the strategy of pointing to the empty box would be successful in winning the candy, whereas pointing to the box that actually contained the candy would result in losing it. Even after many trials, the subjects with autism were unable to point to the empty box, despite the consequences of this strategy. Russell *et al.* (1991) first attributed these results to a perspective-taking deficit that caused an inability to engage in deception. In a follow-up study, Hughes and Russell (1993) demonstrated that significant group differences remained even after the element of social deception was removed from the task. Subjects were simply instructed to point to the empty box to get the candy. Even with no opponent present, the subjects with autism persisted in using the inappropriate strategy. On the basis of these results, Hughes and Russell (1993) reattributed the pattern of performance to a deficit in disengaging from the object and using internal rules to guide behavior, rather than to a social or perspective-taking dysfunction. This work led the way for several other studies that explored the hypothesis that some degree of executive control is necessary for successful performance on theory of mind tasks and, by extension, for the development of theory of mind (Landa & Goldberg, 2005; Moses, 2001; Russell *et al.*, 1999).

The opposite hypothesis – that some level of social awareness is necessary for EF – has also received support. In the WCST, for example, feedback is provided by the examiner after each card is sorted; successful set-shifting requires using this feedback to alter behavior. If, however, feedback supplied in a social context is less salient or more difficult to process for people with autism, they may perform poorly on EF tasks for primarily social reasons. A few studies have contrasted performance on executive tests when they are administered in the traditional manner, by human examiners, to performance when they are administered by computer. Ozonoff (1995) reported that the WCST was significantly easier for individuals with autism when it was given by computer, with group differences considerably smaller in the computer administration than the human administration conditions. In the group with autism, the number of perseverations was cut in half on the computerized version of the task, while performance did not differ across conditions in the typically developing control group (Ozonoff, 1995). This finding was replicated by an independent research group (Pascualvaca *et al.*, 1998). This suggests that the format of the executive task, particularly the nature of the feedback (social vs. nonsocial), may have a much greater impact on performance for people with autism than has previously been appreciated. Thus, it has been difficult to tease apart the relative primacy of EF and mentalizing or other social deficits in the chain of cognitive impairments that are involved in autism.

It has also become clear through recent research that other non-EF skills, such as language and intelligence, may contribute to EF deficits. Liss *et al.* (2001) gave a battery of EF tests to children with high-functioning autism and a control group of children with developmental language disorders. The only group difference – more perserverative errors on the WCST by the autism group – disappeared when Verbal IQ was statistically controlled. Ozonoff has also identified significant contributions of IQ to EF performance in people with autism (Miller & Ozonoff, 2000; Ozonoff & McEvoy, 1994; Ozonoff & Strayer, 2001). Perner and Lang (2002) reported a pair of large studies of typically developing preschool children in which the correlation between EF and a language task was just as high as its correlation with a false-belief task.

Although there remain many important questions about EF to be answered, much progress has been made since the first edition of this book. Robust findings of EF deficits in older children and adults with autism, relative to appropriate clinical and typical controls, have been tempered by the discovery of more complex patterns of EF development in very young children with autism. And there are indications of significant correlations between EF abilities and core social impairments of autism, intelligence, and language, but the causal directions and specific nature of these relationships are as yet unknown.

Central coherence

A third theory put forth as an integrative explanation for the pattern of symptoms seen in autism is that of weak central coherence (Frith, 1989; Frith & Happe, 1994). This theory suggests that the core psychological impairment in autism is the failure to process information in context. The information processing of typically developing individuals is motivated by a "drive" to achieve higher-level meaning and a preference for global processing. Frith (1989) first introduced the idea that it is this drive for central coherence that is missing in autism, resulting instead in detail-focused processing. Central coherence theory predicts that people with autism will perform poorly on tasks that require integration of constituent parts into coherent wholes, but perform normally (or even in a superior fashion) on tasks that require a focus on detail or "local processing." They should also show preserved or enhanced performance on tasks in which the typical tendency to use contextual information actually interferes with performance, since central coherence theory predicts that people with autism would be relatively impervious to context effects. An essential feature of central coherence theory is that the detail orientation of autism is a *consequence* of a deficit in global processing.

Central coherence theory has intuitive appeal, as it appears to explain both the neuropsychological deficits and the particular cognitive strengths of people with autism (Happe, 1999). It also has potential to account for some behavioral symptoms of the condition that other theories have failed to explain, such as repetitive and stereotyped behaviors. For example, weak central coherence could explain the focus on technicalities and trivia seen in the circumscribed interests of people with autism spectrum disorders, as well as their insistence on sameness in the environment.

Several studies have supported the central coherence theory of autism. The first empirical test of the theory used the Embedded Figures Test, in which a small form is embedded within a larger, complex picture. Frith and colleagues found that children with autism were significantly more accurate in discovering the hidden figures than controls matched on mental and chronological age (Shah & Frith, 1983). This research team also found evidence that weak central coherence played a role in the strong performance of people with autism on the Wechsler Block Design subtest (Shah & Frith, 1993). They found that presegmenting the designs significantly improved performance for participants without autism (both with typical development and mental retardation), presumably because of the strong tendency to process the unsegmented designs as a gestalt. The performance of people with autism was not, however, enhanced in this way by presegmentation, suggesting that this group had a natural tendency to see the stimuli in terms of parts rather than as a whole and did not need the parts to be explicitly highlighted.

Other supportive evidence of central coherence deficits in autism came from verbal tasks. Several studies have shown that individuals with autism fail to use sentence context to determine the correct pronunciation of homographs (words with one spelling but two meanings; Frith & Snowling, 1983; Happe, 1997; Jolliffe & Baron-Cohen, 2000).

Later studies have not fully confirmed these results, however. Several subsequent investigations have used the Embedded Figures Test, with one study finding no superiority in accuracy (Ozonoff *et al.*, 1991b), another failing to replicate the accuracy results, but demonstrating significantly faster reaction time on the part of people with autism spectrum disorders (Jolliffe & Baron-Cohen, 1997), and a third failing to find superiority in either accuracy or reaction time (Rodgers, 2000). A prediction of central coherence theory is that there should be little difference in performance when the context within which the shape is embedded is meaningful or nonmeaningful, since the deficit in global processing leads to little or no encoding of context. Two studies used adaptations of the Embedded Figures Test in which the meaningfulness of the context was manipulated. Both investigations found that the performance of participants with autism was affected by the contextual information in the same manner as the controls (Brian & Bryson, 1996; Lopez & Leekam, 2003). Brian and Bryson (1996) also examined memory for the contextual information and found that it was as good as controls, demonstrating that the context *was* being actively processed and encoded.

Global–local tasks have also been used in several experiments to test central coherence theory. Such tasks use stimuli (usually either letters or numbers) that are composed of smaller similar stimuli (also letters or numbers), which can be the same as or different from the larger pattern. For example, in Navon's original task (1977), a large letter H is composed of either small Hs (compatible condition) or small Ss (incompatible condition). Participants are instructed to examine either the large or the small letters and determine if it is an H or an S. In typical development, there is usually a global advantage; that is, typical subjects respond both more quickly and more accurately when asked to identify the large letters than the small letters. There is also typically interference from the global to the local level, so that small letters that are incompatible with the larger stimulus are responded to more slowly and less accurately than those that are compatible. In contrast, the prediction for autism would be the opposite: there should be a local advantage and no global interference. Mixed results have been obtained across studies, however. While one study (Rinehart *et al.*, 2000) confirmed both predictions, other investigations have found the typical global advantage as well as global interference on local processing (Mottron *et al.*, 1999; Ozonoff *et al.*, 1994) or failed to find the predicted local superiority (Rodgers, 2000). In an elegant experimental design, Plaisted *et al.* (1999) demonstrated that administration procedures have large effects on performance and could account for the inconsistent pattern of results across studies. They found normal global processing in autism using a selective attention procedure, in which participants focused on only one level (either global or local) for long blocks of stimulus presentation, but a local advantage in autism during a divided attention procedure, in which participants had to shift between global and local levels from trial to trial. This suggests that the necessity of switching attention (an executive or attentional deficit) may be part of poor performance and argues against a purely central coherence explanation for the deficit found on such global–local tasks.

Findings have been similarly inconsistent using other paradigms. Happe (1996) first reported that individuals with autism were much less likely than control participants to succumb to visual illusions, which are dependent upon context. However, Ropar and Mitchell (1999) failed to replicate this nonsusceptibility, using the same illusions employed in the Happe study. They also reported low and nonsignificant correlations among visual illusion susceptibility and several visuospatial tasks also thought to measure weak central coherence (e.g. Block Design, Embedded Figures Test; Ropar & Mitchell, 2001), further questioning the construct and its selective association with autism.

These nonreplications, particularly the repeated findings that individuals with autism do appear to use context and perceive gestalts (Brian & Bryson, 1996; Lopez & Leekam, 2003; Mottron et al., 1999; Ozonoff et al., 1994; Ropar & Mitchell, 1999), have suggested a modified version of central coherence theory. It has been proposed that the cognition of people with autism does involve some "local bias" or preference for detail-oriented processing, but that this is not due to a deficit in global processing. Several recent investigations have supported this notion. Plaisted and colleagues found that a group of participants with autism demonstrated enhanced ability to identify individual features of a stimulus, but also were as good as controls at integrating these features to see the significance of the configuration of the features (Plaisted et al., 2003). This pattern was also found in the auditory modality, with the autism group performing better than a comparison group at detecting small changes in the pitch (a local feature) of melodies, but also performing as well as controls at detecting changes in the contour (a global feature) of melodies (Mottron et al., 2000).

In a final study of interest, weak central coherence was found to be more common in a group of high-functioning adolescents with autism than developmental norms for the tests would predict, but was far from universal, with half of those with autism demonstrating performance across several tests indicative of *strong* central coherence (Teunisse et al., see also Pellicano et al., 2006).

Conclusion

While aspects of the central coherence theory describe well the cognition of autism, it has fared similarly to the EF and theory of mind accounts in failing as a grand theory, capable of organizing the behavioral and cognitive strengths and weaknesses of autism within one unifying theory. Perhaps the only theory that remains relatively successful in this endeavor is one that by its very nature is a much more general theory. Minshew has proposed that the central cognitive deficit in autism is one of complex information processing (Minshew *et al.*, 1997, 2002). Any neuropsychological task, be it perceptual, spatial, verbal, or motor, that requires less information processing will be spared, according to this account, while those that require higher-order information processing will be impaired. The review of the literature in this chapter, across many neuro-psychological domains, provides quite a lot of support for this theory. We have summarized the relative sparing of simple language processes (e.g. phonology, syntax), simple executive functions (e.g. inhibition), simple attentional processes (e.g. selective and focused attention), and simple memory functions (e.g. rote and recognition), with complementary dysfunction in each of these domains at the level of more complex processes (e.g. language pragmatics, cognitive flexibility, abstraction, attention shifting, working memory). Neurological theories have been proposed to explain this neuropsychological profile, such as reduced integration of local neural networks (Brock *et al.*, 2002). Recent findings of enlarged brains (Courchesne *et al.*, 2001) with increased numbers of cortical columns, of reduced size and density (Casanova *et al.*, 2002), are consistent with significant disruptions in neural networks and perhaps increased "noise" and thus lower efficiency of information processing. It remains to be seen if these theories will hold up as further empirical research is conducted.

Regardless, this is an exciting time to be conducting neuropsychological research in autism, as we hope this chapter attests. The last decade has been an exceedingly productive one in further honing our understanding of the cognition of people with autism. We are beginning to see the potential of this neuro-psychological work to provide a bridge between descriptions of symptoms and findings of neurological investigations that we anticipate will be similarly productive in coming decades.

REFERENCES

Abrahamsen, E. P. and Mitchell, J. R. (1990). Communication and sensorimotor functioning in children with autism. *Journal of Autism and Developmental Disorders*, **20**, 75–85.

Adolphs, R., Sears, L., and Piven, J. (2001). Abnormal processing of social information from faces in autism. *Journal of Cognitive Neuroscience*, **13**, 232–40.

Allen, G. and Courchesne, E. (2001). Attention function and dysfuntion in autism. *Frontiers in Bioscience*, **6**, 105–19.

Allen, G. and Courchesne, E. (2003). Differential effects of developmental cerebellar abnormality on cognitive and motor functions in the cerebellum: an fMRI study of autism. *American Journal of Psychiatry*, **160**, 262–73.

Allen, M. H., Lincoln, A. J., and Kaufman, A. S. (1991). Sequential and simultaneous processing abilities of high-functioning autistic and language-impaired children. *Journal of Autism and Developmental Disorders*, **21**, 483–502.

American Psychiatric Association (1994). *Diagnostic and Statistical Manual of Mental Disorders*, 4th edn (DSM-IV). Washington, DC: American Psychiatric Association.

Asarnow, R. F., Tanguay, P. E., Bott, L., and Freeman, B. J. (1987). Patterns of intellectual functioning in non-retarded autistic and schizophrenic children. *Journal of Child Psychology and Psychiatry*, **28**, 273–80.

Asperger, H. (1944). "Autistic psychopathy" in childhood. *Archiv für Psychiatrie und Nervenkrankheiten*, **117**, 76–136.

Attwood, A. (1998). *Asperger's Syndrome: A Guide for Parents and Professionals*. Philadelphia: Kingsley.

Aylward, E. H., Minshew, M. J., Goldstein, G. *et al.* (1999). MRI volumes of amygdala and hippocampus in non-mentally retarded autistic adolescents and adults. *Neurology*, **52**, 2145–50.

Bachevalier, J. (1994). Medial temporal lobe structures and autism: a review of clinical and experimental findings. *Neuropsychologia*, **32**, 627–48.

Baddeley, A. D. (1986). *Working Memory*. Oxford: Clarendon Press.

Baddeley, A. D. and Warrington, E. K. (1970). The distinction between long- and short-term memory. *Journal of Verbal Learning and Verbal Behavior*, **9**, 176–89.

Bailey, A., Phillips, W., and Rutter, M. (1996). Autism: towards an integration of clinical, genetic, neuropsychological, and neurobiological perspectives. *Journal of Child Psychology and Psychiatry*, **37**, 89–126.

Bar-Haim, Y., Shulman, C., Lamy, D., and Reuveni, A. (2006). Attention to eyes and mouth in high-functioning children with autism. *Journal of Autism and Developmental Disorders*, **36**, 131–7.

Baron-Cohen, S. (1988). Social and pragmatic deficits in autism: cognitive or affective? *Journal of Autism and Developmental Disorders*, **18**, 379–402.

Baron-Cohen, S. (1989a). Joint-attention deficits in autism: towards a cognitive analysis. *Development and Psychopathology*, **1**, 185–9.

Baron-Cohen, S. (1989b). Perceptual role taking and protodeclarative pointing in autism. *British Journal of Developmental Psychology*, **7**, 113–7.

Baron-Cohen, S. (1989c). The autistic child's theory of mind: a case of specific developmental delay. *Journal of Child Psychology and Psychiatry*, **30**, 285–97.

Baron-Cohen, S. (1991a). Do people with autism understand what causes emotion? *Child Development*, **62**, 385–95.

Baron-Cohen, S. (1991b). The theory of mind deficit in autism: how specific is it? *British Journal of Developmental Psychology*, **9**, 301–14.

Baron-Cohen, S., Ring, H., Wheelwright, S. *et al.* (1999). Social intelligence in the normal and autistic brain: an fMRI study. *European Journal of Neuroscience*, **11**, 1891–8.

Baron-Cohen, S., Ring, H. A., Bullmore, E. T. *et al.* (2000). The amygdala theory of autism. *Neuroscience and Biobehavioral Review*, **24**, 355–64.

Barth, C., Fein, D., and Waterhouse, L. (1995). Delayed match-to-sample performance in autistic children. *Developmental Neuropsychology*, **11**, 53–69.

Bauman, M. and Kemper, T. L. (1985). Histoanatomic observations of the brain in early infantile autism. *Neurology*, **35**, 866–74.

Bauman, M. and Kemper, T. L. (1988). Limbic and cerebellar abnormalities: consistent findings in infantile autism. *Journal of Neuropathology and Experimental Neurology*, **47**, 369.

Bennetto, L. (1999). A componential analysis of imitation and movement deficits in autism. *Dissertation Abstracts International: The Sciences and Engineering*, **60**, (2-B).

Bennetto, L., Pennington, B. F., and Rogers, S. J. (1996). Impaired and intact memory functions in autism: a working memory model. *Child Development*, **67**, 1816–35.

Beversdorf, D. Q., Smith, B. W., Crucian, G. P. *et al.* (2000). Increased discrimination of "false memories" in autism spectrum disorder. *Proceedings of the National Academy of Sciences*, **97**, 8734–7.

Biro, S. and Russell, J. (2001). The execution of arbitrary procedures by children with autism. *Development and Psychopathology*, **13**, 97–110.

Bishop, D. V. M. (1989). Autism, Asperger's syndrome and semantic–pragmatic disorder: where are the boundaries? *British Journal of Disorders of Communication*, **24**, 107–21.

Bishop. D. and Rosenbloom L. (1987). Childhood language disorders: classification and overview. In W. Yule and M. Rutter, eds., *Language Development and Disorders*. London: MacKeith Press, pp. 16–41.

Boelte, S. and Poustka, F. (2002). The relation between general cognitive level and adaptive behaviour domains in individuals with autism with and without co-morbid mental retardation. *Child Psychiatry and Human Development*, **33**, 165–72.

Bondy, A. and Frost, L. (1994). The Picture Exchange Communication System. *Focus on Autistic Behaviour*, **9**, 1–19.

Bormann-Kischkel, C., Vilsmeier, M., and Baude, B. (1995). The development of emotional concepts in autism. *Journal of Child Psychology and Psychiatry*, **36**, 1243–59.

Boucher, J. (1981). Immediate free recall in early childhood autism: another point of behavioral similarity with the amnesic syndrome. *British Journal of Psychology*, **72**, 211–15.

Boucher, J. and Warrington, E. K. (1976). Memory deficits in early infantile autism: some similarities to the amnesic syndrome. *British Journal of Psychology*, **67**, 73–87.

Boucher, J., Lewis, V., and Collis, G. (1998). Familiar face and voice matching and recognition in children with autism. *Journal of Child Psychology and Psychiatry*, **39**, 171–81.

Bowler, D. M. (1992). "Theory of mind" in Asperger's syndrome. *Journal of Child Psychology and Psychiatry*, **33**, 877–93.

Braverman, M., Fein, D., Lucci, D., and Waterhouse, L. (1989). Affect comprehension in children with pervasive developmental disorders. *Journal of Autism and Developmental Disorders*, **19**, 301–16.

Brian, J. A. and Bryson, S. E. (1996). Disembedding performance and recognition memory in autism/PDD. *Journal of Child Psychology and Psychiatry*, **37**, 865–72.

Brian, J. A., Tipper, S. P., Weaver, B., and Bryson, S. E. (2003). Inhibitory mechanisms in autism spectrum disorders: typical selective inhibition of location versus facilitated perceptual processing. *Journal of Child Psychology and Psychiatry*, **44**, 552–60.

Brock, J., Brown, C. C., Boucher, J., and Rippon, G. (2002). The temporal binding deficit hypothesis of autism. *Development and Psychopathology*, **14**, 209–24.

Brook, S. L. and Bowler, D. M. (1992). Autism by another name? Semantic and pragmatic impairments in children. *Journal of Autism and Developmental Disorders*, **22**, 61–81.

Buchsbaum, M. S., Siegel, B. V., Wu, J. C. *et al.* (1992). Attention performance in autism and regional brain metabolic rate assessed by positron emission tomography. *Journal of Autism and Developmental Disorders*, **22**, 115–25.

Buitelaar, J. K., van Engeland, H., de Kogel, K. H., de Vries, H., and van Hooff, J. A. R. A. M. (1991). Differences in the structure of social behaviour of autistic children and non-autistic retarded controls. *Journal of Child Psychology and Psychiatry*, **32**, 995–1015.

Buitelaar, J. K., van der Wees, M., Swaab-Barneveld, H., and van der Gaag, R. J. (1999a). Theory of mind and emotion-recognition functioning in autistic spectrum disorders and in psychiatry control and normal children. *Development and Psychopathology*, **11**, 39–58.

Buitelaar, J. K., van der Wees, M., Swaab-Barneveld, H., and van der Gaag, R. J. (1999b). Verbal memory and performance IQ predict theory of mind and emotion recognition ability in children with autistic spectrum disorders and in psychiatric control children. *Journal of Child Psychology and Psychiatry*, **40**, 869–81.

Burd, L., Fisher, W., Knowlton, D., and Kerbeshian, J. (1987). Hyperlexia: a marker for improvement in children with pervasive developmental disorder? *Journal of the American Academy of Child and Adolescent Psychiatry*, **26**, 407–12.

Capps, L., Yirmiya, N., and Sigman, M. (1992). Understanding of simple and complex emotions in non-retarded children with autism. *Journal of Child Psychology and Psychiatry*, **33**, 1169–82.

Capps L., Kehres J., and Sigman M. (1998). Conversational abilities among children with autism and children with developmental delays. *Autism*, **2**, 325–44.

Carpentieri, S. C. and Morgan, S. B. (1994). Brief report: a comparison of patterns of cognitive functioning of autistic and nonautistic retarded children on the Stanford–Binet–Fourth edition. *Journal of Autism and Developmental Disorders*, **24**, 215–23.

Casanova, M. F., Buxhoeveden, D. P., Switala, A. E., and Roy, E. (2002). Minicolumnar pathology in autism. *Neurology*, **58**, 428–32.

Casey, B. J., Gordon, C. T., Mannheim, G. B., and Rumsey, J. M. (1993). Dysfunctional attention in autistic savants. *Journal of Clinical and Experimental Neuropsychology*, **15**, 933–46.

Celani, G., Battacchi, M. W., and Arcidiacono, L. (1999). The understanding of the emotional meaning of facial expressions in people with autism. *Journal of Autism and Developmental Disorders*, **29**, 57–66.

Chakrabarti, S. and Fombonne, E. (2001). Pervasive developmental disorders in preschool children. *Journal of the American Medical Association*, **285**, 3093–9.

Charman, T. (2003). Why is joint attention a pivotal skill in autism? *Philosophical Transactions of the Royal Society of London*, **358**, 315–24.

Charman, T., Drew, A., Baird, C., and Baird, G. (2003). Measuring early language development in preschool children with autism spectrum disorder using the MacArthur Communicative Development Inventory. *Journal of Child Language*, **30**, 213–36.

Courchesne, E., Townsend, J., Akshoomoff, N. A. *et al.* (1994). Impairment in shifting attention in autistic and cerebellar patients. *Behavioral Neuroscience*, **108**, 848–65.

Courchesne, E., Karns, C. M., Davis, B. S. *et al.* (2001). Unusual brain growth patterns in early life in patients with autistic disorder: an MRI study. *Neurology*, **57**, 245–54.

Dahlgren, S. and Trillingsgaard, A. (1996). Theory of mind in nonretarded children with autism and Asperger's syndrome. A research note. *Journal of Child Psychology and Psychiatry*, **37**, 759–63.

Dalton, K. M., Nacewicz, B. M., Johnstone, T. *et al.* (2005). Gaze fixation and the neural circuitry of face processing in autism. *Nature Neuroscience*, **8**, 519–26.

Damasio, A. R. and Maurer, R. G. (1978). A neurological model for childhood autism. *Archives of Neurology*, **35**, 777–86.

Davies, S., Bishop, D., Manstead, A. S. R., and Tantam, D. (1994). Face perception in children with autism and Asperger's syndrome. *Journal of Child Psychology and Psychiatry*, **35**, 1033–57.

Dawson, G., Meltzoff, A., Osterling, J., Rinaldi, J., and Brown, E. (1998). Children with autism fail to orient to naturally occurring social stimuli. *Journal of Autism and Developmental Disorders*, **28**, 479–85.

Dawson, G., Osterling, J., Rinaldi, J., Carver, L., and McPartland, J. (2001). Brief report: recognition memory and stimulus–reward associations. Indirect support for the role of ventromedial prefrontal dysfunction in autism. *Journal of Autism and Developmental Disorders*, **31**, 337–41.

Dawson, G., Carver, L., Meltzoff, A. N. *et al.* (2002). Neural correlates of face and object recognition in young children with autism spectrum disorder, developmental delay, and typical development. *Child Development*, **73**, 700–17.

DeLong, G. R. (1992). Autism, amnesia, hippocampus, and learning. *Neuroscience and Biobehavioral Reviews*, **16**, 63–70.

DeMyer, M. (1976). Motor, perceptual-motor and intellectual disabilities of autistic children. In L. Wing, ed., *Early Childhood Autism: Clinical, Educational and Social aspects*, 2nd edn. Oxford: Pergamon Press.

DeMyer, M. K., Barton, S., and Norton, J. A. (1972). A comparison of adaptive, verbal and motor profiles of psychotic and non-psychotic subnormal children. *Journal of Autism and Childhood Schizophrenia*, **2**, 359–77.

DeMyer, M. K., Barton, S., Alpern, G. D. *et al.* (1974). The measured intelligence of autistic children. *Journal of Autism and Childhood Schizophrenia*, **4**, 42–60.

DeMyer, M. K., Hingtgen, J. N., and Jackson, R. K. (1981). Infantile autism reviewed: a decade of research. *Schizophrenia Bulletin*, **7**, 388–451.

Dennis, M., Lockyer, L., Lazenby, A. L. *et al.* (1999). Intelligence patterns among children with high-functioning autism, phenylketonuria, and childhood head injury. *Journal of Autism and Developmental Disorders*, **29**, 5–17.

Dissanayake, C. and Crossley, S. A. (1996). Proximity and sociable behaviors in autism: evidence for attachment. *Journal of Child Psychology and Psychiatry*, **37**, 149–56.

Duncan, J. (1986). Disorganization of behaviour after frontal lobe damage. *Cognitive Neuropsychology*, **3**, 271–90.

Eaves, L. C. and Ho, H. H. (1997). School placement and academic achievement in children with autistic spectrum disorders. *Journal of Developmental and Physical Disabilities*, **9**, 277–91.

Eisenmajer, R. and Prior, M. (1991). Cognitive linguistic correlates of "theory of mind" ability in autistic children. *Journal of Autism and Developmental Disorders*, **9**, 351–64.

Emery, N. J. (2000). The eyes have it: the neuroethology, function and evolution of social gaze. *Neuroscience and Biobehavioral Reviews*, **24**, 581–604.

Fein, D., Waterhouse, L., Lucci, D., and Snyder, D. (1985). Cognitive subtypes in developmentally disabled children: a pilot study. *Journal of Autism and Developmental Disorders*, **15**, 77–95.

Fein, D., Lucci, D., Braverman, M., and Waterhouse, L. (1992). Comprehension of affect in context in children with pervasive developmental disorders. *Journal of Child Psychology and Psychiatry*, **33**, 1157–67.

Freeman, B. J., Ritvo, E. R., Needleman, R., and Yokota, A. (1985). The stability of cognitive and linguistic parameters in autism: a five-year prospective study. *Journal of the American Academy of Child Psychiatry*, **24**, 459–64.

Freeman, B. J., Rahbar, B., Ritvo, E. R. *et al.* (1991). The stability of cognitive and behavioural parameters in autism: a twelve-year prospective study. *Journal of the American Academy of Child and Adolescent Psychiatry*, **30**, 479–82.

Freeman, B. J., Del'Homme, M., Guthrie, D., and Zhang, F. (1999). Vineland Adaptive Behavior Scale scores as a function of age and initial IQ in 210 autistic children. *Journal of Autism and Developmental Disorders*, **29**, 379–84.

Frith, U. (1989). *Autism: Explaining the Enigma*. Oxford: Basil Blackwell.

Frith, U. (1991). *Autism and Asperger Syndrome*. Cambridge: Cambridge University Press.

Frith, U. and Happe, F. (1994). Autism: beyond theory of mind. *Cognition*, **50**, 115–32.

Frith, U. and Snowling, M. (1983). Reading for meaning and reading for sound in autistic and dyslexic children. *British Journal of Developmental Psychology*, **1**, 329–42.

Fyffe, C. and Prior, M. (1978). Evidence for language recoding in autistic, retarded and normal children: a re-examination. *British Journal of Psychology*, **69**, 393–402.

Garfield, J., Peterson, C., and Perry, T. (2001). Social cognition, language acquisition, and the development of the theory of mind. *Mind and Language*, **16**, 494–541.

Garretson, H. B., Fein, D., and Waterhouse, L. (1990). Sustained attention in children with autism. *Journal of Autism and Developmental Disorders*, **20**, 101–14.

Gepner, B., Deruelle, C., and Grynfeltt, S. (2001). Motion and emotion: a novel approach to the study of face processing by young autistic children. *Journal of Autism and Developmental Disorders*, **31**, 37–45.

Ghaziuddin, M., Butler, E., Tsai, L., and Ghaziuddin, N. (1994). Is clumsiness a marker for Asperger syndrome? *Journal of Intellectual Disability Research*, **38**, 519–27.

Gillberg, I. C. and Gillberg, C. (1989). Asperger syndrome: some epidemiological considerations. A research note. *Journal of Child Psychology and Psychiatry*, **30**, 631–8.

Goldstein, G., Minshew, N. J., and Siegel, D. J. (1994). Age differences in academic achievement in high-functioning autistic individuals. *Journal of Clinical and Experimental Neuropsychology*, **16**, 671–80.

Goldstein, G., Johnson, C. R., and Minshew, N. J. (2001a). Attentional processes in autism. *Journal of Autism and Developmental Disorders*, **31**, 433–40.

Goldstein, G., Beers, S. R., Siegel, D. J., and Minshew, N. J. (2001b). A comparison of WAIS-R profiles in adults with high-functioning autism or differing subtypes of learning disability. *Applied Neuropsychology*, **8**, 148–54.

Grandin, T. (1995). How people with autism think. In E. Schopler and G. B. Mesibov, eds., *Learning and Cognition in Autism*. New York: Plenum Press, pp. 137–56.

Green, L., Fein, D., Joy, S., and Waterhouse, L. (1995). Cognitive functioning in autism: an overview. In E. Schopler and G. B. Mesibov, eds., *Learning and Cognition in Autism*. New York: Plenum Press, pp. 13–31.

Green, D., Baird, G., Barnett, A. *et al.* (2002). The severity and nature of motor impairment in Asperger's syndrome: a comparison with Specific Developmental Disorder of Motor Function. *Journal of Child Psychology and Psychiatry*, **43**, 655–68.

Griffith, E. M., Pennington, B. F., Wehner, E. A., and Rogers, S. J. (1999). Executive functions in young children with autism. *Child Development*, **70**, 817–32.

Grossman, J. B., Klin, A., Carter, A., and Volkmar, F. R. (2000). Verbal bias in recognition of facial emotions in children with Asperger syndrome. *Journal of Child Psychology and Psychiatry*, **41**, 369–79.

Hale, C. and Tager-Flusberg, H. (2005). Social communication in children with autism. *Autism*, **9**(2), 157–78.

Happe, F. G. E. (1994a). Annotation: current psychological theories of autism. The "Theory of Mind" account and rival theories. *Journal of Child Psychology and Psychiatry*, **35**, 215–29.

Happe, F. G. E. (1994b). Wechsler IQ profile and theory of mind in autism: a research note. *Journal of Child Psychology and Psychiatry*, **35**, 1461–71.

Happe, F. G. E. (1994c). An advanced test of theory of mind: understanding of handicapped and normal children and adults. *Journal of Autism and Developmental Disorders*, **24**, 129–54.

Happe, F. (1995). The role of age and verbal ability in the theory of mind task performance of subjects with autism. *Child Development*, **66**, 843–55.

Happe, F. G. E. (1996). Studying weak central coherence at low levels: children with autism do not succumb to visual illusions. A research note. *Journal of Child Psychology and Psychiatry*, **37**, 873–7.

Happe, F. G. E. (1997). Central coherence and theory of mind in autism: reading homographs in context. *British Journal of Developmental Psychology*, **15**, 1–12.

Happe, F. (1999). Autism: cognitive deficit or cognitive style? *Trends in Cognitive Sciences*, **3**, 216–22.

Happe, F. and Frith, U. (1995). Theory of mind in autism. In E. Schopler and G. B. Mesibov, eds., *Learning and Cognition in Autism*. New York: Plenum Press, pp. 177–97.

Harris, S. L. (1975). Teaching language to non-verbal children with emphasis on problems of generalization. *Psychological Bulletin*, **82**, 565–80.

Harris, S. L. (1989). The autistic child's impaired conception of mental states. *Development and Psychopathology*, **1**, 191–5.

Harris, S. L. and Handleman, J. S. (2000). Age and IQ at intake as predictors of placement for young children with autism: a four- to six-year follow-up. *Journal of Autism and Developmental Disorders*, **30**, 137–42.

Harris, S. L., Handleman, J. S., and Burton, J. L. (1990). The Stanford–Binet profiles of young children with autism. *Special Services in the Schools*, **6**, 135–43.

Henderson, S. E., Barnett, A., and Henderson, L. (1994). Visuospatial difficulties and clumsiness: on the interpretation of conjoined deficits. *Journal of Child Psychology and Psychiatry*, **35**, 961–9.

Hermelin, B. (2001). *Bright Splinters of the Mind: A Personal Story of Research with Autistic Savants*. London: Jessica Kingsley.

Hermelin, B. and Frith, U. (1971). Psychological studies of childhood autism: can autistic children make sense of what they see and hear? *Journal of Special Education*, **5**, 107–17.

Hermelin, B. and O'Connor, N. (1967). Remembering of words by psychotic and subnormal children. *British Journal of Psychology*, **58**, 213–18.

Hermelin, B. and O'Connor, N. (1970). *Psychological Experiments with Autistic Children*. New York: Pergamon.

Hermelin, B. and O'Connor, N. (1991). Talents and preoccupations in idiot-savants. *Psychological Medicine*, **21**, 959–64.

Hertzig, M. E., Snow, M. E., and Sherman, M. (1989). Affect and cognition in autism. *Journal of the American Academy of Child and Adolescent Psychiatry*, **28**, 195–9.

Hetzler, B. E. and Griffin, J. L. (1981). Infantile autism and the temporal lobe of the brain. *Journal of Autism and Developmental Disorders*, **11**, 317–30.

Hobson, R. P. (1986a). The autistic child's appraisal of expressions of emotion. *Journal of Child Psychology and Psychiatry*, **27**, 321–42.

Hobson, R. P. (1986b). The autistic child's appraisal of expressions of emotion: a further study. *Journal of Child Psychology and Psychiatry*, **27**, 671–80.

Hobson, R. P. (1989). Beyond cognition: a theory of autism. In G. Dawson, ed., *Autism: Nature, Diagnosis and Treatment*. New York: Guilford, pp. 22–48.

Hobson, R. P. (1991). Methodological issues for experiments on autistic individuals' perception and understanding of emotion. *Journal of Child Psychology and Psychiatry*, **32**, 1135–58.

Hobson, R. P. and Lee, A. (1989). Emotion-related and abstract concepts in autistic people: evidence from the British Picture Vocabulary Scale. *Journal of Autism and Developmental Disorders*, **19**, 601–23.

Hobson, R. P., Ouston, J., and Lee, A. (1988a). Emotion recognition in autism: coordinating faces and voices. *Psychological Medicine*, **18**, 911–23.

Hobson, R. P., Ouston, J., and Lee, A. (1988b). What's in a face? The case of autism. *British Journal of Psychology*, **79**, 441–53.

Hobson, R. P., Ouston, J., and Lee, A. (1989a). Naming emotion in faces and voices: abilities and disabilities in autism and mental retardation. *British Journal of Developmental Psychology*, **7**, 237–50.

Hobson, R. P., Ouston, J., and Lee, A. (1989b). Recognition of emotion by mentally retarded adolescents and young adults. *American Journal on Mental Retardation*, **93**, 434–43.

Holder, H. B. and Kirkpatrick, S. W. (1991). Interpretation of emotion from facial expressions in children with and without learning disabilities. *Journal of Learning Disabilities*, **24**, 170–7.

Howlin, P. (1989). Changing approaches to communication training with autistic children. *British Journal of Disorders of Communication*, **24**, 151–68.

Howlin, P. (2003). Longer term educational and employment outcomes. In M. Prior, ed., *Learning and Behavior Problems in Asperger Syndrome*. New York: Guilford Press, pp. 269–294.

Howlin, P. and Rutter, M. (1987). *The Treatment of Autistic Children*. Chichester: Wiley.

Hughes, C. and Russell, J. (1993). Autistic children's difficulty with mental disengagement from an object: its implications for theories of autism. *Developmental Psychology*, **29**, 498–510.

Hughes, C., Russell, J., and Robbins, T. W. (1994). Evidence for executive dysfunction in autism. *Neuropsychologia*, **32**, 477–92.

Jolliffe, T. and Baron-Cohen, S. (1997). Are people with autism and Asperger syndrome faster than normal on the embedded figures test? *Journal of Child Psychology and Psychiatry*, **38**, 527–34.

Jolliffe, T. and Baron-Cohen, S. (2000). Linguistic processing in high-functioning adults with autism or Asperger's syndrome: is global coherence impaired? *Psychological Medicine*, **30**, 1169–87.

Jones, V. and Prior, M. (1985). Motor imitation abilities and neurological signs in autistic children. *Journal of Autism and Developmental Disorders*, **15**, 37–46.

Joseph, R. M. and Tanaka, J. (2003). Holistic and part-based faced recognition in children with autism. *Journal of Child Psychology and Psychiatry*, **44**, 529–42.

Kanner, L. (1943). Autistic disturbances of affective content. *Nervous Child*, **2**, 217–50.

Kasari, C., Sigman, M., and Yirmiya, N. (1993). Focused and social attention of autistic children in interactions with familiar and unfamiliar adults: a comparison of autistic, mentally retarded, and normal children. *Development and Psychopathology*, **5**, 403–14.

Klin, A. (1991). Young autistic children's listening preferences in regard to speech: a possible characterization of the symptom of social withdrawal. *Journal of Autism and Developmental Disorders*, **21**, 29–42.

Klin, A., Volkmar, F. R., and Sparrow, S. S. (1992). Autistic social dysfunction: some limitations of the theory of mind hypothesis. *Journal of Child Psychology and Psychiatry*, **33**, 861–76.

Klin, A., Volkmar, F. R., Sparrow, S. S., Cicchetti, D. V., and Rourke, B. P. (1995). Validity and neuropsychological characterization of Asperger syndrome: convergence with nonverbal learning disabilities syndrome. *Journal of Child Psychology and Psychiatry*, **36**, 1127–40.

Klin, A., Sparrow, S. S., de Bildt, A. *et al.* (1999). A normed study of face recognition in autism and related disorders. *Journal of Autism and Developmental Disorders*, **29**, 499–510.

Klin, A., Jones, W., Schultz, R., Volkmar, F., and Cohen, D. (2002). Visual fixation patterns during viewing of naturalistic social situations as predictors of social competence in individuals with autism. *Archives of General Psychiatry*, **59**, 809–16.

Konstantareas, M. M., Homatidis, S., and Busch, J. (1989). Cognitive, communication, and social differences between autistic boys and girls. *Journal of Applied Developmental Psychology*, **10**, 411–24.

Landa, R. and Goldberg, M. (2005). Language, social, and executive functions in high-functioning autism: a continuum of performance. *Journal of Autism and Developmental Disorders*, **35**(5), 557–73.

Leekam, S. R. (1993). Children's understanding of mind. In M. Bennett, ed., *The Child as Psychologist*. London: Harvester Wheatsheaf, pp. 26–61.

Leekam, S. R. and Perner, J. (1991). Do autistic children have a metarepresentational deficit? *Cognition*, **40**, 203–18.

Leekam, S. R. and Prior, M. (1994). Can autistic children distinguish lies from jokes? A second look at second-order belief attribution. *Journal of Child Psychology and Psychiatry*, **35**, 901–15.

Leekam, S. and Ramsden, C. (2006). Dyadic orienting and joint attention in preschool children with autism. *Journal of Autism and Developmental Disorders* (in press; available online).

Leslie, A. M. (1987). Pretence and representation: the origins of "Theory of Mind." *Psychological Review*, **94**, 412–26.

Lincoln, A. J., Courchesne, E., Kilman, B. A., Elmasian, R., and Allen, M. (1988). A study of intellectual abilities in high-functioning people with autism. *Journal of Autism and Developmental Disorders*, **18**, 505–24.

Lincoln, A. J., Allen, M. H., and Kilman, A. (1995). The assessment and interpretation of intellectual abilities in people with autism. In E. Schopler and G. B. Mesibov, eds., *Learning and Cognition in Autism*. New York: Plenum, pp. 89–117.

Liss, M., Fein, D., Allen, D. *et al.* (2001). Executive functioning in high-functioning children with autism. *Journal of Child Psychology and Psychiatry*, **42**, 261–70.

Lopez, B. and Leekam, S. R. (2003). Do children with autism fail to process information in context? *Journal of Child Psychology and Psychiatry*, **44**, 285–300.

Lord, C. and Paul, R. (1997). Language and communication in autism. In D. Cohen and F. Volkmar, eds., *Handbook of Autism and Pervasive Developmental Disorders*, 2nd edn. New York: John Wiley, pp. 195–225.

Lord, C. and Schopler, E. (1985). Differences in sex ratios in autism as a function of measured intelligence. *Journal of Autism and Developmental Disorders*, **15**, 185–93.

Lord, C. and Schopler, E. (1988). Intellectual and developmental assessment of autistic children from preschool to schoolage: clinical implications of two follow-up studies. In E. Schopler and G. B. Mesibov, eds., *Diagnosis and Assessment in Autism*. New York: Plenum, pp. 167–81.

Lord, C. and Schopler, E. (1989). The role of age at assessment, developmental level, and test in the stability of intelligence scores in young autistic children. *Journal of Autism and Developmental Disorders*, **19**, 483–99.

Losche, G. (1990). Sensorimotor and action development in autistic children from infancy to early adulthood. *Journal of Child Psychology and Psychiatry*, **31**, 749–61.

Lotter, V. (1974). Factors related to outcome in autistic children. *Journal of Autism and Childhood Schizophrenia*, **4**, 263–77.

Lovaas, O. I. (1987). Behavioural treatment and normal educational and intellectual functioning in young autistic children. *Journal of Consulting and Clinical Psychology*, **55**, 3–9.

Lovaas, O. I., Koegel, R. L., and Schreibman, L. (1979). Stimulus overselectivity in autism: a review of research. *Psychological Bulletin*, **86**, 1236–54.

Loveland, K. A., Tunali-Kotoski, B., Chen, Y. R. *et al.* (1997). Emotion recognition in autism: verbal and nonverbal information. *Development and Psychopathology*, **9**, 579–93.

MacDonald, H., Rutter, M., Howlin, P. *et al.* (1989). Recognition and expression of emotional cues by autistic and normal adults. *Journal of Child Psychology and Psychiatry*, **30**, 865–77.

Manjiviona, J. (2003). The assessment of Specific Learning Difficulties in children with Asperger Syndrome. In M. Prior, ed., *Learning and Behavior Problems in Asperger Syndrome*, pp. 55–84. New York: Guilford Press.

Manjiviona, J. and Prior, M. (1995). Comparison of Asperger syndrome and high-functioning autistic children on a test of motor impairment. *Journal of Autism and Developmental Disorders*, **25**, 23–39.

Mann, T. A. and Walker, P. (2003). Autism and a deficit in broadening the spread of visual attention. *Journal of Child Psychology and Psychiatry*, **44**, 274–84.

Mayes, S. and Calhoun, S. (2003a). Ability profiles in children with autism: Influence of age and IQ. *Autism*, **6**, 83–98.

Mayes, S. and Calhoun, S. (2003b). Relationships between Asperger Syndrome and high functioning autism. In M. Prior, ed., *Learning and Behavior Problems in Asperger Syndrome*. New York: Guilford Press, pp. 15–34.

Mayes, S., Calhoun, S., and Crites, D. (2001). Does DSM-IV Asperger's disorder exist? *Journal of Abnormal Child Psychology*, **29**, 263–72.

McEvoy, R. E., Rogers, S. J., and Pennington, B. F. (1993). Executive function and social communication deficits in young autistic children. *Journal of Child Psychology and Psychiatry*, **34**, 563–78.

Miller, J. and Ozonoff, S. (1997). Did Asperger's cases have Asperger's disorder? A research note. *Journal of Child Psychology and Psychiatry*, **38**, 247–51.

Miller, J. N. and Ozonoff, S. (2000). The external validity of Asperger disorder: lack of evidence from the domain of neuropsychology. *Journal of Abnormal Psychology*, **109**, 227–38.

Minshew, N. J. and Goldstein, G. (1993). Is autism an amnesic disorder? Evidence from the California Verbal Learning Test. *Neuropsychology*, **7**, 209–16.

Minshew, N. J. and Goldstein, G. (2001). The pattern of intact and impaired memory functions in autism. *Journal of Child Psychology and Psychiatry*, **42**, 1095–101.

Minshew, N. J., Goldstein, G., Taylor, H. G., and Siegel, D. J. (1994). Academic achievement in high-functioning autistic individuals. *Journal of Clinical and Experimental Neuropsychology*, **16**, 261–70.

Minshew, N. J., Goldstein, G., and Siegel, D. J. (1997). Neuropsychologic functioning in autism: profile of a complex information processing disorder. *Journal of the International Neuropsychological Society*, **3**, 303–16.

Minshew, M. J., Sweeney, J., and Luna, B. (2002). Autism as a selective disorder of complex information processing and underdevelopment of neocortical systems. *Molecular Psychiatry*, **7**, S14–S15.

Morgan, S. B., Cutter, P. S., Coplin, J. W., and Rodrigue, J. R. (1989). Do autistic children differ from retarded and normal children in Piagetian sensorimotor functioning? *Journal of Child Psychology and Psychiatry*, **30**, 857–64.

Moses, L. J. (2001). Executive accounts of theory-of-mind development. *Child Development*, **72**, 688–90.

Mottron, L. and Burack, J. (2001). Enhanced perceptual functioning in the development of autism. In J. Burack, T. Charman, N. Yirmiya, and P. Zelazo, eds., *The Development of Autism: Perspectives from Theory and Research*. London: Lawrence Erlbaum Associates, pp. 131–48.

Mottron, L., Burack, J. A., Stauder, J. E. A., and Robaey, P. (1999). Perceptual processing among high-functioning persons with autism. *Journal of Child Psychology and Psychiatry*, **40**, 203–11.

Mottron, L., Peretz, I., and Menard, E. (2000). Local and global processing of music in high-functioning persons with autism: beyond central coherence? *Journal of Child Psychology and Psychiatry*, **41**, 1057–65.

Mottron, L., Morasse, K., and Belleville, S. (2001). A study of memory functioning in individuals with autism. *Journal of Child Psychology and Psychiatry*, **42**, 253–60.

Mundy, P. and Sigman, M. (1989a). The theoretical implications of joint-attention deficits in autism. *Development and Psychopathology*, **1**, 173–84.

Mundy, P. and Sigman, M. (1989b). Second thoughts on the nature of autism. *Development and Psychopathology*, **1**, 213–18.

Mundy, P., Sigman, M., Ungerer, J., and Sherman, T. (1987). Play and nonverbal communication correlates to language development in autistic children. *Journal of Autism and Developmental Disorders*, **17**, 349–63.

Mundy, P., Sigman, M., and Kasari, C. (1990). A longitudinal study of joint attention and language development in autistic children. *Journal of Autism and Developmental Disorders*, **20**, 115–28.

Nation, K., Clarke, P., Wright, B. J., and Williams, C. (2006). Patterns of reading ability in children with autism spectrum disorder. *Journal of Autism & Developmental Disorders* (in press).

Noterdaeme, M., Amorosa, H., Mildenberger, K., Sitter, S., and Minow, F. (2001). Evaluation of attention problems in children with autism and children with a specific language disorder. *European Child and Adolescent Psychiatry*, **10**, 58–66.

Noterdaeme, M., Mildenberger, K., Minow, F., and Amorosa, H. (2002). Evaluation of neuromotor deficits in autism and children with a specific speech and language disorder. *European Child and Adolescent Psychiatry*, **11**, 219–25.

Novic, J., Luchins, D. J., and Perline, R. (1984). Facial affect recognition in schizophrenia: is there a differential deficit? *British Journal of Psychiatry*, **144**, 533–7.

O'Connor, N. (1989). The performance of the 'idiot-savant': implicit and explicit. *British Journal of Disorders of Communication*, **24**, 1–20.

O'Connor, N. and Hermelin, B. (1967). Auditory and visual memory in autistic and normal children. *Journal of Mental Deficiency Research*, **11**, 126–31.

O'Connor, N. and Hermelin, B. (1984). Idiot savant calendrical calculators: maths or memory? *Psychological Medicine*, **14**, 801–6.

Ohta, M. (1987). Cognitive disorders of infantile autism: a study employing the WISC, spatial relationships, conceptualization and gesture imitations. *Journal of Autism and Developmental Disorders*, **17**, 45–62.

Ozonoff, S. (1995). Reliability and validity of the Wisconsin Card Sorting Test in studies of autism. *Neuropsychology*, **9**, 491–500.

Ozonoff, S. and McEvoy, R. E. (1994). A longitudinal study of executive function and theory of mind development in autism. *Development and Psychopathology*, **6**, 415–31.

Ozonoff, S. and Strayer, D. L. (1997). Inhibitory function in nonretarded children with autism. *Journal of Autism and Developmental Disorders*, **27**, 59–77.

Ozonoff, S. and Strayer, D. L. (2001). Further evidence of intact working memory in autism. *Journal of Autism and Developmental Disorders*, **31**, 257–63.

Ozonoff, S., Pennington, B. F., and Rogers, S. J. (1990). Are there emotion perception deficits in young autistic children? *Journal of Child Psychology and Psychiatry*, **31**, 343–61.

Ozonoff, S., Rogers, S. J., and Pennington, B. F. (1991). Asperger's syndrome: evidence of an empirical distinction from high-functioning autism. *Journal of Child Psychology and Psychiatry*, **32**, 1107–22.

Ozonoff, S., Pennington, B. F., and Rogers, S. J. (1991). Executive function deficits in high-functioning autistic individuals: relationship to theory of mind. *Journal of Child Psychology and Psychiatry and Allied Disciplines*, **32**, 1081–105.

Ozonoff, S., Strayer, D. L., McMahon, W. M., and Filloux, F. (1994). Executive function abilities in autism: an information processing approach. *Journal of Child Psychology and Psychiatry*, **35**, 1015–31.

Ozonoff, S., Cook, I., Coon, H. *et al.* (2004). Performance on CANTAB subsets sensitive to frontal lobe function in people with autistic disorder: evidence from the CPEA network. *Journal of Autism and Developmental Disorders*, **34**, 139–50.

Pascualvaca, D. M., Fantie, B. D., Papageorgiou, M., and Mirsky, A. F. (1998). Attentional capacities in children with autism: is there a general deficit in shifting focus? *Journal of Autism and Developmental Disorders*, **28**, 467–78.

Pellicano, E., Maybery, M., Durkin, K., and Maley, A. (2006). Multiple cognitive capabilities / deficits in children with an autism spectrum disorder: "weak" central coherence and its relationship to theory of mind and executive control. *Development and Psychopathology*, **18**, 77–98.

Pelphrey, K. A., Sasson, N. J., Reznick, J. S. *et al.* (2002). Visual scanning of faces in autism. *Journal of Autism and Developmental Disorders*, **32**, 249–61.

Pennington, B. F. (1991). *Diagnosing Learning Disorders: A Neuropsychological Framework*. New York: Guilford Press.

Pennington, B. F. and Ozonoff, S. (1996). Executive functions and developmental psychopathologies. *Journal of Child Psychology and Psychiatry Annual Research Review*, **37**, 51–87.

Perner, J. and Lang, B. (2002). What causes 3-year-olds' difficulty on the dimensional change card sorting task? *Infant and Child Development*, **11**, 93–105.

Peterson, C. C. and Siegal, M. (1995). Deafness, conversation and theory of mind. *Journal of Child Psychology and Psychiatry*, **36**, 459–74.

Peterson, C. C. and Siegal, M. (1998). Changing focus on the representational mind. *British Journal of Developmental Psychology*, **16**, 301–20.

Plaisted, K., O'Riordan, M., and Baron-Cohen, S. (1998). Enhanced discrimination of novel, highly similar stimuli by adults with autism during a perceptual learning task. *Journal of Child Psychology and Psychiatry*, **39**, 765–76.

Plaisted, K., Swettenham, J., and Rees, L. (1999). Children with autism show local precedence in a divided attention task and global precedence in a selective attention task. *Journal of Child Psychology and Psychiatry*, **40**, 733–42.

Plaisted, K., Saksida, L., Alcantara, J., and Weisblatt, E. (2003). Towards an understanding of the mechanisms of weak central coherence effects: experiments in visual configural learning and auditory perception. *Philosophical Transactions of The Royal Society of London. Series B, Biological Sciences*, **358**, 375–86.

Posner, M. I. (1980). Orienting of attention. *Quarterly Journal of Experimental Psychology*, **32**, 3–25.

Pring, L., Hermelin, B., and Heavey, L. (1995). Savants, segments, art and autism. *Journal of Child Psychology and Psychiatry*, **36**, 1065–76.

Prior, M. R. (1977). Psycholinguistic disabilities of autistic and retarded children. *Journal of Mental Deficiency Research*, **21**, 37–45.

Prior, M. R. (1979). Cognitive abilities and disabilities in infantile autism: a review. *Journal of Abnormal Child Psychology*, **7**, 357–80.

Prior, M. (2003). What do we know and where should we go? In M. Prior, ed., *Learning and Behavior Problems in Asperger Syndrome*, pp. 295–319. New York: Guilford Press.

Prior, M. R. and Chen, C. S. (1976). Short-term and serial memory in autistic, retarded, and normal children. *Journal of Autism and Childhood Sczophrenia*, **6**, 121–31.

Prior, M. R. and Hoffmann, W. (1990). Neuropsychological testing of autistic children through an exploration with frontal lobe tests. *Journal of Autism and Developmental Disorders*, **20**, 581–90.

Prior, M., Perry, D., and Gajzago, C. (1975). Kanner's syndrome or early-onset psychosis: a taxonomic analysis of 142 cases. *Journal of Autism and Childhood Schizophrenia*, **5**, 71–80.

Prior, M., Dahlstrom, B., and Squires, T. L. (1990). Autistic children's knowledge of thinking and feeling states in other people. *Journal of Child Psychology and Psychiatry*, **31**, 587–601.

Quill, K. A. (1995). *Teaching Children with Autism: Strategies to Enhance Communication and Socialization*. New York: Delmar.

Rapin, I. (1996). Developmental language disorders: a clinical update [practitioner review]. *Journal of Child Psychology and Psychiatry*, **37**, 643–55.

Renner, P., Klinger, L. G., and Klinger, M. R. (2000). Implicit and explicit memory in autism: is autism an amnesic disorder? *Journal of Autism and Developmental Disorders*, **30**, 3–14.

Rimland, B. (1978). Inside the mind of the autistic savant. *Psychology Today*, August, 69–80.

Rinehart, N. J., Bradshaw, J. L., Moss, S. A., Brereton, A. V., and Tonge, B. J. (2000). Atypical interference of local detail on global processing in high-functioning autism and Asperger's disorder. *Journal of Child Psychology and Psychiatry*, **41**, 769–78.

Rodgers, J. (2000). Visual perception and Asperger syndrome: central coherence deficit of hierarchization deficit? *Autism*, **4**, 321–9.

Rodrigue, J. R., Morgan, S. B., and Geffken, G. R. (1991). A comparative evaluation of adaptive behaviour in children and adolescents with autism, Down's syndrome, and normal development. *Journal of Autism and Developmental Disorders*, **21**, 187–96.

Rogers, S. J. (1998). Empirically supported comprehensive treatments for young children with autism. *Journal of Clinical Child Psychology*, **27**, 167–78.

Rogers, S. J. and DiLalla, D. L. L. (1990). Age of symptom onset in young children with pervasive developmental disorders. *Journal of the American Academy of Child and Adolescent Psychiatry*, **29**, 863–72.

Rogers, S. J. and Williams, J. H. (2006). *Imitation and the Social Mind: Autism and Typical Development*. New York: The Guilford Press.

Rogers, S. J., Ozonoff S., and Maslin-Cole, C. (1991). A comparative study of attachment behaviour in young children with autism or other psychiatric disorders. *Journal of the American Academy of Child and Adolescent Psychiatry*, **30**, 483–8.

Rogers, S., Bennetto, L., McEvoy, R., and Pennington B. (1996). Imitation and pantomime in high-functioning adolescents with autism spectrum disorders. *Child Development*, **67**, 2060–73.

Ropar, D. and Mitchell, P. (1999). Are individuals with autism and Asperger's syndrome susceptible to visual illusions? *Journal of Child Psychology and Psychiatry*, **40**, 1287–93.

Ropar, D. and Mitchell, P. (2001). Susceptibility to illusions and performance on visuospatial tasks in individuals with autism. *Journal of Child Psychology and Psychiatry*, **42**, 539–49.

Rumsey, J. M. (1985). Conceptual problem-solving in highly verbal, nonretarded autistic men. *Journal of Autism and Developmental Disorders*, **15**, 23–36.

Rumsey, J. M. and Hamburger, S. D. (1990). Neuropsychological divergence of high-level autism and severe dyslexia. *Journal of Autism and Developmental Disorders*, **20**, 155–68.

Russell, J., Mauthner, N., Sharpe, S., and Tidswell, T. (1991). The "windows task" as a measure of strategic deception in preschoolers and autistic subjects. [Special Issue: Perspectives on the child's theory of mind: II.] *British Journal of Developmental Psychology*, **9**, 331–49.

Russell, J., Jarrold, C., and Henry, L. (1996). Working memory in children with autism and with moderate learning difficulties. *Journal of Child Psychology and Psychiatry*, **37**, 673–86.

Russell, J., Saltmarsh, R., and Hill, E. (1999). What do executive factors contribute to the failure on false belief tasks by children with autism? *Journal of Child Psychology and Psychiatry*, **40**, 859–68.

Rutter, M. (1983). Cognitive deficits in the pathogenesis of autism. *Journal of Child Psychology and Psychiatry*, **24**, 513–32.

Rutter, M. (1984). Autistic children growing up. *Developmental Medicine and Child Neurology*, **26**, 122–9.

Saitoh, O., Karns, C. M., and Courchesne, E. (2001). Development of the hippocampal formation from 2 to 42 years: MRI evidence of smaller area dentata in autism. *Brain*, **124**, 1317–24.

Salmond, C. H., de Haan, M., Friston, K. J., Gadian, D. G., and Vargha-Khadem, F. (2003). Investigating individual differences in brain abnormalities in autism. *Philosophical Transactions of The Royal Society of London. Series B, Biological Sciences*, **358**, 405–413.

Schopler, E. and Mesibov, G. B. (1992). *High Functioning Individuals with Autism*. New York: Plenum Press.

Schultz, R. T., Gauthier, I., Klin, A., *et al.* (2000). Abnormal ventral temporal cortical activity during face discrimination among individuals with autism and Asperger syndrome. *Archives of General Psychiatry*, **57**, 331–40.

Serra, M., Minderaa, R. B., van Geert, P. L. C., *et al.* (1995). Emotional role-taking abilities of children with a pervasive developmental disorder not otherwise specified. *Journal of Child Psychology and Psychiatry*, **36**, 475–90.

Shah, A. and Frith, U. (1983). An islet of ability in autistic children. A research note. *Journal of Child Psychology and Psychiatry*, **24**, 613–20.

Shah, A. and Frith, U. (1993). Why do autistic individuals show superior performance on the block design task? *Journal of Child Psychology and Psychiatry*, **34**, 1351–64.

Shaked, M. and Yirmiya, N. (2003). Understanding social difficulties. In M. Prior, ed., *Learning and Behavior Problems in Asperger Syndrome*. New York: Guilford Press, pp. 104–125.

Shapiro, T. and Hertzig, M. E. (1991). Social deviance in autism: a central integrative failure as a model for social non-engagement. *Psychiatric Clinics of North America*, **14**, 19–32.

Shu, B. C., Lung, F. W., Tien, A. Y., and Chen, B.C. (2001). Executive function deficits in non-retarded autistic children. *Autism*, **5**, 165–74.

Siegel, D. J., Minshew, N. J., and Goldstein, G. (1996). Wechsler IQ profiles in diagnosis of high-functioning autism. *Journal of Autism and Developmental Disorders*, **26**, 389–406.

Sigman, M. (1998). Change and continuity in the development of children with autism. *Journal of Child Psychology and Psychiatry*, **39**, 817–28.

Sigman, M. and Ungerer, J. (1984). Cognitive and language skills in autistic, mentally retarded and normal children. *Developmental Psychology*, **20**, 293–302.

Sigman, M., Mundy, P., Sherman, T., and Ungerer, J. (1986). Social interactions of autistic, mentally retarded and normal children and their caregivers. *Journal of Child Psychology and Psychiatry*, **27**, 647–56.

Sigman, M. D., Kasari, C., Kwon, J., and Yirmiya, N. (1992). Responses to the negative emotions of others by autistic, mentally retarded, and normal children. *Child Development*, **63**, 796–807.

Silberberg, N. and Silberberg, M. (1967). Hyperlexia: specific word recognition skills in young children. *Exceptional Children*, **34**, 41–2.

Smith, I. (2000). Motor functioning in Asperger syndrome. In A. Klin, F. Volkmar, and S. Sparrow, eds., *Asperger Syndrome*. New York: Guilford Press, pp. 97–124.

Smith, I. M. and Bryson, S. E. (1994). Imitation and action in autism: a critical review. *Psychological Bulletin*, **116**, 259–73.

Stevens, M. C., Fein, D. A., Dunn, M. *et al.* (2000). Subgroups of children with autism by cluster analysis: a longitudinal examination. *Journal of the American Academy of Child and Adolescent Psychiatry*, **39**, 346–52.

Stone, W. L. and Caro-Martinez, L. M. (1990). Naturalistic observations of spontaneous communication in autistic children. *Journal of Autism and Developmental Disorders*, **20**, 437–53.

Swanson, J. M., Posner, M., Potkin, S. G. *et al.* (1991). Activating tasks for the study of visual–spatial attention in ADHD children: a cognitive anatomic approach. *Journal of Child Neurology*, **6**, 119–27.

Szatmari, P., Bartolucci, G., Bremner, R., Bond, S., and Rich, S. (1989). A follow-up study of high-functioning autistic children. *Journal of Autism and Developmental Disorders*, **19**, 213–25.

Szatmari, P., Tuff, L., Finlayson, A. J., and Bartolucci, G. (1990). Asperger's syndrome and autism: neurocognitive aspects. *Journal of the American Academy of Child and Adolescent Psychiatry*, **29**, 130–6.

Szatmari, P., Archer, L., Fisman, S., Streiner, D. L., and Wilson, F. (1995). Asperger's syndrome and autism: differences in behavior, cognition, and adaptive functioning. *Journal of the American Academy of Child and Adolescent Psychiatry*, **34**, 1662–71.

Tager-Flusberg, H. (1981). On the nature of linguistic functioning in early infantile autism. *Journal of Autism and Developmental Disorders*, **11**, 45–56.

Tager-Flusberg, H. (1982). Pragmatic development and its implications for social interaction in autistic children. In D. Park, ed., *Proceedings of the 1981 International Conference on Autism*. Washington, DC: NSAC, pp. 103–7.

Tager-Flusberg, H. (1989). A psycholinguistic perspective on language development in the autistic child. In G. Dawson, ed., *Autism: Nature, Diagnosis and Treatment*. New York: Guilford Press, pp. 92–115.

Tager-Flusberg, H. (1991). Semantic processing in the free recall of autistic children: further evidence for a cognitive deficit. *British Journal of Developmental Psychology*, **9**, 417–30.

Tager-Flusberg, H. (1992). Autistic children's talk about theory of mind. *Child Development*, **63**, 161–72.

Tager-Flusberg, H. (1993). What language reveals about the understanding of minds in children with autism. In S. Baron-Cohen, H. Tager-Flusberg, and D. J. Cohen, eds., *Understanding Other Minds: Perspectives from Autism*. Oxford: Oxford University Press, pp. 138–57.

Tager-Flusberg, H. (2001a). Understanding the language and communicative impairments in autism. *International Review of Research in Mental Retardation*, **23**, 185–205.

Tager-Flusberg, H. (2001b). A re-examination of the Theory of Mind hypothesis of Autism. In J. Burack, T. Charman, N. Yirmiya, and P. Zelazo, eds., *The Development of Autism: Perspectives from Theory and Research*. London: Lawrence Erlbaum Associates, pp. 173–93.

Tager-Flusberg, H. (2003). Language and communicative deficits and their effects on learning and behavior. In M. Prior, ed., *Learning and Behavior Problems in Asperger Syndrome*. New York: Guilford Press, pp. 55–103.

Tager-Flusberg, H. and Anderson, M. (1991). The development of contingent discourse ability in autistic children. *Journal of Child Psychology and Psychiatry*, **32**, 1123–34.

Tager-Flusberg, H. and Joseph, R. M. (2003). Identifying neurocognitive phenotypes in autism. *Philosophical Transactions of The Royal Society of London. Series B, Biological Sciences*, **358**, 303–14.

Tager-Flusberg, H. and Sullivan, K. (1994). Predicting and explaining behaviour: a comparison of autistic, mentally retarded and normal children. *Journal of Child Psychology and Psychiatry*, **35**, 1059–75.

Teunisse, J. P., Cools, A. R., van Spaendonck, K. P. M., Aerts, F. H. T. M., and Berger, H. J. C. (2001). Cognitive styles in high-functioning adolescents with autistic disorder. *Journal of Autism and Developmental Disorders*, **31**, 55–66.

Tirosh, E. and Canby, J. (1993). Autism with hyperlexia: a distinct syndrome? *American Journal on Mental Retardation*, **98**, 84–92.

Toichi, M. and Kamio, Y. (2002). Long-term memory and levels-of-processing in autism. *Neuropsychologia*, **40**, 964–9.

Townsend, J. and Courchesne, E. (1994). Parietal damage and narrow "spotlight" spatial attention. *Journal of Cognitive Neuroscience*, **6**, 220–32.

Townsend, J., Courchesne, E., and Egaas, B. (1996). Slowed orienting of covert visual–spatial attention in autism: specific deficits associated with cerebellar and parietal abnormality. *Development and Psychopathology*, **8**, 563–84.

Townsend, J., Courchesne, E., Covington, J. *et al.* (1999). Spatial attention deficits in patients with acquired or developmental cerebellar abnormality. *The Journal of Neuroscience*, **19**, 5632–43.

Turner, M. (1997). Towards an executive dysfunction account of repetitive behavior in autism. In J. Russell, ed., *Autism as an Executive Disorder*. New York: Oxford University Press, pp. 57–100.

Van Lancker, D., Cornelius, C., and Needleman, R. (1991). Comprehension of verbal terms for emotions in normal, autistic, and schizophrenic children. *Developmental Neuropsychology*, **7**, 1–18.

Vellutino, F. R. (1979). *Dyslexia: Theory and Research*. Cambridge, MA: MIT Press.

Venter, A., Lord, C., and Schopler, E. (1992). A follow-up study of high-functioning autistic children. *Journal of Child Psychology and Psychiatry*, **33**, 489–507.

Volden, J. and Lord, C. (1991). Neologisms and idiosyncratic language in autistic speakers. *Journal of Autism and Developmental Disorders*, **21**, 109–30.

Volkmar, F. R., Sparrow, S. S., Rende, R. D., and Cohen, D. J. (1989). Facial perception in autism. *Journal of Child Psychology and Psychiatry*, **30**, 591–8.

Volkmar, F., Carter, A., Grossman, J., and Klin, A. (1997). Social development in autism. In D. Cohen and F. Volkmar, eds., *Handbook of Autism and Pervasive Developmental Disorders*, 2nd edn. New York: John Wiley, pp. 173–94.

Wainwright-Sharp, J. A. and Bryson, S. E. (1993). Visual orienting deficits in high-functioning people with autism. *Journal of Autism and Developmental Disorders*, **23**, 1–13.

Walker, E., McGuire, M., and Bettes, B. (1984). Recognition and identification of facial stimuli by schizophrenics and patients with affective disorders. *British Journal of Clinical Psychology*, **23**, 37–44.

Walters, A. S., Barrett, R. P., and Feinstein, C. (1990). Social relatedness and autism: current research, issues, directions. *Research in Developmental Disabilities*, **11**, 303–26.

Weeks, S. J. and Hobson, R. P. (1987). The salience of facial expression for autistic children. *Journal of Child Psychology and Psychiatry*, **28**, 137–51.

Welsh, M. C., Pennington, B. F., and Rogers, S. J. (1987). Word recognition and comprehension skills in hyperlexic children. *Brain and Language*, **32**, 76–96.

Wetherby, A. M. (1986). Ontogeny of communicative functions in autism. *Journal of Autism and Developmental Disorders*, **16**, 295–316.

Wetherby, A., Prizant B., and Schuler A. (2000). Understanding the nature of communication and language impairments. In A. Wetherby and B. Prizant, eds., *Autism Spectrum Disorders: A Transactional Perspective. Vol. 9. Communication and Language Intervention Series*. Baltimore: Paul Brookes Publishing, pp. 109–42.

Whalen, C. and Schreibman, L. (2003). Joint attention training for children with autism using behavior modification procedures. *Journal of Child Psychology and Psychiatry*, **44**, 456–68.

White, C. P. and Rosenbloom, L. (1992). Temporal lobe structures and autism. *Developmental Medicine and Child Neurology*, **34**, 556–9.

Williams, D. L., Goldstein, G., and Minshew, N. J. (2006). The profile of memory function in children with autism. *Neuropsychology*, **20**, 21–9.

Wing, L. (1976). *Early Childhood Autism: Clinical, Educational and Social Aspects*, 2nd edn. Oxford: Pergamon Press.

Wing, L. (1981). Asperger's syndrome: a clinical account. *Psychological Medicine*, **11**, 115–29.

Wing, L. (1996). *The Autistic Spectrum: A Guide for Parents and Professionals*. London: Constable.

Wing, L. and Gould, J. (1979). Severe impairments of social interaction and associated abnormalities in children: epidemiology and classification. *Journal of Autism and Developmental Disorders*, **9**, 11–29.

Yirmiya, N., Erel, O., Shaked, M., and Solomonica-Levi, D. (1998). Meta-analyses comparing theory of mind abilities of individuals with autism, individuals with mental retardation, and normally developing individuals. *Psychological Bulletin*, **124**, 283–307.

4

Communication and its development in autism spectrum disorders

Rhea Paul

Southern Connecticut State University and Yale Child Study Center

Introduction

Communication deficits are one of the core symptoms of autism spectrum disorders (ASDs). People with ASD can be slow to begin talking, or may not learn to talk at all; others may learn to produce words and sentences but have difficulty using them effectively to accomplish social interactive goals. In this chapter we will discuss the course of the development of communication in ASD and will outline how communication deficiencies in this population are identified and treated. Before we do, however, we should be clear about three important terms we will be using, which are illustrated in Figure 4.1.

The term "communication" is the broadest of this trio. It refers to all forms of sending and receiving messages, not only with language, but in other ways, such as with gestures, body language, even the way we dress. Animals can also communicate by means of their vocalizations to alert others to danger, for example. That's why the largest circle in Figure 4.1 represents communication. Within the realm of communication, language represents a specific type, so it is enclosed within the larger circle of communication in the figure. Language involves the creation of a potentially infinite set of never-before-conveyed messages through the combination of words in rule-governed ways that allow the formation of sentences to express meaning to others. Only humans are truly generative users of language. Figure 4.1 represents speech as contained within language because speech represents a particular mode of language, its expression through the use of sounds produced by oral movements and gestures. There are other ways to express ideas in language, such as through writing for example, that are not speech. It will be helpful to keep these distinctions in mind as we discuss communication in ASD.

Autism and Pervasive Developmental Disorders, 2nd edn, ed. Fred R. Volkmar.
Published by Cambridge University Press. © Cambridge University Press 2007.

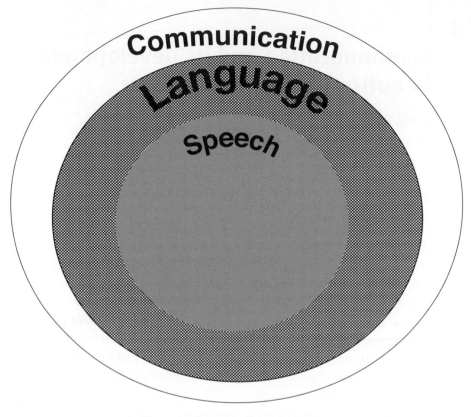

Figure 4.1 Domains of communication.

To help organize our discussion, we will further subdivide the domain of language into the three major categories identified by Bloom and Lahey (1978), as illustrated in Figure 4.2. Language *form* includes the rules for combining sounds to form words (phonology) and combining words to form sentences (syntax). Examples include:

(1)   rules that tell us that "ng" can appear as the last sound in a word in English (*ring*) but not as a first sound (∼*ngir*), although this combination is acceptable in some languages (e.g. Vietnamese);

(2)   rules that tell us how to form sentence variants, such as questions, so that when we want to change *You are invited* to a question, we move the helping verb, *are*, to the beginning of the sentence to form *Are you invited*?

Language *content* refers to the rules for relating words to meaning. For example, our knowledge of the word "bachelor" includes the fact that a man referred to with this term is not married, so this condition does not need to be stated (e.g.

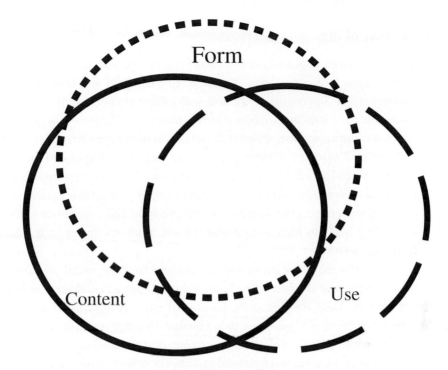

Figure 4.2 Domains of language.

to say "The unmarried bachelor" would be a violation of a rule for language content or *semantics*)

Language *use* is often called *pragmatics*. Both terms refer to the rules for using language appropriately in social situations. For example, pragmatic rules dictate that we must speak politely, even if that means compromising the directness with which we state what we mean. If I ask at dinner, "Would you be kind enough to pass the salt?" I am not really inquiring about the degree of your compassion; I am just saying "Pass the salt," but doing so in a way that conforms to conventions of politeness. In typical communication, these aspects of language interact to enable cooperative expression of meaning across speakers. However, in autism, these aspects can sometimes become dissociated. These dissociations can affect speech, which is the usual output modality for language. Moreover, in ASD there are deficits not only in speech and language, but also in broader aspects of communication.

To better understand how deficits and dissociations in development affect communicative function in ASD, we will review each stage of typical development in order to examine similarities and differences in the course of communicative acquisition between normal children and those with forms of autism.

The first year of life

Typical children begin communicating long before they can talk. Very young babies enjoy looking at faces (Kagan & Lewis, 1965) and listening to voices (Butterfield & Siperstein, 1972), and will inhibit their movements to "listen" when someone is talking to them (Owens, 2004). They begin smiling during their first few months, and use smiles to attract and hold people's attention (LaBarbera *et al.*, 1976). These early abilities to produce, attend, and respond to social stimuli are interpreted by adults as an eagerness to socialize and they engage adults in extended interactions, from which infants not only establish positive affective relations with others, but also acquire information and experience in the social world that leads to increasing sophistication in interacting with it (Mundy & Burnette, 2005).

One of the earliest signs of ASD is a failure to show social preferences and responsiveness in the first year of life. Although not all children who later have autism lack these abilities, many parents of children with ASD report that as babies they were very quiet and didn't babble, that they sometimes seemed deaf and did not respond to voices or their name, that they did not spend much time looking at faces, tried less frequently to attract others' attention, and were less eager to engage in early social games, such as "pat-a-cake," that involve smiling at others and vocalizing (see Volkmar *et al.*, 2005, for review). All these deficits are related to a basic problem in communicating with others, even before language becomes the most important means of communication.

In the second half of their first year, typical infants increase their ability to respond to communication, and begin producing some of their own communicative acts. They respond to their name by 6 months, and by 9 months can follow a pointing gesture to look at what the adult points to (Lempers, 1976). By 10 months they begin making sounds that closely resemble words, and using these sounds to get others' attention and maintain interactions (Oller, 1978). They express a range of intentions such as requesting objects, rejecting proffered actions, calling attention to objects or events (joint attentional acts), commenting on their appearance, and greeting or showing off to initiate social interaction (Bates, 1976; Carpenter *et al.*, 1998), with joint attention and social interaction acts predominating in frequency over requesting and rejecting (Paul & Shiffer, 1991). These intents are expressed first with simple gestures, such as reaching to indicate a request or pushing away to indicate rejection, then by more complex gestures such as pointing in order to request, or shaking the head to mean "no"; and gradually accompanied by, and eventually replaced by, vocalization and speech (Acredolo & Goodwyn, 1988; Adamson & Bakeman, 1991; Bloom 1993).

Children who were later diagnosed with ASD have been found at this age to be less responsive and to pay less attention to people in their environment and to show a lower frequency of looking at objects shown to them by others. They may begin to produce some communication, but their acts are usually for the purpose of getting others to do or not do things (regulatory acts) than for the purpose of sharing and social interaction that characterizes the majority of communicative acts of typical toddlers (Mundy *et al.*, 1994; Wetherby, 1986; Wetherby *et al.*, 2004). Even when they do communicate, their rates are lower and they are less likely to engage people visually or direct their acts to the communication partners with gaze (Chawarska & Volkmar, 2005; Mundy & Burnette, 2005). Moreover, they tend to use unusual gestures, such as pushing an adult's hand towards a desired object, rather than pointing or showing in a more conventional way (Stone & Caro-Martinez, 1997).

The toddler years

During the second and third years of life, typical children begin understanding what particular words mean. At first, a few words associated with games such as "pat-a-cake" or "so big" will be recognized. Infants gradually become more active responders to these routines (Bruner, 1975). By 12 months, merely saying the words ("Let's play pat-a-cake!" or "Show me your nose") in a familiar context will often elicit a spontaneous action from the child such as clapping or touching the nose (Huttenlocher, 1974; Tomasello & Kruger, 1992). Also, around 12 months of age, typical babies begin using words to get things they want and to share experiences with important people in their lives, gradually replacing earlier gestural and vocal forms of communication with words. By 16 to 19 months infants are able to use nonverbal cues, such as an adult's eye gaze, to make quite fine distinctions between an object that an adult is naming and another object that happens to be present (Baldwin, 1991), suggesting that they can now understand the intentions of others within language contexts.

Word learning is slow at first. Average expressive vocabulary size at 12 months is 3 words, at 15 months it is 10 words (Fenson *et al.*, 1994). But at some point during the second year, children go through what is called a "vocabulary spurt," when they suddenly begin learning many new words very quickly, so that average expressive vocabulary size at 18 months is over 100 words and children are beginning to produce some simple 2-word sentences ("My truck!"); at 24 months it is over 300 words and most productions contain word combinations rather than single words (Stoel-Gammon, 1998). Both form and content development are beginning to emerge at this stage, with children learning the meanings for specific words, and beginning to put words together with consistent word order (producing "My truck" consistently and not "Truck my"). Moreover, these new form and content achievements are being quickly integrated for use within the range of communicative acts that emerged preverbally. By 24 months of age, average children are using words and word combinations more frequently than gestures or preverbal vocalizations.

Parents of children with ASD often report that the second year of life was the time they became seriously concerned about their affected child's development. Children with ASD in their second year often fail to show responsiveness to words. Paul *et al.* (2004) and Bruinsma *et al.* (2004) found that comprehension skills are depressed relative to production in the second year of life, while the gap tends to narrow, with receptive skills moving closer to expressive levels in the third to fourth year. Moreover, these children continue to be less attentive and responsive to voices during their second year, and this lack of responsiveness is related to later language development (Rutter *et al.*, 1992).

Parents' most pressing concerns in the child's second year, though, are typically around the child's speech, usually because the child failed to begin saying words, or because he or she learned a few words and never went farther, or lost the early words acquired. About 20% of children who end up on the autism spectrum experience a regression in skills, usually loss of the ability to say words, during their second year (Hoshino *et al.*, 1987; Kobayashi & Murata, 1998; Kurita, 1985; Rogers & DiLalla, 1990; Tuchman & Rapin, 1997). In total, about 40–50% of children with ASD never develop the ability to speak beyond a few single words (Tager-Flusberg *et al.*, 2005). Even those who do speak are often very slow to develop words and word combinations, and speak very little until late in the preschool years.

Delays in language in the early preschool years are not specific to autism, however (Cantwell *et al.*, 1980). In fact, delay in language development is the most common presenting problem for preschool children referred for special educational or psychiatric evaluations (American Speech–Language–Hearing Association, 2002). Moreover, a minority of children with ASD do not show any delays in language development; on the contrary, they may be precocious in their acquisition of words and sentences. These children may turn out to have Asperger's syndrome, a variant of ASD in which children show normal cognitive and language development, but significant difficulties in social uses of language and social interaction (Klin & Volkmar, 1997). The existence of this syndrome suggests that, even though abnormalities in communication are a core feature of pervasive developmental disorders (PDDs), slower language acquisition is neither necessary nor sufficient for a diagnosis within the autism spectrum. To determine that a child has ASD, we need to look for problems beyond the slow growth of language, at more basic issues of communication including gestures, gaze, and vocalization. We know now that language in autism is variable and that there are likely to be subgroups of individuals within the autism spectrum that have distinct language profiles (Tager-Flusberg & Joseph, 2003).

Preschool development

The preschool period (from 3 to 5 years of age) is the time during which the typical child's language evolves from simple word combinations to fully grammatical forms. In addition to rapidly acquiring new vocabulary, the child also goes through a process of approximating more and more closely the grammatical form of the language spoken in the home. There is evidence of the child's active role as a hypothesis generator in the frequent occurrence of overgeneralized forms, such as "goed," "comed," and "mouses" (Cazden, 1968; Pinker, 1999). These errors are taken as evidence that the child is indeed acquiring a rule-governed system, rather than learning these word endings by imitation or on a word-by-word basis.

As the child's grammar becomes more complex, sentence length increases (Brown, 1973; Loban, 1976; Miller & Chapman, 1981) and children begin to use a variety of sentence forms including statements, negatives, and questions. As language form in simple sentences approaches the adult model, complex sentences using embedded clauses ("Whoever wins can go first") and conjoined clauses ("Then it broke and we didn't have it any more") emerge (Paul, 1981).

In addition to expanding their sentence forms, typically developing preschoolers learn to articulate and combine the sounds of their language to produce speech that is understandable to their listeners. Although preschoolers may still make some articulation errors, such as saying *wabbit* for *rabbit*, in general listeners can understand almost all of what they say by the time they reach 4 years of age (Weiss *et al.*, 1987).

In addition to changing their use of grammatical and phonological forms, children between 3 and 5 years of age also change the content that they express in their sentences. Earlier utterances generally described actions and objects that were immediately present, in the "here and now." During later preschool years, sentence content expands to allow for reference to events that are remote in time and space, "there and then" (Chapman, 2000).

Children also begin to use their language in more diverse ways at this time (Dore, 1978) to include imaginative, nonliteral, interpretive, and logical functions. A variety of more advanced conversational uses also emerge and become refined. Children increase their ability to maintain and add new information to the conversational topic; to clarify and request clarification of misunderstood utterances; to make their requests or comments using polite or indirect forms; and to choose the appropriate speech style on the basis of the speaker's role and the listener's status (Bates, 1976; Chapman, 2000). Children also begin to engage in different types of discourse including story-telling, recounting events, and personal narratives, all of which follow cultural conventions.

For children with ASDs, there is considerable variability in the rate at which language progresses among those children who do acquire some speech at this time (Lord *et al.*, 2004). Certain preverbal skills, especially the frequency of initiating joint attention and imitation, are strong predictors of the onset of speech for children with ASD (Charman *et al.*, 2003; Rogers *et al.*, 2003; Sigman & Ruskin, 1999), and there is also often a relationship between IQ and language outcomes (Lord & Rutter, 1994), although higher levels of nonverbal IQ are not always associated with higher-level language skills (Howlin *et al.*, 2004; Kjelgaard & Tager-Flusberg, 2001).

Although few longitudinal studies of language acquisition among verbal children with autism have been conducted, the research suggests that progress in learning language form and content follows pathways similar to those seen in typical development (e.g. Tager-Flusberg *et al.*, 1990). For example, studies have shown that verbal children with autism use semantic groupings (e.g. *bird, boat, food*) in typical ways to categorize and to retrieve words (Boucher, 1988; Minshew & Goldstein, 1993; Tager-Flusberg, 1985). They also increase sentence length and complexity in much the same sequence as do other children (Tager-Flusberg *et al.*, 1990). Generally, articulation development is on a par with mental age (Bartolucci *et al.*, 1976), although distortions of late-developing speech sounds tend to persist more frequently in this population than in typical development (Gibbon *et al.*, 2004; Shriberg *et al.*, 2001). Although many children with ASD who learn to speak eventually acquire forms and meanings that are more or less appropriate for their overall developmental level, some continue to show deficits in the areas relative to nonverbal functioning (Tager-Flusberg & Joseph, 2003).

However, there are some special features of language form and content that appear when children with ASD begin to talk. One feature that is sometimes noted is *pronoun reversal* (Fay, 1969), usually in the form of substituting *you* for *I* (e.g. "Pick you up!"). Although this was originally thought to represent a failure of ego development, Fay (1971) pointed out that, rather than actually reversing pronouns, children with ASD were *failing* to reverse them; preserving the pronoun used in speaking to them when speaking themselves (Adult: "Do you want me to pick you up?" Child: "Pick you up!"). Tager-Flusberg (1994) found that many young children with autism went through a stage of reversing pronouns, though as they got older the more linguistically advanced children stopped making these errors. We now see pronoun reversal as an instance of another feature of early language in ASD: echolalia.

Echolalia is the repetition, with similar intonation, of words or phrases that someone else has said. It can be immediate, for example, a child might repeat the teacher's greeting, "Hi, Sammy," exactly as it was said to him. Echolalia can also be delayed, as in the case of a child who approaches his mother and says, "It's time for you to go outside now" as a signal that he wants to play outdoors, repeating a phrase he has heard his parents say in the past. Echolalia was once viewed as an undesirable, dysfunctional behavior (Lovaas, 1977), but we now see it as a strategy the child uses to attempt to communicate (Tager-Flusberg *et al.*, 2005). McEvoy *et al.* (1988) found that immediate echolalia was most frequent in children with autism who had minimal expressive language.

When children with autism do echo, they often use echolalia for a variety of communicative purposes (Prizant & Duchan, 1981). Shapiro (1977) and Carr *et al.* (1975) found that children with autism were most likely to echo questions and commands that they did not understand or for which they did not know the appropriate response. Although echolalia is one of the most classic symptoms of autism (Kanner, 1946), not all children with autism echo, nor is echoing seen only in autism. It also occurs in blind children, in children with other language impairments, in older people with dementia, and in some normally developing children at early stages of communication (Yule & Rutter, 1987). For all children, including those with autism, echolalia declines over the course of development. It appears to function primarily to help children maintain communication with others, especially when they have very little ability to express their own intentions through spontaneous language. As expressive ability grows, echoing decreases.

Another area of special difficulty for children with autism who speak is the use of prosody. Prosody includes features such as vocal quality, intonation, and stress patterns, which are frequently noted to be unusual in individuals with ASDs (Rutter *et al.*, 1992). Ricks and Wing (1976) carried out one of the first studies in this area, looking at parents' identification of the meaning of the prelinguistic vocalizations of young children with ASD. They found that parents of children with autism were unable to understand the preverbal vocalizations of other children with autism, even though they could understand their own child's messages. In contrast, parents of typically developing children could understand vocalizations of typical children who were not their own, as well as those of their own child. Sheinkopf and his colleagues conducted a detailed examination of the vocal behavior of young preverbal children with autism and a group of comparison children with developmental delays (Sheinkopf *et al.*, 2000) and found that children with ASD showed significant impairments in vocal quality. In addition to their odd intonation, vocalizations of children with autism were less likely to be paired with other nonverbal communication, such as shifts in gaze or gesture or changes in facial expression than they were for the other children (Hellreigel *et al.*, 1995). These findings suggest that the source of the difference between the vocalizations of the young children with autism and those of other young, nonverbal children was in both social intent and in a more basic aspect of the form of the vocalization.

In children with ASD who speak, intonation or "tone of voice" differences are also often reported. The most frequently cited tone is monotony, but Fay and Schuler (1980) also describe a subset of autistic individuals who used an exaggerated sing-song rather than flat pattern. Goldfarb *et al.* (1956) and Pronovost *et al.* (1966) found unusually high pitch levels in speakers with ASD. Other voice disorders, such as hoarseness, harshness, and hypernasality, have also been reported, as well as poor control of volume, with unexplained fluctuations (Pronovost *et al.*, 1966). Fay (1969) reported frequent whispering among children who echo.

Research on Asperger's syndrome suggests that these abnormalities in intonation and prosody may be more prevalent for these speakers (Eisenmajer *et al.*, 1996). But Shriberg and colleagues (Shriberg *et al.*, 2001) analyzed speech samples collected from speakers with autism or Asperger's syndrome and found few differences in prosody between the two groups. They reported that about half of their sample expressed prosodic abnormalities, particularly in the areas of stress or emphasis, and nasal voice quality. Like echolalia, prosodic difficulty is not exclusive to autism; it is also seen in children with mental retardation (Shriberg & Widder, 1990) and specific language disorders (Hargrove, 1997), as well as in adults with certain kinds of brain damage (Patel *et al.*, 1998). Moreover, Shriberg *et al.* (2001) and Baltaxe (1977) found that prosodic deficits were not universal among speakers with ASD, appearing in about half of the individuals in the samples studied. Nonetheless, Paul *et al.* (2005) showed that when prosodic deficits are present they affect listeners' perceptions of the speakers' social and communication competence. Although there are few formal assessments or treatment programs for prosodic disorders, this remains a significant area of impairment for many speakers with ASD.

By far, however, the greatest number of difficulties in the language of speakers with ASD are in the area of language use. Unlike typically developing age mates, who are expanding and elaborating their forms and functions of communication during the preschool period, children with ASD show less frequent and less varied speech acts in free play or more open-ended situations, even when their responses to highly structured situations were similar to those of control groups (Landry & Loveland, 1989; Mermelstein, 1983; Wetherby & Prutting, 1984). Preschool children with autism rarely use language for comments, showing off, acknowledging the listener, initiating social interaction, or requesting information. The speech acts that are missing or rarely used in the conversations of children with autism all have in common an emphasis on social rather than regulatory uses of language (Wetherby, 1986).

Some children with autism never acquire functional language. Early estimates of the prevalence of muteness in ASD were in the range of 40–50% (Lord & Paul, 1997). However, recent longitudinal studies of children referred for possible autism at early ages have suggested that the proportion of children with ASD who do not use words to speak is less than 20% by school age (Lord et al., 2004). This change may be due to recent improved access to early intervention (Goldstein, 2002). However, current research suggests that children who have not begun speaking during the preschool or early school years have a much reduced likelihood of developing speaking after this point (Bryson et al., 1988; Paul & Cohen, 1984). Moreover, many of these children have very low nonverbal IQ scores (Lord & Rutter, 1994). For these nonspeakers with ASD, again, problems go beyond not talking to include difficulty in attending to and understanding language, in initiating communication to share attention and emotion, in using normal vocal quality (even preverbal vocalization), in directing communication to others with gaze, and in using conventional gestures to get messages across (Tager-Flusberg et al., 2005).

Efforts to provide children with ASD with alternative forms of communication, such as Sign language or pictures, afford some help in increasing the child's ability to express wants and needs, but they rarely result in fluent and fully functional use of the alternative system, as is seen, for example, in the use of Sign by children who are deaf. However, very little is known about communication development in nonspeaking children with autism, since very little research has focused on these children.

Later language development

During the school-age and adolescent years, the main changes that take place in typical language development involve:

(1) an increase in the use of language forms that are more abstract and formal, such as those used in written rather than spoken language;

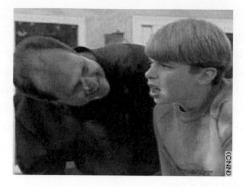

Figure 4.3 Communication is a universal deficit in children with autism spectrum disorder.

(2)   an increase in vocabulary specific to topics, such as those taught in the school curriculum, e.g. science, social studies, math;

(3)   increases in the ability to handle figurative language and multiple or ambiguous meanings of words and sentences;

(4)   a great expansion in the flexibility of language used to accomplish a wider range of interpersonal goals, as children move beyond the family to interact more intensively with peers, teachers, and other adults.

Individuals with autism continue to make progress in language and related developmental domains well beyond the preschool years. Paul and Cohen (1984) found that both comprehension and expressive abilities continued to improve in these populations through adolescence and adulthood, although expressive language showed greater rates of improvement than understanding. In another series of follow-up studies in Britain, almost all of the participants with autism showed substantial improvements in formal aspects of language into adulthood (Cantwell & Baker, 1989). However, the group with autism who had serious receptive language deficits in early childhood, remained more severely language delayed as a whole (Rutter *et al.*, 1992).

The 20–30% of people with ASD who have IQs in the normal range – individuals with high-functioning autism (HFA) and Asperger's syndrome – often have large vocabularies and a rich knowledge of words (Fein & Waterhouse, 1979; Jarrold *et al.*, 1997; Kjelgaard & Tager-Flusberg, 2001) by the time they reach school age. They have age-appropriate language forms and may show a "bookish" (Wing, 1981), "high-falutin'," pedantic style of speech (Ghaziuddin *et al.*, 1992) that can sound odd to peers, and lead adults to refer to them as "little professors." They often appear more comfortable, and are more easily accepted by adults than by typical age mates. McHale and Colleagues (1980) showed that autistic students communicated more in the presence of their teachers than in their absence, and directed their communication to adults more than to peers.

Many of these children can achieve normally in many areas of academics, particularly those that require little social knowledge, such as mathematics and science. They often read at grade level although there is frequently a disconnect between their ability to decode words and their ability to comprehend what they read. Some children with ASD show hyperlexia, an unusual, precocious ability to decode words, often acquired without instruction, but with very little understanding of what is read (Grigorenko *et al.*, 2003). More commonly, though, basic reading comprehension is present, but students with ASD have trouble understanding reading material that requires the understanding of motives, plans, goals, and deceit that are often found in school literature selections (Westby, 2005).

In these higher-functioning individuals it is also common to see a large degree of dissociation between the form and function of their oral language (Tager-Flusberg, 1994). Despite their expansive vocabularies and complex sentences, their ability to use language to establish and maintain interaction can be severely limited, as is their use of language to explain or describe events in a conversational context (Ziatas *et al.*, 2003). The rate of initiation of spontaneous communication can be very low. In a study by Stone and Caro-Martinez (1990), the frequency of communication in school was two or three spontaneous acts per child per hour, only half of the children ever directed a communication to a peer. Moreover, understanding language in conversational and other discourse contexts remains a significant challenge for students with both HFA and Asperger's Syndrome because so much communication among older children and teenagers involves slang, sarcasm, jokes, and other nonliteral forms of language.

Despite these deficits in language use, most speakers with ASD do attempt to use their language to communicate even if only in limited ways. They attempt to use language to offer new information, to communicate with different people, and are more likely than children without speech to address some communication to peers as well as adults, though rates are still low (Stone and Caro-Martinez, 1990). Bernard-Opitz (1982) showed that the communicative performance of one child with autism showed some pragmatic variation with different interlocutors and in different settings, indicating some social awareness in his use of language. Still, difficulties in listening, selfdirected speech, problems in following rules of politeness, irrelevant remarks, difficulties in keeping the cooperative back-and-forth flow of topics in conversation going, and in supplying new information relevant to a listener's purposes are common in many high-functioning speakers with ASD (Baltaxe, 1977; Rumsey *et al.*, 1985). In general, the strategies used by individuals with ASD to maintain conversation are less advanced than formal language ability would predict.

An additional conversational problem seen in this population is the ability to infer and respond appropriately to the interlocutor's implicit intentions. As mentioned earlier, typical speakers sometimes need to trade directness for politeness and this can lead them to use forms of language that can be difficult for the person with HFA or Asperger's syndrome to interpret. A person with ASD who is asked, "Can you tell me the time?" might answer, simply, "Yes," for example. Paul (1987) related the example of a young man with ASD who was asked by a shoe store clerk whether the shoes he was trying on were too big and "slipped up and down on his feet." The young man replied, "No." After a few moments however, he clarified his response by saying, "They slip *down* and *up*." This high degree of literalness in interpreting conversational language can lead the young person with ASD into various kinds of difficulties in trying to understand others' underlying intentions, when they neither say exactly what they mean, nor mean exactly what they say.

Many investigators believe that these overly literal interpretations, and other problems seen in social communication in ASD, are related to deficits in what is called "theory of mind" (ToM), the ability to understand that other people can have mental states that might differ from our own, or from reality (such as when a mother believes that her keys are on the kitchen table but they are not, in fact, because her teenager took them without asking). A large body of research has shown that in tasks that require speakers with ASD to solve problems involving theories of mind and false beliefs, they do less well than we would predict based on their language and cognitive levels (see Tager-Flusberg, 2000, for discussion). This finding highlights the need for high levels of integration among language, thought, and social knowledge that are required in even the most ordinary day-to-day interactions, and the degree of handicap that results from failures in the development and integration of these systems even in very intelligent speakers with ASD.

There are few differences in the language characteristics of subjects with HFA and Asperger's syndrome. However, people with Asperger's do show a greater tendency to be verbose. Ghaziuddin and Gerstein (1996) report that people with Asperger's syndrome often talk too much and have trouble taking turns in conversation (Ramberg *et al.*, 1996), and Shriberg *et al.* (2001) reported a significantly higher rate of utterances per minute in Asperger's syndrome than in HFA. In general, though, an important difference between speakers with ASD and other populations with language impairments has been that, in most groups with language impairment, the more a child talks, the less likely it is that the language will have unusual characteristics. In contrast, two studies with autistic children and adolescents showed that subjects' unusual aspects of language and lack of cohesiveness increased with the amount of speech (Caplan *et al.*, 1994; Volden & Lord, 1991).

The tendency toward a pedantic language style, although it may be present in speakers with any ASD, is also especially strong in young people with Asperger's syndrome, who often, in addition, have obsessive interests in narrow, idiosyncratic topics, such as dead-end roads or deep-fat fryers, about which they can amass a startling amount of knowledge and will discuss at length without regard to their listener's interest (Klin *et al.*, 2000).

Older nonspeakers with autism spectrum disorder

For individuals with ASD who do not begin using functional speech by the age of six or so, the chances that speech will develop are much reduced. There are case reports of children with ASD who began speaking later in life (Mirenda, 2003; Windsor *et al.*, 1994), but these are the exception rather than the rule. Some older children with ASD may produce speech occasionally, use a few single words, or be able to echo but not produce spontaneous language. None of these would be considered to have functional speech, which means that the person uses a variety of words and sentences routinely to get needs met and engage in social interaction. For people without functional speech, a variety of augmentative and alternative communication (AAC) strategies are often used to attempt to provide a means by which individuals can express themselves. This is especially important because nonspeakers with ASD sometimes adopt maladaptive ways of trying to get their needs met, such as throwing tantrums or hurting themselves to get others to pay attention or to escape from things they do not want to do; AAC strategies can often provide these nonspeakers with more conventional ways to accomplish their goals. Methods that are used to provide a communication system to nonspeakers with ASD include Signs of American Sign Language, pictures on a board or in a book they carry with them to point out what they want, electronic devices that "talk" for them by using either pictures linked to stored words and phrases, or keyboards that "speak" what the user types. Since the great majority of older nonspeakers with ASD have low IQs, few are able to master the literacy skills needed for these more advanced electronic systems, and so Sign or picture systems are most commonly used.

Assessing communication

When individuals are diagnosed with ASD, one of the important elements of their assessment is a detailed description of their communicative strengths and

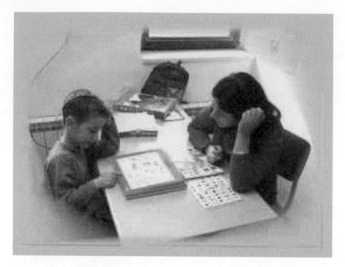

Figure 4.4 Augmentative and alternative communication devices can help nonspeaking children with autism spectrum disorder interact more successfully with others.

needs. Every individual with ASD will have needs in the area of communication, since this is a core deficit in the autism spectrum. But the kinds of needs vary depending on the individual's age, level of function, and individual profile. For this reason, assessment of communication is always part of the diagnostic and educational evaluation for children on this spectrum.

As we have seen, some children with ASD do not talk at all. In these cases it will be especially important to evaluate how they communicate in other ways, such as gestures, gaze, and vocalizations, as well as what they understand of others' communication. Many individuals at this level may be too young or too impaired to engage in standard testing procedures. Less formal procedures that include observing the child responding to "temptations" to communicate (offering a toy contained in a closed jar that the child needs to ask for help to open) are often used to elicit nonverbal communicative behaviors in this population. A sample scoresheet that might be used to summarize an informal evaluation such as this appears in Table 4.1. Comprehension is often assessed by asking these individuals to follow instructions with objects, rather than asking them to point to pictures, since they usually find concrete materials may be more appealing and easier to relate to words heard.

For children who can speak, the usual kinds of tests for assessing language level can be used. However, these will often need to be supplemented with observations of communication behavior in the context of conversation to determine whether there is a disconnect between the elements of language form and

Table 4.1 Summary of communication assessment for preverbal children suspected of autism

Means of communication	Function of communication							
	Request	Protest	Share enjoyment	Comment/joint attention	Pretend	Responds to name	Responds to speech	Identifies objects by name
Gaze to person								
Three-point gaze[a]								
Conventional gesture								
Unconventional gesture								
Typical vocalization								
Unusual vocalization								
Echo								
Spontaneous speech								

[a] Child looks at object, at person, then back at object; or at person, at object, then back at person

meaning that are typically measured in standard tests and the use of language to achieve reciprocity and adequate exchange of information in discourse. Checklists like the one in Box 4.1 are often used to organize these observations, which may take place between the child and parent, clinician, or peer. In addition, areas of language known to be difficult for speakers with autism, such as understanding figurative language, multiple meaning words, and ambiguous sentences can be assessed with tests specially designed to probe these abilities.

Intervention for communication

Most children with ASD will benefit from therapies designed to improve their ability to communicate and engage in social interactions. For young and lower-functioning children, therapy may include highly structured, behaviorist approaches designed to teach a sequence of discrete skills such as vocal imitation, responses to specific words, and single word production (e.g. Sundberg & Michael, 2001). Other approaches can also be used at this stage that include more naturalistic activities, such as withholding a snack or play material until the child requests it in some way (by looking at it and grunting, perhaps), gradually "upping the ante" to include more conventional forms of requesting (such as pointing), eventually working towards words and word combinations (Kaiser et al., 1992). Once words and simple sentences are acquired, longer and more elaborate utterances are encouraged through continued use of similar techniques.

For older, higher-functioning children who master basic elements of language, focused training in social uses of communication is often necessary. Approaches that incorporate typical peers are especially effective (Paul, 2003). These include having the child watch videos of typical peers enacting a social scene, then rehearsing and re-enacting the scene; learning "scripts" for particular social skills such as introducing, asking for a date or requesting homework help and gradually fading the script; and training peers to provide rewards to students with ASD who approach them, greet them, share a conversational topic with them, etc.

For children with ASD who do not acquire speech, again, AAC techniques are taught in much the same way as beginning speech, by rewarding children for making a Sign or pointing to a picture, using either behaviorist techniques or more naturalistic approaches (e.g. Bondy & Frost, 1998). Research to date has not established that one of these techniques is clearly superior to another. Many therapists use a mix of approaches or try to match the child's individual needs and style to an intervention system that seems the best complement.

Box 4.1. Pragmatic checklist

Expresses a variety of communicative intents
Explains	–
Persuades	–
Imagines	–
Others	–

Manages turns and topics in conversation
Takes turn appropriately	–
Allows others appropriate turns	–
Maintains others' topics	–
Initiates topics appropriately	–
Adds relevant info to others' topics	–
Switches topics appropriately	–

Varies speech style
Uses a polite register	–
Talks differently to peers/adults	–
Uses language appropriate for social situation	–

Shows "theory of mind" in conversation
Uses pronouns appropriately	–
Uses ellipsis appropriately	–
Gives adequate information	–
Responds to requests for clarification	–
Sensitive to listener cues for more/less	–
Makes appropriate judgments about listeners prior knowledge	–

Speech and language are clear
Speech is clear and understandable	–
Prosody is typical for age	–
Information is concise and orderly	–
Information is unambiguous	–
Word choice is precise and appropriate	–
Language is not rambling, confusing	–
Ideas are linked coherently	–

Scoring
2 present most of the time
1 present sometimes; emerging
0 hardly ever present or absent

Conclusion

Children with ASD show a range of deficits in communication, which constitutes one of the core deficits of the autism spectrum. Many of these children are slow to begin talking, and for the portion of the population with ASD who do acquire speech, there are features, such as echolalia and use of prosody, that show deviance in addition to delays in development. Whereas many speakers with ASD develop more or less developmentally appropriate forms and meanings for words and sentences, deficits in the use of language for social purposes are universally seen in this population. These deficits can serve as major impediments to successful social adaptation and acceptance, even for very intelligent people on the spectrum, who can show large vocabularies and age appropriate school achievement in many areas. Explicit training in social uses of language can be helpful to reduce these handicaps.

For children with ASD who do not acquire speech, or who show limited language development, intensive instruction and remediation are needed to help the individual reach his or her potential. Often augmentative systems, including Signs, picture communication systems, and electronic aids can be helpful in increasing the ability to communicate and reducing the likelihood of maladaptive forms of communication. These children, too, however, will need help in learning to use whatever communication system they have to engage in spontaneous, meaningful social interactions.

Families, educators, and therapists who work with children with ASD to improve communication skills face a difficult task in attempting to overcome one of the core symptoms of this disorder. However, research has shown that intervention makes a difference, and that early intervention focused on communication and social skills can significantly improve the outlook for individuals on the spectrum (National Research Council, 2001). These findings provide the hope and optimism needed to engage in the long-term, intensive work of opening the channel of communication to children with ASD.

Acknowledgments

Preparation of this chapter was supported by Research Grant P01-03008 funded by the National Institute of Mental Health (NIMH), STAART Center grant U54 MH66494 funded by the National Institute on Deafness and Other Communication Disorders (NIDCD), the National Institute of Environmental Health Sciences (NIEHS), the National Institute of Child Health and Human Development (NICHD), the National Institute of Neurological Disorders and Stroke

(NINDS), and by a MidCareer Development grant to Dr. Paul, K24 HD045576 funded by NIDCD as well as by the National Alliance for Autism Research.

The author wishes to express her appreciation to Professor Helen Tager-Flusberg and Professor Catherine Lord for their contributions to this chapter.

REFERENCES

Acredolo, L. and Goodwyn, S. (1988). Symbolic gesturing in normal infants. *Child Development*, **59**, 450–66.

Adamson, L. B. and Bakeman, R. (1991). The development of shared attention during infancy. In R. Vasta, ed., *Annals of Child Development. Vol. 8*. London: Kingsley, pp. 1–41.

American Speech–Language–Hearing Association (ASHA) (2002). Guidelines for roles and responsibilities for school-based speech-language pathologists. *ASHA 2002 Desk Reference. Vol. 3*. Rockville, MD: ASHA, pp. 240–311.

Baldwin, D. A. (1991). Infants' contribution to the achievement of joint reference. *Child Development*, **62**, 875–90.

Baltaxe, C. (1977). Pragmatic deficits in the language of autistic adolescents. *Journal of Pediatric Psychology*, **2**, 176–80.

Bartolucci, G., Pierce, S., Streiner, D., and Tolkin-Eppel, P. (1976). Phonological investigation of verbal autistic and mentally retarded subjects. *Journal of Autism and Childhood Schizophrenia*, **6**, 303–15.

Bates, E. (1976). *Language in Context*. New York: Academic Press.

Bernard-Opitz, V. (1982). Pragmatic analysis of the communicative behavior of an autistic child. *Journal of Speech and Hearing Disorders*, **47**, 99–109.

Bloom, L. (1993). *The Transition from Infancy to Language: Acquiring the Power of Expression*. Cambridge: Cambridge University Press.

Bloom, L. and Lahey, M. (1978). *Language Development and Language Disorders*. New York: Wiley.

Bondy, A. and Frost, L. (1998). The picture exchange communication system. *Seminars in Speech and Language*, **19**, 373–89.

Boucher, J. (1988). Word fluency in high-functioning autistic children. *Journal of Autism and Developmental Disorders*, **18**, 637–45.

Brown, R. (1973). *A First Language*. Cambridge: Harvard University Press.

Bruinsma, Y., Koegel, R., and Koegel, L. (2004). Joint attention and children with autism: a review of the literature. *Mental Retardation and Developmental Disabilities Research Reviews*, **10**, 169–75.

Bruner, J. S. (1975). The ontogenesis of speech acts. *Journal of Child Language*, **2**, 1–19.

Bryson, S. E., Clark, B. S., and Smith, T. M. (1988). First report of a Canadian epidemiological study of autistic syndromes. *Journal of Child Psychology and Psychiatry*, **29**, 433–45.

Butterfield, E. L. and Siperstein, G. N. (1972). Influence of contingent auditory stimulation upon nonnutritional sucking. In J. Bosma, ed., *Oral Sensation and Perception: The Mouth of the Infant*. Springfield, IL: Charles Thomas, pp. 129–48.

Cantwell, D. P. and Baker, L. (1989). Infantile autism and developmental receptive dysphasia: a comparative follow-up into middle childhood. *Journal of Autism and Developmental Disorders*, **19**, 19–30.

Cantwell, D. P., Baker, L., and Mattison, R. E. (1980). Psychiatric disorders in children with speech and language retardation. *Archives of General Psychiatry*, **37**, 423–6.

Caplan, R. Guthrie, D., Shields, W. D., and Yudovin, S. (1994). Communciation deficits in pediatric complex partial seizure disorders and schizophrenia. *Development and Psychopathology*, **6**, 499–517.

Carpenter, M., Nagell, K., and Tomasello, M. (1998). Social cognition, joint attention, and communicative competence from 9 to 15 months of age. *Monographs of the Society for Research in Child Development*, **63**(4), Serial No. 255.

Carr, E., Shriebman, L., and Lovaas, O. L. (1975). Control of echolalic speech in psychotic children. *Journal of Abnormal Child Psychology*, **3**, 331–51.

Cazden, C. (1968). The acquisition of noun and verb inflections. *Child Development*, **39**, 443–8.

Chapman, R. S. (2000). Children's language learning: an interactionist perspective. *Journal of Child Psychology and Psychiatry*, **41**, 33–54.

Charman, T., Baron-Cohen, S., Swettenham, J. *et al.* (2003). Predicting language outcome in infants with autism and pervasive developmental disorder. *International Journal of Language and Communication Disorders*, **38**, 265–85.

Chawarska, K. and Volkmar, F. (2005). Autism in infancy and early childhood. In F. Volkmar, A. Klin, and R. Paul, eds., *Handbook of Autism and Pervasive Developmental Disorders. Vol. 1* New York: Wiley, pp. 223–46.

Dore, J. (1978). Requestive systems in nursery school conversations: analysis of talk in its social context. In R. Campbell and P. Smith, eds., *Recent Advances in the Psychology of Language*. New York: Plenum, pp. 343–50.

Eisenmajer, R., Prior, M., Leekam, S. *et al.* (1996). Comparison of clinical symptoms in autism and Asperger's disorder. *Journal of the American Academy of Child Adolescent Psychiatry*, **35**, 1523–31.

Fay, W. (1969). On the basis of autistic echolalia. *Journal of Communication Disorders*, **2**, 38–47.

Fay, W. (1971). On normal and autistic pronouns. *Journal of Speech and Hearing Disorders*, **36**, 242–9.

Fay, W. and Schuler, A. L. (1980). *Emerging Language in Autistic Children*. Baltimore: University Park Press.

Fein, D. and Waterhouse, L. (1979). *Autism is not a disorder of language.* Paper presented at the October meeting of the New England Child Language Association, Boston.

Fenson, L., Dale, P., Reznick, J. *et al.* (1994). Variability in early communicative development. *Monographs of the Society for Research in Child Development*, **59**(5), Serial No. 242.

Ghaziuddin, M. and Gerstein, L. (1996). Pedantic speaking style differentiates Asperger syndrome from high-functioning autism. *Journal of Autism and Developmental Disorders*, **26**, 585–95.

Ghaziuddin, M., Tsai, L., and Ghaziuddin, N. (1992). Brief report: a comparison of the diagnostic criteria for Asperger syndrome. *Journal of Autism and Developmental Disorders*, **22**, 643–9.

Gibbon, F., McCann, J., Peppe, S., O'Hare, A., and Rutherford, M. (2004). *Articulation disorders in children with high-functioning autism.* Paper presented at the World Congress of the International Association of Logopedics and Phoniatrics, September, Brisbane, Australia.

Goldfarb, W., Braunstein, P., and Lorge, I. (1956). A study of speech patterns in a group of schizophrenic children. *American Journal of Orthopsychiatry*, **26**, 544–55.

Goldstein, H. (2002). Communication intervention for children with autism: a review of treatment efficacy. *Journal of Autism and Developmental Disorders*, **32**, 373–96.

Grigorenko, E. L., Klin, A., and Volkmar, F. (2003). Hyperlexia: disability or superability? *Journal of Child Psychology and Psychiatry*, **44**, 1079–91.

Hargrove, P. (1997). Prosodic aspects of language impairment in children. *Topics in Language Disorders*, **17**, 76–83.

Hellreigel, C., Tao, L., DiLavore, P., and Lord, C. (1995). *The effect of context on nonverbal social behaviors of very young autistic children.* Paper presented at the biannual meetings of the Society for Research in Child Development, Indianapolis, IN, April.

Hoshino, Y., Kaneko, M., Yashima, Y. *et al.* (1987). Clinical features of autistic children with setback course in their infancy. *Japanese Journal of Psychiatry and Neurology*, **41**, 237–45.

Howlin, P., Goode, S., Hutton, J., and Rutter, M. (2004). Adult outcome for children with autism. *Journal of Child Psychology and Psychiatry*, **45**, 212–29.

Huttenlocher, J. (1974). The origins of language comprehension. In R. L. Solso, ed., *Theories in Cognitive Psychology.* Hillsdale, NJ: Lawrence Erlbaum, pp. 331–68.

Jarrold, C., Boucher, J., and Russell, J. (1997). Language profiles in children with autism: theoretical and methodological implications. *Autism*, **1**, 57–76.

Kagan, J. and Lewis, M. (1965). Studies of attention in the human infant. *Merrill–Palmer Quarterly*, **11**, 95–127.

Kaiser, A., Yoder, P. J., and Keetz, A. (1992). Evaluating milieu teaching. In S. Warren and J. Reichle, eds., *Causes and Effects in Communication and Language Intervention.* Baltimore: Paul H. Brookes, pp. 9–47.

Kanner, L. (1946). Irrelevant and metaphorical language. *American Journal of Psychiatry*, **103**, 242–6.

Kjelgaard, M. and Tager-Flusberg, H. (2001). An investigation of language impairment in autism: implications for genetic subgroups. *Language and Cognitive Processes*, **16**, 287–308.

Klin, A. and Volkmar, F. (1997). Asperger's syndrome. In D. J. Cohen and F. R. Volkmar, eds., *Handbook of Autism and Pervasive Developmental Disorders*, 2nd edn. New York: Wiley, pp. 94–122.

Klin, A., Volkmar, F., and Sparrow, S, eds. (2000). *Asperger Syndrome.* New York: Guilford Press.

Kobayashi, R. and Murata, T. (1998). Setback phenomenon in autism and long-term prognosis. *Actuarial Psychiatry Scandanavia*, **98**, 296–303.

Kurita, H. (1985). Infantile autism with speech loss before the age of 30 months. *Journal of the American Academy of Child Psychiatry*, **24**, 191–6.

LaBarbera, J., Izard, C., Vietze, P., and Parisi, S. (1976). Four and six month old infants' visual responses to joy, anger, and neutral expression. *Child Development*, **47**, 535–8.

Landry, S. H. and Loveland, K. A. (1989). The effect of social context on the functional communication skills of autistic children. *Journal of Autism and Developmental Disorders*, **19**, 283–99.

Lempers, J. (1976). Production of pointing, comprehension of pointing, and understanding of looking behavior. Unpublished doctoral dissertation, University of Minnesota.

Loban, W. (1976). *Language Development: Kindergarten Through Grade 12.* Urbana, IL: National Council of Teachers of English.

Lord, C. and Paul, R. (1997). Language and communication in autism. In D. J. Cohen and F. R. Volkmar, eds., *Handbook of Autism and Pervasive Development Disorders*, 2nd edn. New York: John Wiley, pp. 195–225.

Lord, C. and Rutter, M. (1994). Autism and pervasive developmental disorders. In M. Rutter, L. Hersov, and E. Taylor, eds., *Child and Adolescent Psychiatry: Modern Approaches*, 3rd edn. Oxford: Blackwell, Scientific, pp. 569–93.

Lord, C., Shulman, C., and DiLavore, P. (2004). Regression and word loss in autistic spectrum disorders. *Journal of Child Psychology and Psychiatry*, **45**, 936–55.

Lovaas, O. I. (1977). *The Autistic Child*. New York: Irvington.

McEvoy, R. E., Loveland, K. A., and Landry, S. H. (1988). The functions of immediate echolalia in autistic children: a developmental perspective. *Journal of Autism and Developmental Disorders*, **18**, 657–68.

McHale, S., Simeonsson, R. J., Marcus, L. M., and Olley, J. G. (1980). The social and symbolic quality of autistic children's communication. *Journal of Autism and Developmental Disorders*, **10**, 299–310.

Mermelstein, R. (1983). *The relationship between syntactic and pragmatic development in autistic, retarded, and normal children*. Paper presented at the Eighth Annual Boston University Conference on Language Development, Boston, October.

Miller, J. and Chapman, R. S. (1981). The relation between age and mean length of utterance in morphemes. *Journal of Speech and Hearing Research*, **24**, 154–62.

Minshew, N. J. and Goldstein, G. (1993). Is autism an amnesic disorder? Evidence from the California Verbal Learning Test. *Neuropsychology*, **7**, 209–16.

Mirenda, P. (2003). "He's not really a reader . . .": perspectives on supporting literacy development in individuals with autism. *Topics in Language Disorders*, **23**, 271–82.

Mundy, P. and Burnette, C. (2005). Joint attention and neurodevelopmental models of autism. In F. Volkmar, A. Klin, and R. Paul, eds., *Handbook of Autism and Pervasive Developmental Disorders*. *Vol. 1*. New York: John Wiley, pp. 650–82.

Mundy, P., Sigman, M., and Kasari, C. (1994). Joint attention, developmental level, and symptom presentation in autism. *Development and Psychopathology*, **6**, 389–401.

National Research Council (2001). *Educating Children with Autism* (C. Lord and J. McGee, eds.). Washington, DC: National Academy Press.

Oller, K. (1978). Infant vocalization and the development of speech. *Allied Health and Behavior Sciences*, **1**, 523–49.

Owens, R. E., Jr. (2004). *Language Development: An Introduction*, 5th edn. Needham Heights, MA: Allyn & Bacon.

Patel, A., Peretz, I., Tramo, M., and Lebreque, R. (1998). Processing prosodic and musical patterns: a neuropsychological investigation. *Brain and Language*, **43**, 4–11.

Paul, R. (1981). Complex sentence development. In J. Miller, ed., *Assessing Language Production in Children*. Boston: Allyn & Bacon, pp. 36–44.

Paul, R. (1987). The natural history of infantile autism. In D. Cohen and A. Donnellan, eds., *Handbook of Autism and Pervasive Developmental Disorders*. New York: John Wiley, pp. 121–32.

Paul, R. (2003). Promoting social communication in high-functioning individuals with autistic spectrum disorders. *Child and Adolescent Psychiatric Clinics of North America*, **12**, 87–106.

Paul, R. and Cohen, D. J. (1984). Outcomes of severe disorders of language acquisition. *Journal of Autism and Developmental Disorders*, **14**, 405–22.

Paul, R. and Shiffer, M. (1991). Expression of communicative intention in normal and late-talking toddlers. *Applied Psycholinguistics*, **12**, 416–32.

Paul, R., Chawarska, K., Klin, A., and Volkmar, F. (2004). *Profiles of communication in toddlers with autism spectrum disorders*. Paper presented at the American Psychological Association, Honolulu, Hawaii, August.

Paul, R., Shriberg, L., McSweeney, J. *et al.* (2005). Brief report: relations between prosodic performance and communication and socialization ratings in high functioning speakers with autism spectrum disorders. *Journal of Autism and Developmental Disorders*, **35**, 861–9.

Pinker, S. (1999). How the mind works. *Annals of the New York Academy of Sciences*, **882**, 119–27.

Prizant, B. and Duchan, J. (1981). The functions of immediate echolalia in autistic children. *Journal of Speech and Hearing Disorders*, **46**, 241–9.

Pronovost, W., Wakstein, M., and Wakstein, D. (1966). A longitudinal study of speech behavior and language comprehension in fourteen children diagnosed as atypical or autistic. *Exceptional Children*, **33**, 19–26.

Ramberg, C., Ehlers, S., Nyden, A., Johansson, M., and Gillberg, C. (1996). Language and pragmatic functions in school-age children on the autism spectrum. *European Journal of Disorders of Communication*, **31**, 387–413.

Ricks, D. M. and Wing, L. (1976). Language, communication and use of symbols. In L. Wing, ed., *Early Childhood Autism*. Oxford: Pergamon Press, pp. 93–134.

Rogers, S. J. and DiLalla, D. L. (1990). Age of symptom onset in young children with pervasive developmental disorders. *Journal of the American Academy of Child and Adolescent Psychiatry*, **29**, 863–72.

Rogers, S., Hepburn, S., Stackhouse, T., and Wehner, E. (2003). Imitation performance in toddlers with autism and those with other developmental disorders. *Journal of Child Psychology and Psychiatry*, **44**, 763–81.

Rumsey, J. M., Rapoport, M. D., and Sceery, W. R. (1985). Autistic children as adults: psychiatric, social, and behavioral outcomes. *Journal of the American Academy of Child Psychiatry*, **24**, 465–73.

Rutter, M., Mawhood, L., and Howlin, P. (1992). Language delay and social development. In P. Fletcher and D. Hall, eds., *Specific Speech and Language Disorders in Children: Correlates, Characteristics and Outcomes*. London: Whurr Publishers, pp. 63–78.

Shapiro, T. (1977). The quest for a linguistic model to study the speech of autistic children: studies of echoing. *Journal of the American Academy of Child Psychiatry*, **16**, 608–19.

Sheinkopf, S., Mundy, P., Oller, K., and Steffens, M. (2000). Vocal atypicalities of preverbal autistic children. *Journal of Autism and Developmental Disorders*, **30**, 345–54.

Shriberg, L. and Widder, C. J. (1990). Speech and prosody characteristics of adults with mental retardation. *Journal of Speech and Hearing Research*, **33**, 627–53.

Shriberg, L., Paul, R., McSweeney, J. *et al.* (2001). Speech and prosody characteristics of adolescents and adults with high-functioning autism and AS. *Journal of Speech, Language, and Hearing Research*, **44**, 1097–115.

Sigman, M. and Ruskin, E. (1999). Continuity and change in the social competence of children with autism, Down syndrome and developmental delays. *Monographs of the Society for Research in Child Development*, **64**, Serial No. 256.

Stoel-Gammon, C. (1998). Sounds and words in early language acquisition: the relationship between lexical and phonological development. In R. Paul, ed., *Exploring the Speech–Language Connection*. Baltimore: Paul H. Brookes, pp. 23–45.

Stone, W. L. and Caro-Martinez, L. M. (1990). Naturalistic observations of spontaneous communication in autistic children. *Journal of Autism and Developmental Disorders*, **20**, 437–53.

Sundberg, M. and Michael, J. (2001). The benefits of Skinner's analysis of verbal behavior for children with autism. *Behavior Modification*, **25**, 698–724.

Tager-Flusberg, H. (1985). The conceptual basis for referential word meaning in children with autism. *Child Development*, **56**, 1167–78.

Tager-Flusberg, H. (1994). Dissociations in form and function in the acquisition of language by autistic children. In H. Tager-Flusberg, ed., *Constraints on Language Acquisition: Studies of Atypical Children*. Hillsdale, NJ: Erlbaum, pp. 175–94.

Tager-Flusberg, H. (2000). Language and understanding minds: connections in autism. In S. Baron-Cohen, H. Tager-Flusberg, and D. Cohen, eds., *Understanding Other Minds: Perspectives from Autism and Developmental Cognitive Neuroscience*, 2nd edn. Oxford: Oxford University Press, pp. 297–321.

Tager-Flusberg, H. and Joseph, R. M. (2003). Identifying neurocognitive phenotypes in autism. *Philosophical Transactions of The Royal Society. Series B*, **358**, 303–14.

Tager-Flusberg, H., Calkins, S., Noin, I. *et al.* (1990). A longitudinal study of language acquisition in autistic and Down syndrome children. *Journal of Autism and Developmental Disorders*, **20**, 1–22.

Tager-Flusberg, H., Paul, R., and Lord, C. (2005). Language and communication in autism. In F. Volkmar, A. Klin, and R. Paul, eds., *Handbook of Autism and Pervasive Developmental Disorders*. *Vol. 1*. New York: John Wiley, pp. 335–64.

Tomasello, M. and Kruger, A. C. (1992). Joint attention on actions: acquiring verbs in ostensive and non-ostensive contests. *Journal of Child Language*, **19**, 311–33.

Tuchman, R. F. and Rapin, I. (1997). Regression in pervasive developmental disorders: seizures and epileptiform electroencephalogram correlates. *Pediatrics*, **99**, 560–6.

Volden, J. and Lord, C. (1991). Neologisms and idiosyncratic language in autistic speakers. *Journal of Autism and Developmental Disorders*, **21**, 109–30.

Volkmar, F., Chawarska, K., and Klin, A. (2005). Autism in infancy and early childhood. *Annual Review of Psychology*, **56**, 315–36.

Weiss, C., Gordon, M., and Lillywhite, H. (1987). *Clinical Management of Articulation and Phonological Disorders*. Boston: Williams & Wilkins.

Westby, C. (2005). Assessing and remediating text comprehension problems. In H. Catts and A. Kamhi, eds., *Language and Reading Disabilities*. Boston: Allyn & Bacon, pp. 274–340.

Wetherby, A. (1986). Ontogeny of communication functions in autism. *Journal of Autism and Developmental Disorders*, **16**, 295–316.

Wetherby, A. M. and Prutting, C. A. (1984). Profiles of communicative and cognitive–social abilities in autistic children. *Journal of Speech and Hearing Research*, **27**, 364–77.

Wetherby, A., Woods, J., Allen, L. *et al.* (2004). Early indicators of autism spectrum disorders in the second year of life. *Journal of Autism and Developmental Disorders*, **34**, 473–93.

Windsor, J., Doyle, S., and Siegel, G. (1994). Language acquisition after mutism: a longitudinal case study of autism. *Journal of Speech and Hearing Research*, **37**, 96–105.

Wing, L. (1981). Asperger's syndrome: a clinical account. *Journal of Autism and Developmental Disorders*, **9**, 11–29.

Yule, W. and Rutter, M. (1987). *Language Development and Disorders*. London: MacKeith.

Ziatas, K., Durkin, K., and Pratt, C. (2003). Differences in assertive speech acts produced by children with autism, Asperger syndrome, specific language impairment, and normal development. *Development and Psychopathology*, **15**, 73–94.

5

Genetic epidemiology of autism spectrum disorders

Peter Szatmari

Department of Psychiatry, McMaster University

Marshall B. Jones

Offord Centre for Child Studies, McMaster University

Introduction

Almost 30 years ago Hanson and Gottesman (1976) published a review article entitled "The genetics, if any, of infantile autism and childhood schizophrenia." As the title suggests, the two authors found little evidence of a genetic role in the etiology of autism. "No strong evidence exists," they wrote, "implicating genetics in the development of childhood psychoses that begin before the age of 5." The viewpoint expressed in this article was not idiosyncratic and was generally held to be true at the time. Currently, the general viewpoint regarding autism has reversed itself completely. Autism today is thought to be one of the most heritable of all psychiatric conditions, more so than bipolar disorder or schizophrenia, and much more so than alcoholism or antisocial behavior. The issue today is not whether autism has a genetic basis but what that basis is, the specific genes involved, and how they act.

Several developments were responsible for this reversal. The most influential was a series of twin studies, the first of which appeared a year after the Hanson and Gottesman review. Folstein and Rutter (1977) attempted "to obtain information on all school-age autistic twin pairs (same sex twins at least one of whom was autistic) in Great Britain." This attempt was implemented in a variety of ways, including a list of autistic twin pairs collected over the years by the late Dr. M. Carter, a search of the records of all children known to the National Society for Autistic Children, and a request for cases published in the Society's newsletter. These efforts resulted in 11 monozygotic and 10 dizygotic pairs. Four of the monozygotic pairs were concordant for autism, which yielded a proband wise

Autism and Pervasive Developmental Disorders, 2nd edn, ed. Fred R. Volkmar.
Published by Cambridge University Press. © Cambridge University Press 2007.

concordance rate of 53%. None of the dizygotic pairs was concordant for autism, which, of course, yielded a proband wise concordance rate of 0%.

The next twin study (Ritvo *et al.*, 1985) obtained subjects primarily through an advertisement placed in the newsletter of the National Society for Autistic Children, USA. Unfortunately, this same advertisement also solicited children who came from multiplex sibships, i.e. sibships with more than one affected child. This combined solicitation of both twin and multiplex families could reasonably be expected to skew the twin results toward concordant pairs. Those results were 22 concordant out of 23 monozygotic pairs for a proband wise concordance rate of 98% and 4 concordant out of 17 dizygotic pairs for a proband wise concordance rate of 38%.

In 1988 Smalley and colleagues summarized twin studies of autism to that time. These studies were the Folstein–Rutter and Ritvo studies plus 11 monozygotic and 9 dizygotic pairs from single-case studies. They also corrected all of the results for a well-known ascertainment effect, namely that when searches are made for autistic twins, concordant pairs are roughly twice as likely to be located as discordant pairs. Correcting for this effect, Smalley and colleagues found an overall concordance rate of 64% for the monozygotes and 9% for the dizygotes.

The third study (Steffenburg *et al.*, 1989) was carried out in Denmark, Finland, Iceland, Norway, and Sweden. In Denmark and Sweden, cases were obtained primarily through the twin registers maintained in those two countries. In the remaining three countries (none of which maintained national twin registers) cases were obtained through the National Autistic Societies or through specialists who were contacted and asked if they knew of any autistic twins. These efforts succeeded in locating 11 monozygotic pairs plus a triplet, all three of whom were concordant for autism, and 10 dizygotic pairs. Ten of the monozygotic pairs were concordant for autism which, together with the concordant triplet, yielded a proband wise concordance rate of 96% (23 of 24). None of the dizygotic pairs was concordant so that in this case, as in the Folstein–Rutter study, the concordance rate for dizygotic pairs was 0%.

An extension of the early Folstein–Rutter study has been reported by Bailey *et al.* (1995). The extension includes 23 monozygotic pairs plus 1 triplet. Thirteen of the 23 pairs are concordant and all 3 members of the triplet are autistic, which yields a concordance rate of 73% (29 of 39). The extension also includes 20 dizygotic pairs, none of whom is concordant.

In the same years that these twin studies were being conducted, the analysis of twin data was also developing. For decades concordance rates from twin studies had been made to yield heritability estimates by means of formulas originally advanced by Holzinger (1929). The Holzinger estimates, however, were arbitrary and bore no demonstrable relation to genetic theory. Concordance rates could, however, be related to genetic theory if it were assumed that a person became affected when an underlying, continuous, and normally distributed liability exceeded a threshold value. Falconer (1965), who introduced this formulation, also assumed that the underlying liability constituted a final common path for all determinants of the disorder, environmental as well as genetic. Subsequent papers by Edwards (1969) and Smith (1970, 1974) advanced Falconer's approach.

Estimating heritability by reference to an underlying liability continuum brings into play a consideration that was ignored in the Holzinger estimates, i.e. population risk. In the Falconer approach the same concordance rates for monozygotic and dizygotic twins may give rise to very different heritability estimates, depending on population risk. In general, the rarer a condition is the higher the heritability estimate will be for the same concordance rates. Autism was once thought to be a rare condition. The population risk was generally estimated at between 4 and 10 cases per 10 000. It is now thought to occur at a rate of roughly 16 per 10 000 (Chakrabarti & Fombonne, 2001). Hence taking either population risk into account tends to reinforce the impression one gets from the raw concordance rates that autism is highly heritable. Using the Falconer approach, heritability estimates for autism based on the summary by Smalley *et al.* (1988), the North European study by Steffenburg and associates, or the recent extension of the Folstein–Rutter study are all in excess of 90%.

Hanson and Gottesman (1976) based their conclusion that autism was probably not genetic on the result culled from the literature then available, that "very few siblings of early onset cases are affected." By "early onset cases" the two authors meant "cases where the proband's disorder begins before the age of 5." For this group of probands they quoted a 1.8% rate of "schizophrenia or schizophrenic like childhood psychosis in siblings." Given that "schizophrenia or schizophrenic like," while it might include autism, could also include children with psychoses or developmental delay who were not specifically autistic, the figure of 1.8% should probably be regarded as an upper bound. Even if the true risk to siblings was considerably less than 1.8%, say 1.0%, it would still be greater than the population risk and, in the next two decades, estimates of sibling risk would increase steadily.

In their review of the literature, Smalley *et al.* (1988) summarized six "recent studies" of sibling risk, all published after the Hanson and Gottesman paper and all focused on autism specifically. Their estimate of the sibling risk of autism, based on all six studies, was 2.7%, a substantial increase over the estimate made by Hanson and Gottesman.

About the same time as the Smalley *et al.* review, Jones and Szatmari (1988) pointed out that autistic children tended to be born late in their sibships. In this respect autistic children were similar to children with Down's syndrome or cerebral palsy. They suggested that the explanation was also similar. The parents of children with burdensome conditions that become apparent at birth or in early childhood were less likely to have more children than other parents. They abbreviated their family because the burden of the child they already had was great and they feared, in addition, the probability of having another such child. If every autistic child was the last in his or her sibship, then no sibship could have more than one affected child and the risk to siblings would be zero. The conclusion, however, that autism was not genetic would plainly not be warranted. If the tendency not to have any more children after the birth of an affected child was complete, a condition could be completely determined genetically and the risk to siblings could still be zero.

In the presence of stoppage rules (as the tendency not to have more children is called) the segregation ratio has to be estimated by the recurrence risk, i.e. the risk to children born after the first affected child. This, in turn, requires a population with large families and little tendency to be deterred by the birth of handicapped children. The Mormon population in Utah is such a population. In an apparently complete survey of autism in this population, Ritvo *et al.* (1989) reported a sibling risk of 4.5% and a recurrence risk of 8.6%. The sibling risk is somewhat higher than has been reported in most other studies, so perhaps the recurrence risk may somewhat overestimate the true segregation ratio. Even so, using the recurrence risk (and thereby avoiding an underestimate due to stoppage rules) yields an estimate of the segregation ratio that is twice that given by Smalley *et al.* (1988) and very much larger than the estimate made by Hanson and Gottesman (1976).

As a result of these twin and family studies, six early reviews (Folstein & Rutter, 1977; Pauls, 1987; Reiss *et al.*, 1986; Rutter *et al.*, 1990; Silliman *et al.*, 1989; Smalley *et al.*, 1988) all concluded that a genetic etiology is plausible for autism. Although individually many of the older studies suffered from convenience sampling, poorly standardized diagnostic procedures, nonblind assessments of relatives, etc., the consistency of results across studies is impressive.

This chapter reviews more recent data on the role, rather than the existence or extent, of genetic factors in autism/pervasive developmental disorder (PDD). This involves consideration of issues that are commonly seen in other complex disorders, such as variable expressivity, pleiotropy, and genetic heterogeneity. The chapter concludes with a discussion of a genetic model for autism spectrum disorder (ASD) and several unresolved issues that must be addressed before further progress is possible.

Variable expressivity and pleiotropy

Variable expressivity refers to the phenomenon whereby the genes for a disorder also confer susceptibility to milder or incomplete manifestations of the same disorder, even some that may fall below the threshold for a diagnosis. Variable expressivity is often seen in dominant Mendelian disorders such as tuberous sclerosis and neurofibromatosis, and in complex genetic disorders due to a dynamic mutation such as fragile X syndrome and Huntington's disease.

Several studies taken as a whole indicate that the genes for autism also confer susceptibility to milder or incomplete manifestations of autism. For example, the co-twins of monozygotic autistic probands can have atypical autism or Asperger's syndrome (Bailey et al., 1995; Folstein & Rutter, 1977) and the risk of Asperger's syndrome and atypical autism in the non-twin siblings of autistic probands is roughly 3% (Bolton et al., 1994). Thus the overall risk of both autism and other ASDs to siblings of autistic probands is 5–6% (Szatmari et al., 1993) even without taking account of stoppage. The risk relative to the general population cannot be calculated in this case because systematic data on the population prevalence of the other forms of ASD are not available.

Another type of impairment that has recently been reported to occur in first degree relatives is a "lesser variant" of ASD characterized by similar impairments in reciprocal social interaction, communication and interests but not enough to merit a diagnosis of any form of ASD, even Asperger's syndrome. For example, Piven et al. (1994) report that parents of autistic children were more often rated as aloof, untactful, and unresponsive on a standardized personality interview than parents of Down's syndrome controls. Similarly, Bolton et al. (1994) found that roughly 20% of siblings of autistic probands had social or communication impairments or a restricted pattern of interests compared with 3% of siblings of Down's controls ($p < 0.001$). Similar findings have been reported by Landa et al. (1992) and Narayan et al. (1990) using other measures. In these studies the ratings of social impairment were not conducted blind to proband status and the control group of parents of children with Down's syndrome (in the Piven et al., 1994 and Landa et al., 1992 studies) were ascertained from a parent support group. Such parents might be expected to have better social skills than parents who do not belong to such organizations and this makes the comparison difficult to interpret.

Two controlled studies have looked at the prevalence of milder social impairments in collateral second- and third-degree relatives of ASD probands. This is a useful design as second- and third-degree relatives share genes with autistic children but do not generally live with them. Thus if elevated rates of a condition are found in extended relatives this can be taken as reasonable evidence that the elevated risk in siblings and parents is due to genetic factors, not shared environmental factors. Pickles *et al.* (1995) reported that the lesser variant was found in 6% of male second- and third-degree relatives of autistic probands compared with 3% in similar relatives of children with Down's syndrome. The finding of similar rates in second- and third-degree relatives is inconsistent with a purely genetic model but may have to do with the precision of measurement and low numbers. Szatmari *et al.* (2000) have also investigated rates of this same lesser variant in extended relatives. Families with two or more children affected with ASD were compared with families with a single affected male or female child and families that had either adopted an ASD child or were step-parents to an ASD child. The use of these groups controls for familiarity with ASD among informants and allows for similar sampling procedures in proband and control families. It has been shown, for example, that familiarity with a disease can change rates of other conditions as reported by family history (Chapman *et al.*, 1994; Gibbons *et al.*, 1993). Even with this design, Szatmari *et al.* (2000) found that rates of the lesser variant were more common among biological relatives of ASD probands than among nonbiological relatives, indicating that informant bias is not a major issue.

Based on their twin study, Folstein and Rutter (1977) originally postulated that what is inherited in autism is not so much the disorder itself but rather more broadly based cognitive impairments, particularly in language. While several early family history studies have supported this finding (August *et al.*, 1981; Baird & August, 1985; Minton *et al.*, 1982), more recent studies using direct testing of parents and siblings have failed to confirm this result (Freeman *et al.*, 1989; Gillberg *et al.*, 1992; Szatmari *et al.*, 1993). Previous studies often failed to exclude siblings affected with ASD and so the cognitive impairments reported may have been a part of the siblings' ASD instead of being due to a pure learning disorder. It appears as if persistent cognitive impairments are part of the autism phenotype only if also associated with social–communication problems. It is possible, however, that relatives are at risk of transient language delay that does not lead to chronic language impairment though this hypothesis remains to be tested.

If it is true that variable expressivity exists (but is limited to other forms of ASD and the lesser variant), the next question is whether genetic or environmental factors account for these variations in severity. The best design to answer this question is to see whether concordant monozygous twins are more alike in severity than concordant dizygous twins. This would demonstrate that genetic factors account for variations in severity rather than environmental factors which can be either shared or nonshared. The one twin study with enough concordant dizygous twins did not address this issue (Ritvo *et al.*, 1985). An alternative design is to see whether the variation among affected (non-twin) siblings is less than the variation seen between affected ASD children from different families. The comparison of variation between and within families is estimated using an Intraclass Correlation Coefficient (ICC) (similar to a Pearson correlation). Spiker *et al.* (1994) found very low correlations between affected siblings on IQ and autistic symptoms using a sample of 37 multiple-incidence families with autism. In contrast, MacLean *et al.* (1999) found significant ICCs for measures of nonverbal IQ, communication, and socialization scores in a sample of multiple-incidence families with ASD children. Lower correlations were observed for autistic symptoms (MacLean *et al.*, 1999). Other more recent studies have found positive ICCs for some measures of autistic symptoms from the Autism Diagnostic Interview-Revised (ADI-R) (Silverman *et al.*, 2002). Thus the results from these studies indicate that familial, and presumably genetic, factors account for the variation in severity seen among ASD children. Such high correlations in clinical features are also seen in disorders caused by dynamic mutations because the number of trinucleotide repeats will vary between families but will be similar within a family (Snell *et al.*, 1993). These findings are also seen in disorders with genetic heterogeneity; siblings will share the same genetic mechanism but may have different susceptibility genes than affected children from other families (see below).

Another active area of investigation is whether the genes for autism/ASD confer susceptibility to qualitatively different disorders such as affective disorders or substance abuse. For example, if the genes involved in serotonin transmission are involved in the etiology of autism (Young *et al.*,1982), then these genes may confer susceptibility to other psychiatric disorders that are also associated with serotonin transmission. This is known as pleiotropy.

Several studies have reported that parents and siblings of autistic probands have increased rates of affective and anxiety disorders. Two studies have used control groups and direct interviews of first degree relatives. For example, Piven *et al.* (1991) measured rates of psychiatric disorders using the Schedule of Affective Disorders and Schizophrenia Lifetime version in parents of autistic children compared with parents of children with Down's syndrome. Elevated rates of anxiety disorders were found (23.5% vs. 2.9%). Smalley *et al.* (1995) conducted semistructured psychiatric interviews on the parents and siblings of probands with autism and controls with other neurological disorders. They reported that rates of major depression (32.3% vs. 11.1%), social phobia (20.2% vs. 2.4%), and substance abuse (22.1% vs. 0%) were significantly higher in relatives of the autistic children compared with controls.

The key issue is whether this association is due to genetic or environmental mechanisms. It is possible, for example, that the stress of raising a profoundly handicapped child may, by itself, give rise to these disorders. Indeed, a number of studies have reported that parenting stress generated by the child's handicap correlates with the presence of depression in the mothers (Bristol & Schopler, 1983; Holroyd & McArthur, 1976; Petersen, 1984; Wolf et al., 1989). However, Smalley et al. (1995) reported that the majority (64%) of parents of autistic probands had the onset of their mood disorder prior to the birth of the child with autism, compared with 20% of the parents of controls, which suggests that the affective disorder is not due to stress; however, this result needs to be replicated with a larger sample.

The most informative design to resolve this issue is to use twin or adoption studies. None of the twin studies has reported rates of psychiatric disorders in discordant co-twins and there is only one adoption study in autism (Szatmari et al., 2000). Another informative design involves estimating the risk of psychiatric disorders in collateral relatives who do not live with a handicapped child. If these conditions have a genetic relation to autism, second- and third-degree relatives should also show an increased risk compared with population base rates. In a family history study, Szatmari et al. (1995) did not find that rates of psychiatric symptoms were increased in extended relatives of ASD probands compared with controls. This suggests that the increased rate in parents reported in other studies may be, at least in part, a function of family stress; however, that study reported on rates of symptoms not disorders and used family history not direct interview of relatives.

Conclusion

It seems that there is now some agreement that autism is a strongly genetic disorder and that the genes for autism also confer susceptibility to other forms of ASD such as Asperger's syndrome, atypical autism, and perhaps to milder forms of social impairment that fall below a threshold for a diagnosis of ASD (the lesser variant). It also seems likely that the genes for autism do not confer susceptibility to persistent learning disabilities or mental retardation unaccompanied by ASD-like social impairment. The evidence is not clear whether there is an increased risk for other psychiatric disorders such as affective disorders and social phobia. Further replication of these latter findings is needed as well as twin and adoption studies to determine whether the observed familial aggregation is due to environmental or genetic factors.

Etiological and genetic heterogeneity in ASD

There are several different meanings of the term "heterogeneity" in the context of genetic disorders. Etiological heterogeneity refers to the possibility that a disorder might be caused by both genetic and environmental etiologies. Genetic heterogeneity, on the other hand, refers to the possibility that ASD might be caused either by several mutations at a single genetic locus (intralocus or allelic heterogeneity) or by several genes at different loci (interlocus heterogeneity).

There is, in fact, considerable evidence that autism is both etiologically and genetically heterogeneous. For example, autism occasionally occurs with certain viral diseases such as congenital rubella and cytomegalovirus (Garrow et al., 1984) or as a result of maternal ingestion of anticonvulsants (Moore et al., 2000). Autism can also occur in association with several different chromosomal abnormalities such as duplication of chromosome 15 (Xu et al., 2004) and different genetic diseases, i.e. tuberous sclerosis, neurofibromatosis, phenylketonuria, fragile X syndrome, etc. (Ritvo et al., 1989). Such cases with known disease associations probably only account for 10–15% of the cases of ASD (Xu et al., 2004). Furthermore, the mechanism of the comorbidity in these situations is unclear: is the autism a nonspecific sequela of the mental retardation or is it the direct result of disruption in certain key brain regions?

Another important question is whether genetic heterogeneity exists among the idiopathic cases of ASD. There are several ways in which genetic heterogeneity can be detected (Khoury et al., 1993). If different mutations are associated with different clinical features, heterogeneity can be detected by seeing if certain clinical features run true within families. The Spiker et al. (1994) data, referred to earlier, reported that individual autistic behaviors as assessed by the ADI showed little or no correlation among affected siblings from the same family. However, MacLean et al. (2000) and other studies (Silverman et al., 2002) have found that IQ, severity of impairment, and summary measures of autistic behaviors do appear to run true within families. On the other hand, PDD subtypes do not (MacLean et al., 2000). For example, probands with IQ below 50 tend to have affected siblings with IQ below 50, and probands with IQ above 70 tend to have affected siblings with similar levels of IQ. But if the proband had Asperger's syndrome, the affected sibling is just as likely to have autism. Thus variations in severity, but not necessarily specific autistic behaviors, could be due to genetic heterogeneity; high- and low-functioning ASD probands could arise from separate genetic mechanisms.

Another way of detecting heterogeneity in complex genetic disorders is to see whether there are differences in recurrence risk to relatives associated with certain clinical features of probands. This way of testing for genetic heterogeneity has proved very successful in mapping genes for other complex genetic diseases such as Alzheimer's disease, breast cancer, and diabetes. Ritvo *et al.* (1990) reported a higher risk of autism to siblings of female autistic probands compared with male probands (14% vs. 7%), however, power was too low to test this hypothesis adequately. Bolton *et al.* (1994) reported that the risk of the lesser variant in siblings was higher in nonverbal probands compared with those who were verbal. In contrast, we found that the lesser variant was more common in higher-functioning sib pairs than in those who were lower functioning. There was, however, no difference in risk for the lesser variant by the sex of the proband in both studies.

Conclusion

It is clear that autism can rarely occur as a result of both viral etiologies and several single gene disorders. Among the idiopathic cases of autism, however, the picture is much less clear. There is some tentative evidence which suggests that severity of impairment appears to run true within families. In multiple incidence families, affected siblings tend to show similar levels of functioning. This suggests that perhaps higher- and lower-functioning sib pairs may arise from separate genetic mechanisms. This would be strengthened if there was converging evidence that the risk of the lesser variant of autism was more common in relatives of probands with high- or low-functioning autism. However, there is at present no agreement on this point. Clearly, more studies are needed to pursue the hypothesis that clinical markers can delineate genetic heterogeneity.

Possible genetic models

Both the low risk to sibs and the anomalous sex ratio (approximately four males to every female) are incompatible with any simple Mendelian or single gene inheritance (i.e. autosomal recessive, dominant, or X-linked). These would predict a recurrence risk of at least 25% to sibs, and either an equal sex ratio for autosomal transmission, or an overwhelming number of males compared with females for X-linked recessive transmission. The remaining possible modes of inheritance belong to the spectrum of complex genetic models (Kidd, 1981; Reich *et al.*, 1972; Risch, 1990).

Multilocus models

Multilocus models are often differentiated into polygenic and oligogenic models. The polygenic model proposes that autism is caused by many genes each of very small effect. In contrast, oligogenic models postulate that autism/ASD is caused by a small number of genes. In both cases, the genes may interact in an additive or multiplicative (epistatic) manner.

In a polygenic model, the liability to develop autism is normally distributed in the general population and is determined by the number of "autism" genes that a child inherits from both parents. To be consistent with the skewed sex ratio, separate thresholds can be postulated for males and females. The main problem with polygenic models is that further work at characterizing autism genes would be fruitless as each gene would only contribute a tiny portion of the variance to the disorder. In a sense, polygenic models represent the "null hypothesis" for genetic studies.

The polygenic model is consistent with some but not all aspects of the genetic epidemiology of autism. For example, the relatives of female and low IQ probands should be at higher risk of autism/ASD and the lesser variant than relatives of male probands or those with higher IQ. As reviewed above, there are some limited data to support these predictions. Similarly, a complex segregation analysis performed by Jorde *et al.* (1991) on nuclear families indicated that the mode of transmission of autism within families (particularly the paucity of affected cousins) was most consistent with polygenic transmission. Unfortunately, complex segregation analysis has little power to discriminate among alternative genetic models (Ott, 1990) particularly if the issue of genetic heterogeneity is ignored, as it was in this study.

Another useful way to differentiate polygenic and oligogenic epistatic models that is not affected by heterogeneity is to estimate the relative risk of a disorder in various classes of relatives. Risch (1990) has pointed out that if a disorder is caused by a single gene (and there are no dominance effects), the relative risk should fall by roughly half as one looks at the relative risk in monozygous co-twins, siblings, and second- and third-degree relatives. For example, in a single-gene disorder, the relative risk might fall from 32 in monozygotic co-twins to 16 in first-degree relatives to 8 and 4 in second- and third-degree relatives, respectively. In a polygenic–epistatic model (where many genes each of small effect interact multiplicatively), the risk would fall as a function of the square root of the risk in the previous class of relative. For example, if the relative risk is 16 in first-degree relatives; the risk should be 4 in second-degree relatives; however, if the multiple genes interact in an additive manner, the overall effect will mimic the single-gene pattern (Risch, 1990). In an oligogenic model with epistatic effects, the risk falls more rapidly than for a single gene but more slowly than in a polygenic model.

Although there are data on the rates of autism in twins and siblings, they are much more limited for more distant relatives. Pooling the results of three twin studies with systematic sampling, it is possible to estimate that the risk of autism to monozygotic co-twins is roughly 60%. There were no concordant dizygotic twins found in these three studies so the rate of 3% found in non-twin siblings can be used instead. If the prevalence of autism is taken to be 16 per 10 000 (Chakrabarti & Fombonne, 2001), the relative risk goes from 375 in monozygotic twins to 19 in siblings. Such a large drop is clearly inconsistent with a single-gene model where the relative risk should fall to roughly 200. Under a polygenic (epistatic) model, the relative risk in siblings is much closer to the observed figure. Using family history from a single informant, Pickles *et al.* (1995) were unable to detect any second- and third-degree relatives with autism, a finding that is also consistent with polygenic transmission; however, family history from a single informant will underestimate the true risk to extended relatives.

The data are somewhat different if one focuses on the lesser variant. Pickles *et al.* (1995) reported on rates of this personality characteristic in monozygotic twins, first-, second-, and third-degree relatives. The relative risk of this trait (excluding cases with autism) in monozygotic co-twins and siblings is 6.1 and 3.7, respectively. Model fitting using a latent class analysis with the lesser variant was consistent with a three-gene model. By contrast, the relative risk for autism in this data set is 846 in monozygotic co-twins and 29.2 in siblings, a decrement entirely consistent with polygenic–epistatic transmission. Although latent class analysis can account for a certain extent of measurement error using family history, remaining error is likely to produce a pattern consistent with multiple genes (Szatmari & Jones, 1999). In other words, it is possible that the Pickles *et al.* (1995) result is a conservative one and the true number of genes involved in the lesser variant may be less than three.

Candidate genes and association studies

Given the strength of genetic effects it should be possible to identify autism-susceptibility genes. There are two approaches to gene identifications: association studies of candidate genes and genome-wide linkage scans. Candidate genes are genes that a priori might be involved in the etiology of autism (for example, genes that control serotonin metabolism). In association studies, the frequencies of alleles or genotypes at a candidate locus are compared in children with autism and in unrelated controls. Although such studies are able to detect genes that contribute a relatively small proportion of the variance to a disorder, there is considerable controversy on the use of association studies in complex genetic disorders (Crowe, 1993). A positive association may result from several mechanisms, the marker loci may exist in linkage disequilibrium with susceptibility genes, the measured alleles may be the susceptibility genes themselves, or else the result is a false-positive and reflects population admixture and stratification.

As there is a high rate of false-positive findings with association studies (Hodge, 1995) these results need to be replicated. Furthermore, if replicated, there needs to be evidence that the result is not due to population stratification. This can be accomplished by the use of family-based association studies, which are now the standard design. In recent years, many candidate genes have been found to be associated with autism (for a review, see Folstein & Rosen-Sheidley, 2001; and see also Ingram et al. 2000; Persico et al., 2001; Tordjman et al., 2001; Wassink et al., 2001), but attempts to replicate these have been unsuccessful (Betancur et al., 2002; Li et al., 2001). Perhaps the most promising region identified by association methods is on chromosome 15 where frequent chromosome duplications have been documented. Recent reports using family-based association analyses suggest that the UBE3A locus or a subset of GABA genes in that region may be involved (Martin et al., 2000; Nurmi et al., 2001).

While it is true that the association strategy is more powerful than linkage (Risch & Merikangas, 1996), our understanding of the pathophysiology of autism is probably too incomplete to prioritize the most relevant candidates. Many in the field (for example, Gershon et al., 2001 and Baron, 2001) believe that an approach that begins with a genome scan to localize regions of interest and then utilizes fine mapping to narrow the region probably has greater potential for identifying true "autism" genes.

Genome-wide scans

Linkage studies are based on the concept that if a disorder is caused by genetic factors, affected individuals in a pedigree will share genetic markers more often than by chance alone. If markers are shared and in linkage with the disease locus, they must be close to the actual genes that cause the disorder. Several genome-wide linkage scans have been conducted in autism using an affected sib pair design (dense pedigrees are not available due to stoppage rules and reduced fecundity). As shown in Table 5.1, these reports (Alarcon et al., 2002; Auranen et al., 2000; Barrett et al., 1999; Buxbaum et al., 2001; IMGSAC, 1998, 2001; Liu et al., 2001; Philippe et al., 1999; Risch et al., 1999; Shao et al., 2002) vary with respect to sample size, number of markers, map density, diagnostic instruments, method of diagnosis, and phenotypes analyzed. Of these, variation in the number of sib pairs (range 17–152) and in the diagnostic strategy employed is most marked. The only consistency across studies is in the use of the ADI to identify affected individuals. The use of other phenotypic data is surprisingly limited.

Table 5.1 Review of genome-wide linkage studies of autism

Research group	Year of publication	n. of affected sibling pairs	Chromosome region	Markers	Highest LOD score
IMGSAC,	1998	87	7q	D7S530/D7S684	MLS 2.53
			16p	D16S407/D16S3114	MLS 1.51
			4p	D4S412	MLS 1.55
CLSA,	1999	75	13q	D13S217/D13S1229 13q	MMLS/ het 2.3
			13q	D13S800	MMLS/ het 3.0
			7q	D7S1813	MMLS 2.2
Philippe et al.,	1999	51	6q	D6S283	MMLS 2.23
Risch et al.,	1999	147	1p	D1S1675	MMLS 2.15
Auranen et al.,	2000	17	3p	D353038	MLS 2.39
Buxbaum et al.,	2001	95 total 49 "narrow" definition	2q	D2S364/D2S335	HLOD 1.96
			2q	D2S364/D2S335	NPL 2.39
			2q	D2S364/D2S335	HLOD 2.99
			2q	D2S364/D2S335	NPL 3.32
Liu et al.,	2001	118 total 75 "narrow" definition	5q	D5S2494	MMLS
			Xqter	DXS1047	2.55X-MLS 2.56
			19p	D19S714	MMLS
			Xqter	DXS1047	2.53X-MLS 2.67
			16p	D16S2619	MMLS 1.93M
			19q	D19S587/D19S601	MLS 1.70
			5q	D5S2488	MMLS 1.63
IMGSAC	2001	152 total 127 "strict" definition	2q	D2S2188	MMLS 3.74
			7q	D7S477	MMLS 3.20
			16p	D16S3102	MMLS 2.93
			17q	HTTINT2	MMLS 2.34
			2q	D2S2188	MMLS 4.80
Shao et al.,	2002	99	3p	D3S3680	MLS 1.51
			7q	D7S495	MLS 1.66
			Xq	DXS6789	MLS 2.54
Alarcon et al.,	2002	152	7q	D7S1824	NPL-Z 2.98
Auranen et al.,	2002	38	3q	D3S3037	MLS 4.81
			7q	D7S2462	MLS 3.66
			Xq	DXS7132	MLS 2.75
			1q	D1S1653	MLS 2.63
Yonan et al.,	2003	345	17q	D17S1800	MLS 2.83
			5p	D5S2494	MLS 2.54
			11p	D11S1392/D11S1993	MLS 2.24
			4q	D4S2361/D4S2909	MLS 1.72
			8q	D8S1832	MLS 1.6
Ylisaukko-oja et al.,	2004	17 Asperger's syndrome	1q	D1S484	MLS 3.58
			3p	D3S2432	MLS 2.50
			13q	D13S793	MLS 1.59

CLSA: Collaborative Linkage Studies of Autism; IMGSAC: International Molecular Genetic Study of Autism Consortium; LOD: Log of the Odds Ratio.

Despite this variability, it is encouraging to see that preliminary linkage signals (LOD scores above 1.5) from different scans overlap (see Table 5.1) particularly on 7q, 16p, 17q, and 2q. It is difficult to interpret these results as none of the linkage signals is significant, according to current criteria (Lander & Kruglyak, 1995), and the use of overlapping samples and different markers makes it difficult to conclude that a finding has been truly replicated. What is important though is that the linkage signals from different groups are reasonably consistent. Since the regions identified are too large, and the LOD score peaks too low, to start fine mapping, more work is required to strengthen those signals.

It is interesting to note that "broad" and "narrow" definitions of the ADI phenotype alone make little difference to the linkage signals, suggesting that this approach to dealing with the complexity of autism is insufficient. Bradford *et al.* (2001), Buxbaum *et al.* (2001), and now Shao *et al.* (2002) report that some LOD scores on chromosomes 2, and 7 and 13, increase if the analysis is restricted to sib pairs with language delay. Alarcon *et al.* (2002) report a similar increase in linkage signal on chromosome 7 if the quantitative trait "age at first phrases" is used. The higher-linkage signals associated with these alternative phenotypes suggest that stratification of sib pairs or the use of quantitative phenotypes to deal with possible heterogeneity may be important strategies.

Based on several lines of evidence, perhaps the most promising susceptibility region for autism is on chromosome 7:

(1) the region 7q31–35 contains the recently cloned FOXP2 gene responsible for a type of language disorder (Lai *et al.*, 2001);

(2) most children with autism have a serious language deficit (Kjelgaard & Tager-Flusberg, 2001);

(3) two groups have reported that their LOD scores in this region increase if the phenotype is narrowed by requiring some measure of language delay in probands and relatives (Alarcon *et al.*, 2002; Bradford *et al.*, 2001);

(4) several pedigrees with an autistic proband have been reported with apparent deletions in this region (Yu *et al.*, 2002);

(5) a recent meta-analysis of linkage results concurs that a susceptibility gene might well exist on 7q (Badner & Gershon, 2002).

This enthusiasm must be balanced, however, by several reservations. First, the FOXP2 gene has been ruled out as a major susceptibility gene in autism and in specific language impairment (Newbury *et al.*, 2002). Second, the linkage signals on chromosome 7 are separated by large distances suggesting that perhaps there are several genes in the region or that the most appropriate phenotype has not yet been determined. Narrowing the region on chromosome 7 is not simply a matter of sample size or density of markers; even the study with the largest sample size and the most markers could not resolve this issue (IMGSAC, 2001). We may have reached an impasse on refining the signals on chromosome 7 (and by implication elsewhere) unless the genetic complexity of autism is reduced by defining more specific phenotypes within and between families.

Modifier genes

The term "intrauterine effects" refers to the possibility that the intrauterine environment may play a role in the etiology of autism in conjunction with genetic susceptibility in the child. These intrauterine effects may result from genetic conditions in the mother that place the developing fetus at risk. The classic example of this is phenylketonuria (PKU). The children of mothers with PKU often have developmental disabilities and congenital anomalies not because the children have PKU but because high levels of maternal phenylalanine cross the placenta and affect the developing brain (Stevenson & Huntley, 1967). There is some evidence of an intrauterine effect in autism / ASD. One of the most consistent findings in autism is that affected children have a higher rate of pregnancy and birth complications than their siblings or controls (Piven *et al.*, 1993). These complications could conceivably arise from a genetic condition in the mother that might affect the fetus. In addition, we (Jones *et al.*, 2004) have reported that variation in the maternal dopamine β-hydroxylase and monoamine oxidase genes in the mother were associated with variation in the IQ of the affected children. The joint interaction of genetic susceptibility in the child and a maternal genetic factor that affects the intrauterine environment would look like an epistatic mode of transmission and is therefore consistent with the relative risk data in relatives presented earlier.

Conclusion

It has become abundantly clear that autism is a genetic disorder. The studies reviewed above, however, indicate that there is no consensus on the mode of transmission of autism / ASD. The genetic epidemiology of the disorder is complicated by variable expressivity and heterogeneity which makes it difficult to decide who is affected in a pedigree, and thus to establish firmly the mode of transmission.

It seems clear, however, that the data do not support a single gene model for autism. Therefore, at least two or more genes need to be considered. What is striking about the relative risk data in various classes of relatives is the fact that the pattern of fall in relative risk seems to be different if one focuses on the lesser variant. The decrement in relative risk for autism is consistent with an epistatic polygenic model whereas for the lesser variant the pattern is consistent with a very small number of genes or even a single gene. In other words, the genetic mechanism for the lesser variant may be different from the mechanism for autism. It may be that the lesser variant is caused by a very small number of genes, whereas autism is caused by additional genes or some other mechanism in addition to the genes for the lesser variant. The form of epistasis is unknown and may include gene–gene or gene–environment interactions. This is not dissimilar to the two-hit hypothesis currently considered as the mechanism for many forms of cancer (Knudson, 1971). What is encouraging at this point is that there is no reason to reject an oligogenic model in favor of a purely polygenic–epistatic one.

Given the high heritability and risk to siblings, there is no logical reason that mapping autism genes cannot be successful. Linkage studies, however, need to be conducted on genetically homogeneous families where the disorder is caused by a few major genes. Without such evidence, linkage studies represent a high-risk strategy at best and require very large sample sizes. It is hoped that with more accurate knowledge about the inheritance of the lesser variant and a greater ability to identify more genetically homogeneous subgroups, the prospects for identifying "autism genes" are much more favorable now than they were just a few years ago. Once these genes are identified, it is hoped that a clearer understanding of pathogenesis will be possible and that this will lead to more effective interventions in the future.

REFERENCES

Alarcon, M., Cantor, R. M., Liu, J., Gilliam T. C., and Geschwind, D. H. (2002). Evidence for a language quantitative trait locus on chromosome 7q in multiplex autism families. *American Journal of Human Genetics*, **70**, 60–71.

August, G. J, Stewert, M. A., and Tsai, L. (1981). The incidence of cognitive disabilities in siblings of autistic children. *British Journal of Psychiatry*, **138**, 416–22.

Auranen, M., Nieminen, T., Majuri, S. *et al.* (2000). Analysis of autism susceptibility gene loci on chromosomes 1p, 4p, 6q, 7q, 13q, 15q, 16p, 17q, 19q and 22q in Finnish multiplex families. *Molecular Psychiatry*, **5**, 320–2.

Auranen, M., Vanhala, R., Varilo, T. *et al.* (2002). A genomewide screen for autism-spectrum disorders: evidence for a major susceptibility locus on chromosome 3q25–27. *American Journal of Human Genetics*, **71**, 777–90.

Badner, J. A. and Gershon, E. S. (2002). Regional meta-analysis of published data supports linkage of autism with markers on chromosome 7. *Molecular Psychiatry*, **7**, 56–66.

Bailey, A., Le Couteur, A., Gottesman, I. *et al.* (1995). Autism as a strongly genetic disorder: evidence from a British twin study. *Psychological Medicine*, **25**, 63–77.

Baird, T. D. and August, G. K. (1985). Familial heterogeneity in infantile autism. *Journal of Autism and Developmental Disorders*, **15**, 315–21.

Baron, M. (2001). The search for complex disease genes: fault by linkage or fault by association? *Molecular Psychiatry*, **6**, 143–9.

Barrett, S., Beck, J. C., Bernier, R. *et al.* ((CLSA) 1999). An autosomal genomic screen for autism. *American Journal of Medical Genetics (Neuropsychiatric Genetics)*, **88**, 609–15.

Betancur, C., Corbex, M., Spielewoy, C. *et al.* (2002). Serotonin transporter gene polymorphisms and hyperserotonemia in autistics. *Molecular Psychiatry*, **79**, 67–71.

Bolton, P., Macdonald, H., Pickles, A. *et al.* (1994). A case-control family history study of autism. *Journal of Child Psychology and Psychiatry*, **35**, 877–900.

Bradford, Y., Haines, J., Hutcheson, H. *et al.* (2001). Incorporating language phenotypes strengthens evidence of linkage to autism. *American Journal of Medical Genetics*, **105**, 539–47.

Bristol, M. M. and Schopler, E. (1983). Stress and coping in families of autistic adolescents. In E. Schopler and G. B. Mesibov, eds., *Austism in Adolescents and Adults*. New York: Plenum Press, pp. 251–78.

Buxbaum, J. D., Silverman, J. M., Smith, C. J. *et al.* (2001). Evidence for a susceptibility gene for autism on chromosome 2 and for genetic heterogeneity. *American Journal of Human Genetics*, **68**, 1514–20.

Chakrabarti, S. and Fombonne, E. (2001). Pervasive developmental disorders in preschool children. *Journal of the American Medical Association*, **285**, 3093–9.

Chapman, T. F., Mannuzza, S., Klein, D. F., and Fyer, A. J. (1994). Effects of informant mental disorder on psychiatric family history data. *American Journal of Psychiatry*, **151**, 574–9.

Crowe, R. R. (1993). Candidate genes in psychiatry: an epidemiologic perspective. *American Journal of Medical Genetics (Neuropsychiatric Genetics)*, **48**, 74–7.

Edwards, J. H. (1969). Familial predisposition in man. *British Medical Bulletin*, **25**, 58–64.

Falconer, D. S. (1965). The inheritance of liability to certain diseases estimated for the incidence among relatives. *Annals of Human Genetics*, **29**, 51–76.

Folstein, S. E. and Rosen-Sheidley, B. (2001). Genetics of autism: complex aetiology for a heterogeneous disorder. *Nature Reviews. Genetics*, **2**, 943–55.

Folstein, S. and Rutter, M. (1977). Infantile autism: a genetic study of 21 twin pairs. *Journal of Child Psychology and Psychiatry*, **18**, 297–321.

Freeman, B. J., Ritvo, E., Mason-Brothers, A. *et al.* (1989). Psychometric assessment of first-degree relatives of 62 autistic probands in Utah. *American Journal of Psychiatry*, **146**, 361–4.

Garrow, B., Bartheleng, C., Savage, D., Leddert, I., and Lelord, A. (1984). Comparison of autistic syndromes with and without associated neurological problems. *Journal of Autism and Developmental Disorders*, **14**, 105–11.

Gershon, E. S., Kelsoe J. R., Kendler, K. S., and Watson, J. D. (2001). A scientific opportunity. *Science*, **294**, 957.

Gibbons, L. E., Ponsonby, A. L., and Dwyer, I. A. (1993). Comparison of prospective and retrospective responses on sudden infant death syndrome by case and control mothers. *American Journal of Epidemiology*, **137**, 654–9.

Gillberg, C., Gillberg. I. C., and Steffenburg, S. (1992). Siblings and parents of children with autism: a controlled population-based study. *Developmental Medicine and Child Neurology*, **34**, 389–98.

Hanson, D. R. and Gottesman, I. I. (1976). The genetics, if any, of infantile autism and childhood schizophrenia. *Journal of Autism and Childhood Schizophrenia*, **6**, 209–34.

Hodge, S. E. (1995). An oligogenic disease displaying weak marker associations: a summary of contributions to problem I of GAW9. *Genetic Epidemiology*, **12**, 545–54.

Holroyd, J. and McArthur, D. (1976), Mental retardation and stress on the parents: a contrast between Down's syndrome and childhood autism. *American Journal of Mental Deficiency*, **80**, 431–6.

Holzinger, K. J. (1929). The relative effect of nature and nurture on twin differences. *Journal of Educational Psychology*, **20**, 241–8.

Ingram, J. L., Stodgell, C. J., Hyman, S. L., Figlewicz, D. A., and Weitkamp, L. R. (2000). Discovery of allelic variants of HOXA1 and HOXB1: genetic susceptibility to autism spectrum disorders. *Teratology*, **62**, 393–405.

International Molecular Genetic Study of Autism Consortium (IMGSAC) (1998). A full genome screen for autism with evidence for linkage to a region on chromosome 7q. *Human Molecular Genetics*, **7**, 571–8.

International Molecular Genetic Study of Autism Consortium (IMGSAC) (2001). A genomewide screen for autism: strong evidence for linkage to chromosomes 2q, 7q, and 16p. *American Journal of Human Genetics*, **69**, 570–81.

Jones, B. and Szatmari, P. (1988). Stoppage rules and genetic studies of autism. *Journal of Autism and Developmental Disorders*, **18**, 31–40.

Jones, B., Palmour, M., Zwaigenbaum, L., and Szatmari, P. (2004). Modifier effects in autism at the MAO-A and DBH loci. *American Journal of Medical Genetics (Neuropsychiatric Genetics)*, **126**, 58–65.

Jorde, L. B., Hasstedt, S. J., and Ritvo, E. R. (1991). Complex segregation analysis of autism. *American Journal of Human Genetics*, **49**, 932–8.

Khoury, M. J., Beatty, T. H., and Cohen, B. H. (1993). *Fundamentals of Genetic Epidemiology*. New York: Oxford University Press.

Kidd, K. K. (1981). Genetic models for psychiatric disorders. In E. S. Gershon, S. Mathysse, X. O. Breakfield, and R. Ciaranello, eds., *Gentic Research Strategies for Psychobiology and Psychiatry*. New York: Boxwood Press, pp. 150–7.

Kjelgaard, M. G. and Tager-Flusberg, H. (2001). An investigation of language impairment in autism: implications for genetic subgroups. *Language and Cognitive Processes*, **16**, 287–308.

Knudson, A. G. (1971). Mutation and cancer: statistical study on retinoblastoma. *Proceedings of the National Academy of Science USA*, **68**, 82.

Lai, C. S., Fisher, S. E., Hurst, J. A., Vargha-Khadem, F., and Monaco, A. P. (2001). A forkhead-domain gene is mutated in a severe speech and language disorder. *Nature*, **413**, 519–23.

Landa, R., Piven, J., Wzorek, M. M. *et al.* (1992). Social language use in parents of autistic individuals. *Psychological Medicine*, **22**, 245–54.

Lander, E. and Kruglyak, L. (1995). Genetic dissection of complex traits: guidelines for interpreting and reporting linkage results. *Nature Genetics*, **11**, 241–7.

Li, J., Tabor, H. K., Nguyen, L. *et al.* (2001). *Lack of association between HOXA1, HOXB1, Reelin and WNT-2 gene variants and autism in 110 multiplex families*. Presented at the Annual Meeting of American Society of Human Genetics, San Diego, California, October.

Liu, J., Nyholt, D. R., Magnussen, P. *et al.*, and the Autism Genetic Resource Exchange Consortium (2001). A genomewide screen for autism susceptibility loci. *American Journal of Human Genetics*, **69**, 327–40.

MacLean J. E., Szatmari, P., Jones, M. B. *et al.* (1999). Familial factors influence the severity of pervasive developmental disorder: evidence for genetic heterogeneity. *American Academy of Child and Adolescent Psychiatry*, **38**, 746–53.

MacLean, J. E., Teshima, I. E., Szatmari, P., and Nowaczyk, M. J. (2000). Ring chromosome 22 and autism: report and review. *American Journal of Medical Genetics*, **90**, 382–5.

Martin, E. R., Menold, M. M., Wolpert, C. M. *et al.* (2000). Analysis of linkage disequilibrium in gamma-aminobutyric acid receptor subunit genes in autistic disorder. *American Journal of Medical Genetics*, **96**, 43–8.

Minton, J., Campbell, M., Green, W. L., Jenings, S., and Samet, C. (1982). Cognitive assessment of siblings of autistic children. *Journal of the American Academy of Child Psychiatry*, **21**, 256–61.

Moore, J., Turnpenny, P., Quinn, A. *et al.* (2000). A clinical study of 57 children with fetal anticonvulsant syndromes. *Journal of Medical Genetics*, **37**, 489–97.

Narayan, S., Moyes, B., and Wolff, W. (1990). Family characteristics of autistic children: a further report. *Journal of Autism and Developmental Disorders*, **20**, 523–35.

Newbury, D. F., Bonora E., Lamb, J. A. *et al.*, and the International Molecular Genetic Study of Autism Consortium (2002). FOX P2 is not a major susceptibility gene for autism or specific language impairment. *American Journal of Human Genetics*, **70**, 1315–27.

Nurmi, E. L., Bradford, Y., Chen, Y. *et al.* (2001). Linkage disequilibrium at the Angelman syndrome gene UBE3A in autism families. *Genomics*, **77**, 105–13.

Ott, J. (1990). Invited editorial: cutting a Gordian knot in the linkage analysis of complex human traits. *American Journal of Human Genetics*, **46**, 219–21.

Pauls, D. (1987). The familiality of autism and related disorders: a review of the evidence. In D. Cohen and A. N. Donnellan, eds., *Handbook of Autism and Pervasive Developmental Disorders*. New York: John Wiley, pp. 192–8.

Persico, A. M., D'Agruma, L., Majorano, N., and Totaro, A. (2001). Reelin gene alleles and haplotypes as a factor predisposing to autistic disorder. *Molecular Psychiatry*, **6**, 150–9.

Petersen, P. (1984). Effects of moderator variables in reducing stress outcomes in mothers of children with handicaps. *Journal of Psychosomatic Medicine*, **28**, 337–44.

Philippe, A., Martinez, M. Guilloud-Bataille, M. *et al.* (1999). Genome-wide scan for autism susceptibility genes. Paris Autism Research International Sibpair Study. *Human Molecular Genetics*, **8**, 805–12.

Pickles, A., Bolton, P., Macdonald, H. *et al.* (1995). Latent-class analysis of recurrence risks for complex phenotypes with selection and measurement error: a twin and family history study of autism. *American Journal of Human Genetics*, **57**, 717.

Piven, J., Chase, G. A., Landa, R. *et al.* (1991). Psychiatric disorders in the parents of autistic individuals. *Journal of the American Academy of Child and Adolescent Psychiatry*, **311**, 471–8.

Piven, J., Simon, J., Chase, G. A. *et al.* (1993). The etiology of autism: pre-, peri- and neonatal factors. *Journal of the American Academy of Child and Adolescent Psychiatry*, **32**, 156–63.

Piven, J., Wzorek, M., Landa, R. *et al.* (1994). Personality characteristics of the parents of autistic individuals. *Psychological Medicine*, **24**, 783–95.

Reich, T., James, J. W., and Morris, C. A. (1972). The use of multiple thresholds in determining the mode of transmission of semi-continuous traits. *Annals of Human Genetics*, **36**, 163–83.

Reiss, A. L., Feinstein, C., and Rosenbaum, K. N. (1986). Autism and genetic disorders. *Schizophrenia Bulletin*, **12**, 724–38.

Risch, N. (1990). Linkage strategies for genetically complex traits. I. Multilocus models. *American Journal of Human Genetics*, **46**, 222–8.

Risch, N. and Merikangas K. R. (1996). The future of genetic studies of complex human diseases. *Science*, **273**, 1516–17.

Risch, N., Spiker, D., Lotspeich, L. *et al.* (1999). A genomic screen of autism: evidence for a multilocus etiology. *American Journal of Human Genetics*, **65**, 493–507.

Ritvo, E. R., Freeman, B. J., Mason-Brothers, A., and Ritvo, A. M. (1985). Concordance for the syndrome of autism in 40 pairs of afflicted twins. *American Journal of Psychiatry*, **142**, 74–7.

Ritvo, E. R., Jorde, L. B., Mason-Brothers, A. *et al.* (1989). The UCLA University of Utah epidemiologic survey of autism: recurrence risk estimates and genetic counseling. *American Journal of Psychiatry*, **146**, 1032–6.

Ritvo, E. R., Mason-Brothers, A., Freeman, B. J. *et al.* (1990). The UCLA University of Utah epiderniologic survey of autism: the etiologic role of rare diseases. *American Journal of Psychiatry*, **147**, 1614–21.

Rutter, M., Bolton, P., Harrington, R. *et al.* (1990). Genetic factors in child psychiatric disorders. I. A review of research strategies. *Journal of Child Psychology and Psychiatry and Allied Disciplines*, **31**, 3–37.

Shao, Y., Wolpert, C. M., Raiford, K. L. *et al.* (2002). Genomic screen and follow-up analysis for autistic disorder. *American Journal of Medical Genetics (Neuropsychiatric Genetics)*, **114**, 99–105.

Silliman, E. R., Campbell, M., and Mitchell, R. S. (1989). Genetic influences in autism and assessment of metalinguistic performance in siblings of autistic children. In G. Dawson, ed., *Autism Nature Diagnosis and Treatment*. New York: Guilford Press, pp. 225–9.

Silverman, M., Smith, J. Schmeidlor, J. *et al.*, and the Autism Genetic Research Exchange Consortium (2002). Symptom domains in autism and related conditions: evidence to familiality. *American Journal of Medical Genetics*, **114**, 64–73.

Smalley, S. L., Asarnow, R. F., and Spence, A. (1988). Autism and genetics: a decade of research. *Archives of General Psychiatry*, **45**, 953–61.

Smalley, S. L., McCracken, J., and Tanguay, P. (1995). Autism, affective disorders, and social phobia. *American Journal of Medical Genetics*, **611**, 19–26.

Smith, C. (1970). Heritability of liability and concordance in monozygous twins. *Annals for Human Genetics*, **26**, 85–91.

Smith, C. (1974). Concordance in twins: methods and interpretation. *American Journal of Human Genetics*, **26**, 454–66.

Snell, R. G., MacMillan, J. C., Cheadler, J. P. *et al.* (1993). Relationship between trinucleotide repeat expansion and phenotypic variation in Huntington's disease. *Nature Genetics*, **4**, 393–7.

Spiker, D., Lotspeich, L., Kraemer, H. C. *et al.* (1994). Genetics of autism: characteristics of affected and unaffected children from 37 multiple families. *American Journal of Medical Genetics (Neuropsychiatric Genetics)*, **54**, 27–35.

Steffenburg, S., Gillherg, C., Hellgren, L. *et al.* (1989). A twin study of autism in Denmark, Finland, Iceland, Norway and Sweden. *Journal of Child Psychology and Psychiatry*, **30**, 405–16.

Stevenson, R. E. and Huntley, C. C. (1967). Congenital malformations in offspring of phenylketonuric mothers. *Pediatrics*, **40**, 33–45.

Szatmari, P. and Jones, M. B. (1999). Effects of misclassification on estimates of relative risk in family history studies. *Genetic Epidemiology*, **16**, 368–81.

Szatmari, P., Jones, M. B., Tuff, L. *et al.* (1993). Lack of cognitive impairment in first-degree relatives of children with pervasive developmental disorders. *Journal of the American Academy of Child and Adolescent Psychiatry*, **32**, 1264–73.

Szatmari, P., Jones, M. B., Fisman, S. *et al.* (1995). Parents and collateral relatives of children with pervasive developmental disorders: a family history study. *American Journal of Medical Genetics (Neuropsychiatric Genetics)*, **60**, 282–9.

Szatmari, P., MacLean J. E., Jones, M. B. *et al.* (2000). The familial aggregation of the lesser variant in biological and nonbiological relatives of PDD probands: a family history study. *Journal of Child Psychology and Psychiatry*, **41**, 579–86.

Tordjman, S., Gutknecht, L., Carlier, M. *et al.* (2001). Role of the serotonin transporter gene in the behavioral expression of autism. *Molecular Psychiatry*, **6**, 434–9.

Wassink T. H., Piven, J., Vieland, V. J. *et al.* (2001). Evidence supporting WNT2 as an autism susceptibility gene. *American Journal of Medical Genetics*, **105**, 406–13.

Wolf, L. C., Noh, S., Fisman, S. N., and Speechley, M. (1989). Psychological effects of parenting stress on parents of autistic children. *Journal of Autism and Developmental Disorders*, **19**, 156–66.

Xu, J., Zwaigenbaum, L., Szatmari, P., and Scherer, S. (2004). Molecular cytogenetics of autism. *Current Genomics*, **5**, 347–64.

Ylisaukko-oja, T., Nieminen-von Wendt, T., Kempas, E. *et al.* (2004). Genome-wide scan for loci of Asperger syndrome. *Molecular Psychiatry*, **9**, 161–8.

Yonan, L., Alarcon, M., Cheng, R. *et al.* (2003). A genomewide screen of 345 families for autism-susceptibility loci. *American Journal of Human Genetics*, **73**, 886–97.

Young, J. G., Kavanagh, M. E., Anderson, G. M., Shaywitz, B. A., and Cohen, D. J. (1982). Clinical neurochemistry of autism and associated disorders. *Journal of Autism and Developmental Disorders*, **12**, 147–65.

Yu, C-E., Dawson, G., Munson, J. *et al.* (2002). Presence of large deletions in kindreds with autism. *American Journal of Human Genetics*, **71**, 100–15.

6

The neurobiology of autism

Fritz Poustka

Head, Department of Child and Adolescent Psychiatry, J. W. Goethe University

Introduction

The neurobiology of autism encompasses a wide range of neurophysiological, chemical, neuroimaging, and morphological research data. However, there is no unifying etiological concept from which to deduce and explain biological markers and the various causes and consequences of psychiatric and physical symptoms. For example, hypoactivation of the lateral right fusiform gyrus has been replicated as a neurofunctional marker, but it does not fully explain the social cognitive deficits in autism (Schultz et al., 2003) nor is it unique for autism (Quintana et al., 2003). Thus the relevance of obvious organic etiology to syndrome pathogenesis and the development of the affected child remains unclear. Some medical conditions arise during the course of autism (for example, seizures), whereas others may be present from very early in life and thus probably are more likely relevant to etiology

There are several challenges for reviewing the neurobiological basis of autism. Data are difficult to interpret because of small sample sizes, problems of diagnosis (particularly with severe mental retardation), a lack of reasonable control groups, a lack of replication studies, and contradictory findings due to the use of different classifying schemes and instruments. Examples of the latter are given by Eaves and Milner (1993) where they examine the relationship between two popular screening instruments for autism. Correlations between the Childhood Autism Rating Scale and the Aberrant Behavior Checklist ranged from -0.16 to 0.73 with a median of 0.39 and with a moderate correlation on the nominal classification produced by the two tests. Diagnostic problems in neurobiological research further complicate the issue because the most widely used classification systems in child psychiatry differed in their approach until recently. In The *Diagnostic and Statistical Manual of Mental Disorders* (DSM-III-R), criteria for autism tended

Autism and Pervasive Developmental Disorders, 2nd edn, ed. Fred R. Volkmar.
Published by Cambridge University Press. © Cambridge University Press 2007.

to lead to overdiagnosis compared with the *International Classification of Disease* (ICD-10) (Fombonne, 1992) and DSM-III (Volkmar & Cohen, 1988; Volkmar *et al.*, 1992). Given this, DSM-III-R guidelines work more like a screening test (Szatmari, 1992). Volkmar *et al.* (1992) compared the correlation between DSM-III, DSM-III-R, and the draft criteria of ICD-10, (ICD-10, 1993) in relation to each other and to clinical diagnosis. Since then, DSM-IV and Research Diagnostic Criteria of ICD-10 have moved closer to each other, partly as a result of the DSM-IV autism/pervasive developmental field trial (Volkmar *et al.*, 1994). The data from this field trial supported the ICD-10 approach because they had a better combination of a reasonable balance of sensitivity/specificity with coverage of the range of syndrome expression, and ease of use for clinical and research purposes.

Comorbidity is a major difficulty and source of lack of specificity in research findings. New epidemiological data show the overlap with mental retardation for autism spectrum disorder (ASD) (Chakrabarti & Fombonne, 2001) to be less than previously expected perhaps as a result of better and earlier intervention. Data from genetic studies, particularly the overlap in genomic scanning of attention deficit hyperactivity disorder (ADHD) with autism (Ogdie *et al.*, 2003), is also interesting in clinical studies. Finding commonalities in these different disorders would help resolve many conflicting results, but such work would require a higher number of samples and rigorous trial standards.

All this notwithstanding, if research data were repeated and were not too anecdotal or based in single case reports, they could at least serve to generate a hypothesis.

This review will cover any evidence that may suggest the importance of neurobiological mechanisms in syndrome pathogenesis within various fields, and medical conditions that arise during the course of autism, for example, high rates of seizures. Variants such as Asperger's syndrome and atypical autism will be discussed when appropriate and relevant.

Neurology and related conditions

Neurological dysfunction

Approximately 75% of autistic subjects show abnormalities on neurological examination. These include soft and hard signs (Lisch *et al.*, 1993). Both soft and hard signs correlated with level of intelligence (higher scores in more severely retarded subjects), without significant sex differences if intelligence was taken into account. Four percent had difficulties in the optomotoric activities, 5% in their reflex status, 5% had abnormal extrapyramidal signs, 15% abnormal muscle tones, 60% dysdiadochokinesia and approximately one-third had difficulties with gait or postural positioning. Fifteen percent of the autistic probands who developed some language exhibited problems in articulation and coordination of speech. Sensory deficits were noted as well with small numbers having visual (4%) or hearing (2%) problems. These figures are probably biased by the problem of participant cooperation during the examination. A third of the probands could only be observed during action, and sensory skills could only be checked superficially in about half of the sample. "Clumsiness" in this study did not differentiate high-functioning autism (HFA), Asperger's syndrome, or autism with slight or moderate mental retardation. Similarly, Ghaziuddin et al. (1994b) could not differentiate probands with Asperger's syndrome from those with HFA in regard to clumsiness as measured by tests of coordination (Rinehart et al., 2006).

There are few studies available with carefully controlled investigations in neurological dysfunction. Hallett et al. (1993) studied only five adults with autism. Three showed some gait irregularity, suggesting disturbance of the cerebellum. DeLong and Nohria (1994) reported positive neurological findings in half of the 40 probands with ASD.

Several additional abnormal signs were observed in children with autism. These included tone postural dysfunctions, dominance patterns, dermoglyphic patterns, and perinatal conditions. Kohen-Raz (1991) showed that weight distribution and toe synchronizations are stable from 5 years of age. Kohen-Raz et al. (1992) evaluated postural control in children with autism and mental retardation compared with normal children. Postural patterns differed in children with autism from the other groups and also from adults with vestibular disorders. Postural patterns in children with autism were more variable, less stable with more lateral sway, and this group also had more so-called stressful postures, i.e. putting excessive weight on one foot, toe, or heel. Instability of anteroposterior and total body sway, with some insensitivities to visual perception of environmental motion, were described by Gepner et al. (1995).

Interestingly, age of walking was not delayed in 93% of children with autism nor did age of onset of walking correlate with intellectual disability in a larger study of children with different disabilities (Kokubun et al., 1995)

Hand dominance patterns of parents and other relatives of children with autism showed no increased incidence of left-handiness (Boucher et al., 1990).

In the Basque Country, Arrieta et al. (1990) found different digital and palmar dermatoglyphic patterns in autistic boys compared with controls and other differences in autistic girls, postulating a genetic basis for these differences. However, Wolman *et al.* (1990) failed to establish discriminant patterns in dermatoglyphic analysis among children with autism and various control groups.

In autistic individuals an excess in neurological signs is not necessarily obvious, of course. In a careful study, Skjeldal *et al.* (1998) did find significant clinical differences in, for example, tendon reflexes and mobility problems between children with autism and the control group. Rühl *et al.* (2001) did not find differences in clumsiness between high-functioning and low-functioning autistic probands.

Pre- and perinatal conditions

The aim of many studies since the 1960s was to identify factors that were probably relevant for the etiology of autism. In this context, several studies found significantly increased rates of obstetric complications in pregnancies resulting in the birth of autistic persons compared with different control groups (Deykin & MacMahon, 1980; Knobloch & Pasamanick, 1975; Lobascher *et al.*, 1970). The abnormalities described were manifold and they comprised pre-, peri-, and postnatal complications, such as prolonged time of gestation, neonatal cyanosis, umbilical strangulation, and severe neonatal icterus.

In a Swedish register study (Hultman, 2002), perinatal risk factors linked to early fetal development were evaluated for association with maternal, pregnancy, delivery, and infant characteristics, and risk of infantile autism (according to the ICD-9 classification). This epidemiologically based case-control study for children younger than 10 years of age (born in Sweden 1973–93) compared 408 children with autism (321 boys) with 2040 matched controls. The risk of autism was associated with the mother smoking daily in early pregnancy, cesarean delivery, the baby being small for gestational age, having a five-minute Apgar score below 7 (which suggests an association of asphyxia with autism as a threefold risk factor), and congenital malformations. The threefold risk for autism among children of mothers born outside Europe or North America is probably influenced by selective migration of persons with a genetic vulnerability to autism or lack of immunity during pregnancy to certain viral infections uncommon in the mother's country of origin. No association could be reported for head circumference, maternal diabetes, being a twin, or season of birth. Thus findings suggested that intrauterine and neonatal factors related to deviant intrauterine growth or fetal distress may be important in the pathogenesis of autism and probably reflect not only genetic factors but medication by environmental influences. The results extend previous findings by other studies (e.g. Bolton *et al.*, 1997; Burd, 1999; Nelson *et al.*, 1991).

The study is limited for various reasons (approximately 50% of the cases were found by comparing prevalence data in the 1990s), but the most common comorbid classifications were rather rare (intellectual impairment moderate to severe, uncertainty of the kind of classification in 37 cases, partial–complex epilepsy in 8 cases, and unspecified epilepsy in 7 cases).

The results of these studies were inconsistent and partly contradictory. Today they are difficult to interpret for two reasons. First, the diagnostic criteria they used differ from the criteria used at present (i. e. DSM-IV- and ICD-10). Second, the studies themselves probably used variable diagnostic criteria, for example, including index probands exhibiting severe mental retardation with known etiology (such as rubella or tuberous sclerosis), and inclusion of probands exhibiting early-onset child psychosis.

These observations make us question what the nature and meaning of the increased birth complication rate are, and to what extent these complications could have an etiological function in causing autism. Since the late 1970s, research findings have increasingly highlighted the important role of genetic factors in the etiology of autism, and these findings lead to a change of view regarding the role of birth complications in the etiology of autism. It is important to mention that objective and reliable instruments to register and measure birth complications were available at this time and used for research: the "optimality concept" (Prechtl, 1980, modified by Gillberg, 1983) and the Rochester Obstetric Scale (Sameroff et al., 1982).

One of the first strong hints that genetic factors cause autism was given by the findings of Folstein and Rutter's twin study (1977). They found a highly increased concordance rate for autism in monozygotic (MZ) twins (36%), but not for dizygotic (DZ) twins (0%) (MZ: $n = 11$; DZ: $n = 10$). Steffenburg et al. (1989) found even higher concordance rates for monozygotic twins (60%) in contrast to dizygotic twins (3%).

Interestingly, Folstein and Rutter (1977) had found an increased rate of birth complications for the autistic twins, compared with their nonautistic twin siblings. Obviously twin studies cannot be generalized to singeltons because twinning itself affects a number of birth and malformation complications compared with singletons (Myrianthopoulos & Melnick, 1977) and these also have behavioral influences (Rutter & Redshaw, 1991). This finding can, along with the earlier research findings, suggest perinatal stress may cause significant brain damage for the autistic child and therefore probably may cause autism. However, there exist serious arguments and research findings that contradict this. Birth complications are a relatively nonspecific finding, and they can also be observed in children with autism as well as in nonautistic, healthy children. If birth complications are an etiologically relevant factor, autism would be expected to occur with increased frequency in populations with an increased risk for birth complications, such as in twins and populations with lower socioeconomical status. This seems not to be the case (Steffenburg & Gillberg, 1989). The complication factors observed in autistic probands are mostly quite mild and not usually known to cause severe brain damage or mental retardation (Bryson et al., 1988; Gillberg & Gillberg, 1983; Levy et al., 1988; Tsai & Stewart, 1983). It is not possible to identify one single birth complication factor or group of factors regularly associated with autism (Gillberg & Gillberg, 1983; Rutter, 1988). An increased rate of birth complications can also be found in children with cerebral palsy and severe mental retardation (Miller, 1989; Nelson & Ellenberg, 1986; Rantakallio & von Wendt, 1985), and in children with chromosomal aberrations and genetic disorders (Bailey et al., 1993a,b).

Gillberg and Gillberg (1983) found complications during the course of pregnancy for every autistic proband who later exhibited birth complications, and their conclusion was that birth complications could just have been the consequence of an existing prenatal abnormality. Perinatal complications, such as birth asphyxia, are not associated with autism except for those conditions that are correlated with prenatal complications (Goodman, 1990).

Further research strengthened the presumption that autism is likely to be a genetically determined disorder. An important finding was that the autism rate of first-grade relatives of autistic persons is 50- to 100-fold higher than the normal incidence of the disorder, while second-grade relatives have a normal risk. One conclusion is that several interactive genes must be responsible for the disorder (Risch, 1990a,b; Jorde et al., 1991). With reference to a subpopulation of autistic probands Bolton et al. (1993) found a correlation between the rate of birth complications and several indicators that the disorder was genetically determined.

Juul-Dam et al. (2001) found, in contrast to data from the normal population, a significantly higher incidence of uterine bleeding (but also a lower incidence of maternal vaginal infection, and less maternal use of contraceptives during conception) for autism, and in the pervasive developmental disorder not otherwise specified (PDD-NOS) group a higher incidence of hyperbilirubinemia. Again, no unifying feature could be established. On the basis of these findings, it appears to be quite unlikely that birth complication factors are directly responsible for the etiology of autism. In contrast, the concept of autism as a strongly genetically determined disorder supports the assumption that autism is a condition that produces an increased probability of pregnancy and birth complications.

Future research has to take into account the probable interactive nature of the relationship between autism and birth complications that are likely to influence the phenotype (severity) of the disorder.

EEG abnormalities and seizure disorders in autism

Early research findings reported an increased incidence of EEG abnormalities and seizure disorders in autistic persons (Ornitz, 1978). The prevalence of EEG abnormalities reported in the literature is high and in most studies more than half the autistic subjects have EEG abnormalities regardless of the occurrence of seizures (Tsai et al., 1985); all regions of the cortex, mostly bilateral, are involved (Minshew, 1991).

The incidence of epileptic seizures in autism range from about 25% to 30% by early adulthood (Volkmar & Nelson, 1990; Rutter, 1984, Deykin & MacMahon, 1979). These values are markedly increased compared with the normal population of children and adolescents (0.5%; Rossi et al., 1995) and also increased if compared with other psychiatric populations. Some studies report lower rates. Wong (1993) found only 5% of children with autistic conditions to have epilepsy, the majority of whom had onset of seizures before the age of 1 year.

Volkmar and Nelson (1990) found histories of seizure disorder in 21% of a sample of autistic subjects ($n = 192$). In a retrospective study undertaken by Carod et al. (1995), 47% of the children with autism were seen to exhibit some kind of epileptic syndrome. Using a different approach, Steffenburg et al. (1996) found, in a population of school-age children exhibiting the combination of mental retardation and active epilepsy, that 27% had an autistic disorder. All these findings demonstrate a strong association between autism and EEG abnormalities in seizure disorders.

Tuchman et al. (1991) reported different frequency of seizures according to various comorbid deficits. The major risk factor for epilepsy was severe mental deficiency in combination with motor deficits; 41% of children with autism with severe language delay exhibit autism. In those without language, motor deficits, associated perinatal or medical disorder, or positive family history of epilepsy, seizures occurred in only 6%. This rate was analogous to dysphasic non-children with autism (8%). The higher percentage in autistic girls (24%; 18 of 74) compared to boys (11%; 25 of 228) was in accord with the associated comorbidity mentioned above. Similar associations were seen in a study by Elia et al. (1995), leading to the conclusion that seizures are not related to autism (or the severity of autism) itself. Aman et al. (1995) reported that 19% of autistic subjects (all ages) had had epilepsy, but only 13% were taking anticonvulsant drugs. Nearly 19% had more than one seizure per month, nearly 40% had a 3-year seizure-free interval that could be an indication for anticonvulsant drug withdrawal.

The kind of EEG abnormalities and the types of seizures are various and heterogeneous. EEG abnormalities are described as diffuse or focal spikes, slow waves, and paroxysmal spike-and-wave activity with mixed discharge and mostly bilateral location (Minshew, 1991), and, respectively mostly focal and multifocal and typical of benign childhood partial epilepsy with centrotemporal spikes (Rossi *et al.*, 1995). In a study undertaken by Dawson *et al.* (1995), children with autism exhibited reduced EEG power in the frontal and temporal regions, but not in the parietal region. Differences were more prominent in the left than in the right hemisphere, and subgroups of children with autism displayed distinct patterns of brain activity ("passive" children with autism displayed reduced alpha EEG power in the frontal region, compared to children classified as "active but odd").

Autistic probands exhibit different types of epilepsy, and no particular epileptic syndrome was found to be more frequently correlated to autism (Elia *et al.*, 1995). Autistic individuals had generalized major motor seizures, hypsarrhythmia, absence episodes, and complex partial and myoclonic seizures (Elia *et al.*, 1995; Rossi *et al.*, 1995; Volkmar & Nelson, 1990).

Forty-five per cent of the subjects with autism observed by Rossi *et al.* (1995) had their first seizure after the age of 10 years. There appear to be two peaks of onset: early adulthood and during adolescence (Volkmar & Nelson, 1990). Volkmar and Nelson discuss the possibility that early onset of seizures could reflect a closer relation to pre- and perinatal relationships, and later onset a closer relation to other processes.

Females with autism have seizures more frequently than males (Elia *et al.*, 1995; Tuchman *et al.*, 1991). There is also a higher proportion of probands exhibiting seizures in combination with a lower level of intellectual functioning (Elia *et al.*, 1995), severe mental deficiency, motor deficit, and a positive family history of epilepsy (Tuchman & Rapin, 1991). Tuchman & Rapin (2002) give more evidence that the prevalence of epilepsy in autism is highest in adolescents and young adults with moderate-to-severe mental retardation, motor deficits, and severe receptive language deficits. The association of autism with clinical or subclinical epilepsy might denote common genetic factors in some cases.

Results of these studies suggest that the higher incidence of epilepsy was not related to organic pre-, peri-, and postnatal antecedents or cerebral lesions.

Similarly, severity of autism was not correlated with an increased risk to develop seizures. These findings lead to the conclusion that genetic factors may be responsible for both autism and epilepsy (Rossi *et al.*, 1995).

Neuroanatomy and brain imaging studies

Neuroanatomical findings

Few autopsy studies on autistic brains have been carried out and no neurochemical investigation is available to date. Ritvo *et al.* (1986) reported a decreased number of Purkinje cells in the cerebellum (vermis and hemispheres) in four autistic subjects. Williams *et al.* (1980) found no consistent abnormalities in four autistic brains, but reported a heavier brain weight in one of two idiopathic autistic cases.

Bailey *et al.* (1993b) reported a heavier brain weight in three of four brains of handicapped autistic individuals compared to the normal range in the population. An obvious decrease in neuronal density was not evident. Thus an excess of the number of neurons was suggested due to the epidemiological findings that autistic twins and singletons under the age of 16 years had significantly larger head circumferences in 42% and 37% (respectively) of the cases, suggesting signs of megencephaly as a contributory factor to autism. This suggestion was confirmed in a study (Piven *et al.*, 1995) using magnetic resonance imaging (MRI). Volumes of total brain, total brain tissue, and total lateral ventricle volumes in 22 male autistic individuals were significantly greater than in a control group and after controlling for height and performance IQ (the latter was significantly lower in the autistic individuals). Therefore enlargement of the brain seems to result from both more cerebral parenchyma brain tissue and greater lateral ventricle volume. Enlarged head circumference could be consistent with enlargement of the parietotemporal cortex, which governs visuospatial (splinter) skills. Deutsch and Joseph (2003) found that in a subgroup of children with autism with unevenly developed nonverbal skills, the nonverbal profile was correlated with an unusually large head circumference.

The most comprehensive study of anatomical alterations has been done by Bauman and Kemper. The brains of six patients have been studied systematically so far (Bauman, 1991; Bauman & Kemper, 1985; Kemper & Bauman, 1992; Raymond *et al.*, 1989, 1996). Of these, one was female, three had severe mental retardation, one was of normal intelligence (a 12-year-old boy). Three were younger subjects, aged 9, 10, and 12 years, the remainder were in their twenties. Four had seizures and had been treated with anticonvulsant medication.

No brain showed gross morphological abnormalities. Reduced neuronal cell size and increased cell-packing density, most significantly in the medial, cortical, and central nuclei of the amygdale, were observed in these cases compared to controls. This involved areas of the forebrain (hippocampus, subiculum, entorhinal cortex, amygdala, mammillary body, anterior cingulate cortex, and septum bilaterally). Pyramidal neurons (CA1, CA4) of the hippocampus displayed decreased complexity and extent of the dentric arbors. In the medial septal nucleus cell-packing density was increased and the neuronal size reduced. In the nucleus of the diagonal band of Broca (NDB) the neurons were found to be unusually large in the brains of younger individuals with autism and numbers were adequate; this was not so in the brains of older individuals with autism. The number of neurons of the NDB was reduced and the nucleus small in size. Moreover, all six brains had abnormalities in the cerebellum, and related inferior olive with a significant decrease of Purkinje cells and various decreases in granule cells throughout the cerebellar hemisphere. Further failure of retrograde cell loss and atrophy was seen in the olivary nucleus of the brainstem. Again, the three brains of older persons displayed adequate numbers but small and pale olivary neurons. The three younger brains were significantly enlarged but normal in number and appearance. In summary, these neuroanatomical abnormalities were related to the limbic system, the cerebellum, and the related inferior olive.

Bauman and Kemper (1994) came to several conclusions from these findings. Four patients who had had seizures and had received anticonvulsants showed no different abnormalities in their brains compared with the other two without seizures or medication. No differences were found between the brain of the only case with normal intelligence and the brains of the others. Abnormalities in the cerebellum and the related olivary nucleus suggest an onset prior to birth. The limbic system could present a developmental maturational shortening involving its circuitry. Dysfunction in these circuits may disrupt acquisition and understanding of information. In particular, the substrate of representational memory (involving sensory modalities and mediating of facts, experience, and events, and the integration and generalization of information) and not habit memory is impaired by the significant abnormalities in the hippocampal complex, amygdala, entorhinal cortex, septum, and medial mammillary body. The occurrence of retrograde loss of olivary neurons after cerebellar lesions could be associated with a cerebellar cortical lesion before the thirtieth week of gestation. Differences between brains of different ages may be due to an establishment of postnatal persistence of the prenatal projection to the cerebellar nuclei because of the early lack of availability of an adequate number of Purkinje cells as target cells for the mature inferior olivary projection. The fetal circuit is then unable to be sustained over time. Nevertheless, the etiology of these abnormalities remains unclear. Subsets of phenotypic expression may stem from a similar abnormal anatomical pattern.

The relationship to cerebellar abnormalities and therefore to the dysfunctions in autism is less clear. There is some evidence that cerebellar functions may contribute to autism. For example, the lateral cerebellum is strongly engaged during the acquisition and discrimination of sensory information and is not activated by the control of movement per se. This was confirmed by MRI of the lateral cerebellar output during passive and active sensory tasks in healthy volunteers (Goa et al., 1996). The strongest sensory discrimination occurred when sensory discrimination was paired with finger movements. Bauman and Kemper (1994) discuss the involvement of the cerebellum for higher functions (Schmamann, 1991) and the possibilities of disturbances of emotions, behavior, and learning due to cerebellar lesions. However, Peterson (1995) in his review concludes that findings on the cerebellum in autism (in neuroimaging studies) could be an epiphenomenon of early pathophysiological impairment during the development of the central nervous system, i.e. a correlate rather than an immediate cause (see below).

Findings of brain imaging studies
Cerebellum and MRI studies
Besides the discussion about cerebellar abnormalities in anatomical autopsy studies, the findings of MRI studies on alterations of cerebellar regions seemed to heighten the evidence that there could be some gross markers for autism. After investigations by the research group of Courchesne et al. (1988) showed hypoplasia of cerebellar vermian lobules VI and VII in children with autism, adolescents, and adults, Hashimoto et al. (1995) reported similar results. Courchesne et al. (1994a) provided a meta-analysis on vermal area measures of 78 patients with autism from four separate studies. Results showed the majority (85–92%) to have cerebellar hypoplasia and 8–16% to have hyperplasia. A similar distribution was reported by Courchesne et al. (1994b). They compared 50 patients with autism (aged 2–40 years) with a control group of 43 and found that 16% had cerebellar lobules VI and VII with a smaller area than in the control group. Six had 34% larger (hyperplastic) areas than the controls. Courchesne (1991) and Courchesne et al. (1994c) postulated that these findings are related to an impairment in the ability of autistic individuals to shift their attention rapidly between auditory and visual stimuli.

However, these findings could not be replicated by others and remain somewhat inconclusive for various reasons (Peterson, 1995). In their MRI study of the cerebellar vermis in 102 patients with a variety of neurogenetic abnormalities against 125 normal controls, Schaefer *et al.* (1996) concluded hypoplasia of cerebellar vermal lobules VI and VII to be a nonspecific anatomical marker in autism. This nonspecificity is underlined in the studies of Reiss *et al.* (1988, 1991), who found a significantly decreased area of the cerebellar vermis in fragile X syndrome.

In various samples of different sizes heterogeneous or no results on cerebellar volume measures were reported (Ciesielski & Knight, 1994; Ekman *et al.*, 1991; Hashimoto *et al.*, 1992a; Holttum *et al.*, 1992; Kleiman *et al.*, 1992; Nowell *et al.*, 1990; Piven *et al.*, 1990, 1992). In the study of Piven *et al.* (1992), cerebellar lobules VI–VII were found not to be smaller in autistic subjects compared to a control group of age- and IQ-comparable male volunteers. No differences were found after multivariate analysis adjusting for midsagittal brain area (MSBA), age, and IQ (MSBA was significantly larger than that for subjects in various control groups). This exemplifies the difficulties in interpreting the studies available so far. The source of the frequently conflicting results could be attributable to the selection criteria for control groups and autistic individuals (Holttum *et al.*, 1992) which should take into consideration developmental variation, IQ, age, socioeconomic status, maternal age, and other possibly underlying medical conditions. In a review of structural MRI studies Brambilla *et al.* (2003) concluded that there should be rigorous matching between patients with autism and normal controls based on a checklist developed by Strakowski *et al.* (2002). Courchesne *et al.* (1994b) retrospectively reanalyzed four MRI studies and reported that the majority of patients had hypoplasia of vermal lobules VI–VII. Abell *et al.* (1999) found increased vermis pyramis gray matter density in young adults with HFA compared to matched normal controls. Studies on cerebellar hemispheres remain contradictory in well-designed studies (Brambilla *et al.*, 2003).

Other brain abnormalities in MRI studies

The significance of earlier findings of an enlarged ventricular system, mainly based on computed tomography studies have been complicated to understand and results are conflicting. The relation to developmental delay and regression, use of medication, seizures, and the often poorly controlled relation to a general enlargement of the ventricular system all increase the difficulties in interpreting associations (Minshew & Dombrowski, 1994). Piven *et al.* (1995) also observed larger lateral ventricles in autistic probands but also greater brain volume (see above). Increased brain volume in younger children in contrast to older children and age-matched controls were found in studies by Sparks *et al.* (2002) and Courchesne *et al.* (2001). Aylward *et al.* (2002) discovered an increase of brain volume in children under 12 years, with slight decrease in children over 12 years, compared to a carefully matched control group, suggesting an accelerated growth in early life as both age groups had abnormal head sizes.

A significantly smaller size of the brainstem (midbrain and medulla oblongata) in high-functioning children with autism was observed by Hashimoto *et al.* (1993) regardless of their developmental quotient or IQ (Hashimoto *et al.*, 1992). The size of the pons did not differ from controls, in contrast to an earlier report by Hashimoto *et al.* (1991) where it had been found to be significantly smaller. Hsu *et al.* (1991) could not find differences in the sizes of the midbrain and pons between normal children and those with autism. These results show no unique problems in the pathway to and from the cerebellum. Midbrain abnormalities would also suggest some associations to the neurotransmitter system.

In a study by Courchesne *et al.* (1993) parietal lobes were abnormal in appearance in 9 of 21 patients with autism due to cortical volume loss with some extension to superior frontal and occipital loss. As the size of the corpus callosum in the posterior subregions was observed to be reduced in 51 patients with autism of various levels of mental retardation and ages (against a control group matched for age and sex), Egaas *et al.* (1995) postulated an involvement of the parietal lobe over projection fibers in autism. Saitoh *et al.* (1995) found no malformation in the hippocampal region in autistic cases with cerebellar vermian lobules VI and VII or in the posterior portion of the corpus callosum. Cody *et al.* (2002) postulated that findings of a reduction in the size of the corpus callosum (discrepant due to enlargement of brain volume) may serve as an indication of an overall disconnectivity in autism or that only selected layers contribute axons that cross at the corpus callosum.

Observations of cortical malformations are seldom reported. Piven *et al.* (1990) found cerebral cortical malformations in a controlled study of 13 high-functioning male autistic cases consisting of polymicrogyria, macrogyria, and schizencephaly. They postulated neuronal defects of migration during the first 6 months of gestation. Berthier *et al.* (1990) described left frontal macrogyria and bilateral opercular polymicrogyria in two cases with Asperger's syndrome. Focal pachygyria was seen in 3 of 13 children with autism, which also suggests neuronal migration abnormalities in a study by Schifter *et al.* (1994). Kates *et al.* (2004) described differences between twins concordant versus discordant for autism. Discordant twin pairs showed lower frontal, temporal, and occipital volumes than in the compared subjects. A computerized analysis by Casanova *et al.* (2002) showed greater neuronal dispersion and normal cell density in the brains of patients with autism, and more and less compact minicolumns in the frontal and temporal cerebral lobes, possibly influencing information processing.

Functional abnormalities in the brain (fMRI, PET, and SPECT studies)

Siegel *et al.* (1995) compared 14 autistic adults with 25 with schizophrenia and 20 normal controls in the continuous performance test, and correlated glucose metabolic rate (GMR) using positron emission tomography (PET) in selected regions. In patients with autism, negative correlation of the medial frontal cortical GMR with attentional performance was observed, in contrast to the control groups. Glucose metabolic rate asymmetry was observed in an earlier study by Siegel *et al.* (1992). Autistic adult patients had a greater left than right anterior rectal gyrus GMR, in contrast to the control group's right-less-than-left asymmetry in the same region. Low GMR in the left posterior putamen and high GMR in the right posterior calcaric cortex in the autistic cases was also reported. Schifter *et al.* (1994) (see above) also found hypometabolic abnormalities in 4 of 13 children with autism who also had abnormalities in magnetic resonance imaging (MRI). This suggests that it would be fruitful to search for subtle abnormalities using MRI techniques after findings of regional metabolic aberration are revealed by PET.

Gillberg *et al.* (1993) studied the regional cerebral blood flow (rCBF) using ^{99m}Tc SPECT 26 (single photon emission computed tomography) in patients with autism plus an additional six patients with autistic-like conditions; there was no control group. The main finding in the patients without epilepsy was temporal hypofusion, mostly bilateral, but most pronounced on the left side. Nine of 16 patients had also displayed hypoperfused prefrontal and frontal areas. This was most pronounced in patients without mental retardation and often unilateral, but with no special side preference. This study is partly in agreement with George *et al.* (1992) who studied a small group of four young autistic adults and controls using high-resolution brain SPECT. The total brain perfusion and the regional flow were significantly reduced in the right lateral temporal and in the right, left, and midfrontal lobes as compared with the controls.

Minshew *et al.* (1993) reported clinical deficits and correlating alterations in high-energy phosphate and membrane phospholipid metabolism in the dorsal prefrontal brain of 11 high-functioning autistic subjects (aged 12–36 years). The control group was carefully matched for age, sex, IQ, race, and socioeconomic status. When the energy status of the brain (*in vivo* ^{31}P nuclear magnetic resonance spectroscopy) was compared within groups using neuropsychological and language test scores, a number of significant correlations were observed in the autistic group but not in the control group. Selected scores that correlated with alterations in high-energy phosphate and membrane phospholipid metabolism were drawn from the Wisconsin Card Sorting Test, from Test of Language Competence, semantic language comprehension, and secondary memory (delayed recall scores from the California Verbal Learning Test). Correlations followed a consistent pattern in parallel with the severity of autism. These findings were reported to be consistent with a hypermetabolic energy state and with under-synthesis and enhanced degradation of brain membranes.

Metabolic maturation delay was seen in the study using SPECT by Zilbovicius et al. (1995) after reporting a negative result earlier (Zilbovicius et al., 1992). Frontal hypoperfusion was found in five children with autism at age 3–4 years, corresponding to a pattern found in much younger normal children. Three years later, normalization of perfusion was seen in the same children. Regional cerebral blood flow (^{99m}Tc SPECT) was observed predominantly in the temporal and parietal lobes with more left abnormalities than right in six children with autism. In a small, controlled SPECT study, Wilcox et al. (2002) found significant hypoperfusion in the prefrontal areas of autistic individuals. Changes in perfusion over time correlated with language development. A deficiency in prefrontal areas could be associated with word identification and language formation skills.

The neuronal integrity of the prefrontal lobe, which is related to severity of clinical symptoms, was studied in a proton magnetic resonance spectroscopy of 14 probands with Asperger's syndrome and 18 matched controls. Murphy et al. (2002) revealed significantly higher prefrontal lobe concentration of N-acetylaspartate (which was significantly correlated with obsessional behavior), phosphocreatine, and choline (which was also significantly correlated with obsessional behavior).

Right temporal hypoperfusion in one, diffusely decreased right hemispheric uptake in another, and decreased frontal and occipital uptake in the third patient with Asperger's syndrome aged 12–16 years was found by McKelvey et al. (1995). In a PET study by Boddaert et al. (2002) of 21 autistic and 10 age-matched non-children with autism, significant bilateral temporal hypoperfusion was revealed in the associative auditory cortex (superior temporal gyrus) and multimodal cortex (superior temporal sulcus) in the autistic group, and temporal hypoperfusion was detected individually in 77% of the children with autism. Hypoperfusion of the temporal lobe in children with ASD was found in several other studies (Boddaert et al., 2002).

Chiron et al. (1995) also reported lack of normal hemispheric asymmetry. Eighteen children with autism, aged 4–17 years, were compared with 10 age-matched controls. They displayed higher left than right rCBF for the total hemispheres, and sensorimotor and language-related cortex to be independent of handiness, sex, and age, which suggests a left-hemispheric dysfunction. Children with autism with deficits in the theory of mind performed significantly worse than a control group of children on the ability to recognize mental-state terms in a word list (Baron-Cohen *et al.*, 1994). Subsequently, in a second experiment, increased cerebral blood flow in the right orbitofrontal cortex during the mental-state recognition task was observed in normal adult volunteers. This suggests that the right orbitofrontal cortex serves as the basis of this ability.

In a PET study (Castelli *et al.*, 2000), 10 able adults with autism or Asperger's syndrome and 10 matched controls watched interactively moving triangles, which were seen as animation (mentalizing) by the controls but not by the autistic group. The normal group showed increased activation in the "mentalizing network" (medial prefrontal cortex, superior temporal sulcus – STS – at the temporoparietal junction and temporal poles). The autism group showed less activation than the normal group in all these regions, but both groups showed activation of the extrastriate cortex, with, in the autism group, reduced functional connectivity with the superior temporal sulcus at the temporoparietal junction (an area associated with the processing of biological motion as well as with mentalizing).

The authors postulate that the difficulty in understanding mentalizing animation in the autism group is due to reduced activation in the STS, and normal activation in the inferior occipital gyrus (V3) in autism as a failure to transmit important information about the motion of the triangle from V3 to STS. This may reflect a lack of feedback from the temporal pole and/or medial prefrontal cortex to STS, resulting in an inability to perceive the social meaning of movements.

More sensitive functional (fMRI) measurements of brain activity during specific cognitive task responses have revealed a remarkably stable neurobiological marker (Schultz *et al.*, 2003). Abnormal activations are found for amygdale and frontotemporal regions for perception of emotions from eye expression, and in temporal and fusiform gyri during face discrimination (Baron-Cohen *et al.*, 1999; Critchley *et al.*, 2000; Hubl *et al.*, 2003; Pierce *et al.*, 2001; Schultz, 2000). In contrast to normal control groups, individuals with ASD activate other brain regions than the facial fusiform gyrus, revealing a predisposition to local rather than global modes of information processing (Hubl *et al.*, 2003). Similar activations can be shown in schizophrenia, so these abnormalities seem not to be specific to autism (Quintana *et al.*, 2003).

In an fMRI study, five adolescent and adult individuals with HFA were intensively trained in basic emotion detection over a period of five weeks, while a remaining five did not receive any comparable intervention (Boete *et al.*, 2004). Compared to the control group, the sample of trained subjects showed marked improvements on both behavioral measures, which were accompanied by higher signals in the right medial occipital gyrus and superior parietal lobule. No marked activation changes in the fusiform gyrus were found. These fMRI results may indicate that the observed improvements in facial emotion recognition on the behavioral level correlate on the neurobiological level with enhanced compensatory mechanisms rather than with a reutilization of face-specific cortical areas.

Neurochemistry

In his review, Cook (1990) emphasized the important body of work on neurochemistry in autism. In particular, hyperserotonemia shows a familial pattern and is found consistently in over 25% of children and adolescents with autism. The role in autism of the neurotransmitter serotonin (as well as the serotonin precursor tryptophan and tryptophan depletion) was studied in urine, serum, plasma platelets, cerebrospinal fluid (CSF) concentrations, and brain imaging studies.

Biochemical research in autism has two possible goals. One is to define a basis for treatment (as with selective serotonin receptor inhibitors); the other is to find markers for genetic "susceptibility" by examining receptor genes or changes of certain gene products such as neurotransmitters and their receptors.

Support for the hypothesis of a maturation defect of monoaminergic systems was seen by Martineau et al. (1992a) in an age-matched controlled study of 156 children with autism from 2–12 years of age, along with mentally retarded non-children with autism and normal children. Children with autism had high serotonin levels in the urine, but so did the non-children with autism. In all three groups the serotonin levels decreased with age. Similar results were seen for dopamine (DA) and its metabolite and for norepinephrine (NE) and epinephrine.

One possible effect of maturation on altering serotonin blood level was ruled out by Tordjman et al. (1995). Though levels of testosterone and whole-blood serotonin are significantly negatively correlated, no differences were found in the variation of androgen secretion (testosterone and dehydroepiandrosterone sulfate) between prepubertal and postpubertal in autistic and normal subjects.

Serotonin

Most of the more recent studies since Schain and Freedman's original report (1961) have shown elevation of blood serotonin in autistic subjects (Anderson et al., 1987; Minderaa et al., 1987; Naffah-Mazzacoratti et al., 1993). Rolf et al. (1993) investigated platelet levels of serotonin and the amino acids aspartic acid, glutamine, glutamic acid, and γ-aminobutyric acid. Serotonin levels were increased and amino acids decreased in autistic subjects compared with a healthy match control group. Piven *et al.* (1991) suggested an autosomal recessive defect as the reason for the hyperserotonemia. This could be a negative influence on fetal brain development (Buznikov, 1984). This result raises the importance of familial patterns of serotonemia. Furthermore, some investigations are studying the correlation of hyperserotonemia with symptom patterns related to autism. The whole blood serotonin (5HT), in contrast to plasma NE, was significantly positively correlated between children with autism and their parents and sibs in a replicated study by Leventhal *et al.* (1990). Twenty-three of 47 families had at least one additional member with hyperserotonemia and, of these, 10 families had two or more hyperserotonemic members with 5HT more than 270 ng/ml. Family members had a heightened risk for hyperserotonemia if the autistic child also had raised levels of blood 5HT. In the study by Piven *et al.* (1991) children with autism had the highest hyperserotonemia compared to their sibs. Serotonin levels in platelet-rich plasma were higher in autistic subjects who had affected siblings (affected with either autism or PDD) compared with those autistic probands without affected sibs. The latter had also significantly higher serotonin levels compared with normal controls.

Two groups investigated serotonin involvement in autism compared with other neuropsychiatric disorders and healthy control groups. Singh *et al.* (1990) studied lymphocyte binding of $[^3H]$-serotonin and found no difference between autistic and healthy children. Yuwiler *et al.* (1992) found no close relationship between elevated blood serotonin and inhibition of serotonin binding to human cortical membranes by antibody-rich blood fractions for autism (in contrast with multiple sclerosis).

The variation of serotonin level in autism may be explained by different binding and uptake mechanisms. Cook *et al.* (1993a) postulated subgroups for increased serotonin (5HT) uptake and decreased $5HT_2$ binding respectively. The affinity for $[^3H]$-paroxetine binding was higher in the normoserotonemic group, whereas the density (B_{max}) of platelet $5HT_2$ receptor-binding sites was significantly lower in the hyperserotonemic group. The two groups consisted of 12 hyperserotonemic and 12 normoserotonemic carefully matched relatives of autistic probands. Earlier findings by Perry *et al.* (1991) observed a correlation of density of platelet $5HT_2$-binding sites between autistic boys and their fathers. Norepinephrine seemed also to be involved in the heterologous regulation of $5HT_2$ receptors in the platelet due to a negative correlation of NE and B_{max}.

Elevated levels of serotonin seem to correlate with psychopathological symptoms in family members of autistic subjects. The same research group as above (Cook *et al.*, 1994) compared parents who had autistic offspring with parents of children with Down's syndrome. Hyperserotonemic parents of an autistic child scored significantly higher on a depression scale and on an obsessive–compulsive inventory than parents of children with Down's syndrome, and both groups of parents had lower depression scores when blood serotonin was not raised.

One investigation by Cuccaro et al. (1993) (limited by a possible bias attributable to race) of an association between cognitive (especially verbal expressive abilities) of autistic probands and first-degree relatives showed a substantial variance of cognitive performance correlated to whole-blood serotonin level adjusted for race and familial classification. Cook et al. (1990) also found a negative correlation between vocabulary performance and whole-blood serotonin in their study on children with autism, their sibs, and parents. This was also true for plasma NE. Moreover self-injurious behavior and decreased pain sensitivity – often reported in autistic probands (Lisch et al., 1993) – was not correlated with whole-blood serotonin or plasma NE level.

A significantly lower serum tryptophan to large neutral amino-acids ratio was observed by D'Eufemia et al. (1995) compared to normal controls. In approximately a third of the 40 children with autism in this study, this ratio was two standard deviations below the mean value of the control group. This would suggest a low brain tryptophan availability. This observation is strongly supported by the effects of tryptophan depletion in adults with autistic disorders (McDougle et al., 1996). Short-term tryptophan depletion exacerbated a number of behavior variables, such as stereotyped movements. Moreover, autistic subjects were more anxious and significantly less calm and happy after short-term tryptophan depletion compared with sham testing. These behavior changes occurred in parallel to a significantly reduced plasma-free and total tryptophan. No significant changes could be detected in social relationships, effectual reactions, sensory responses, language, or repetitive thinking and behavior. The lack of effects on repetitive thinking may be due to the short duration of the depletion.

However, it is not clear whether serotonin only has an effect on the many symptoms often associated with autism (aggression, motoric stereotype symptoms, aggression, impulsivity) rather than the core features of autism as such (communication and reciprocal social interaction). Disturbances of serotonergic pathways have been implicated in many neuropsychiatric disorders that include anxiety, depression, schizophrenia, alcoholism, migraine, aggression, and suicidal behavior (Erdmann et al. 1995; Heath & Hen, 1995; Lappalainen et al., 1995). Moreover, it is unclear whether tryptophan depletion affects neuropeptides, second messenger systems, receptor synthesis, or the balance with other neurotransmitter systems such as DA and NE (McDougle et al., 1996). Haarmann *et al.* (1998) found decreased values of the amino acids, such as glutamic acid, glutamine, aspartic acid, and γ-aminobutyric acid, as well as hyperserotonemia, and therefore presumed there was an imbalance between these neurotransmitters.

The difficulties in understanding the extent and kind of involvement of the serotonin neurotransmitter system, especially in autism, can be underlined by studies of the CSF. The central metabolite of serotonin (5-hydroxyindolacetic acid, 5-HIAA) was examined in the CSF of eight autistic subjects. Anderson *et al.* (1988) did not find any increase when compared to the normal population. Narayan *et al.* (1993) also did not find marked alterations of serotonin metabolite (5HIAA) CFS concentration (or of the dopamine metabolite homovanillic acid, HVA).

McBride *et al.* (1989) found a reduced amount of receptor-binding sites in the brain of autistic individuals and suggested this could be due to an autoimmune reaction, until now a mere hypothesis (Root-Bernstein & Westall, 1990; Todd *et al.* 1988). In a sample of 62 autistic subjects and 122 of their first-degree relatives (compared to age- and sex-matched controls) Leboyer *et al.* (1999) found familial hyperserotoninemia in autism, as mothers (51%), fathers (45%), and siblings (87%) had elevated levels of 5HT measured by radioenzymology.

Serotonin synthesis changes during developmental stages – it declines after the age of 5 years. In children with autism, serotonin synthesis capacity increases gradually between the ages of 2–15 years to values 1.5 times the adult normal values and shows no sex difference (in normal girls these values decline earlier than in normal boys). Data suggest that humans undergo a period of high brain serotonin synthesis capacity during childhood, and that this developmental process is disrupted in children with autism (Chugani *et al.*, 1999). In a small study of 13 male, post-pubertal, Caucasian patients with autism (age 12–18 years with IQs greater than 55) and 13 matched volunteers, Croonenberghs *et al.* (2000) found the serotonergic and noradrenergic markers showed significantly lower plasma concentrations of tryptophan in patients with autism than in the controls, and no significant differences in the serum concentrations of 5HT, or the 24-hour urinary excretion of 5HIAA, adrenaline, noradrenaline, and DA. They also found highly significant positive correlations between age and 24-hour urinary excretion of 5HIAA and serum tryptophan. The authors suggested that while serotonergic disturbances, such as defects in the 5HT transporter system and lowered plasma tryptophan, may play a role in the pathophysiology of autism, autism is not associated with alterations in the noradrenergic system, and the metabolism of serotonin in humans undergoes significant changes between the ages of 12–18 years. Thus the reported findings so far reveal still somewhat unclear results.

Dopamine

Another line of work has focused on the involvement of brain catecholamine dysfunction in the development and/or expression of autism. As with dopamine metabolism, high urinary levels of the metabolite HVA of children with autism were reported by different authors (Barthelemy et al., 1988; Garnier et al., 1986; Garreau et al., 1988). Narayan et al. (1993) (see above) and others have not found abnormal levels of CSF HVA in autism. In a study to measure melatonin concentration (because of the association with inhibition of calcium-dependent DA release from amacrine cells), Ritvo et al. (1993) reported preliminary results of daytime melatonin in the urine of 10 autistic subjects and family members and a (poorly matched) control group of normals. The autistic subjects, and some of their parents and unaffected sibs, showed a persistence of melatonin into the daylight hours in contrast to the control group. Nocturnal melatonin production did not differ.

In the meantime most of the receptor genes of DA could be localized (among them the D_2-receptor locus by Comings et al. (1991)) but none proved to be a primary etiologic agent for the autistic disorder. In 1989, Buckle et al. found a subunit of the GABA(3) receptor on Xq28, which Cohen related to autism (Cohen et al., 1991). Derry and Bernard (1991) found a further receptor gene on the short arm of the X chromosome, namely Xp21.3, the GABA A α3-subunit gene. However, definite links to autistic phenotypes have not been established yet.

Opioid peptides

Several studies have linked neuropeptides such as the endogenous opioids to autism (Gillberg, 1995; Lensing et al., 1992; Nagamitsu, 1993). In the Nagamitsu study patients with autism showed no significant difference of the CSF β-endorphin concentration compared with the controls. A higher level was found in Rett's syndrome and infections involving the central nervous system. Therapeutic studies in autism using the opioid antagonist naltrexone are inconclusive. Willemsen-Swinkels et al. (1995) found no, or a worsening, effect of symptoms in autistic adults and no effect on self-injury behavior.

Adrenergic function and stress

Other studies tried to exclude or include the role of further biochemical agents in autism. An elevation of epinephrine and NE in blood was found by Launay et al. (1987) and Barthelemy et al. (1988). Possible abnormalities of dopaminergic and noradrenergic neurotransmission were reported by Realmuto et al. (1990). In contrast, Minderaa et al. (1994) found no marked abnormalities when they investigated plasma levels and urinary excretion of NE, epinephrine and their central and peripheral metabolites respectively (MHPG, vanillylmandelic acid, VMA). Thus, basal noradrenergic functioning seems not to play an important role in autism.

Richdale and Prior (1992) studied cortisol circadian rhythm and dexamethasone suppression test effects in children with autism. No clear effects were found other than a tendency towards a cortisol hypersecretion during the day in children with autism who were integrated into the normal school system, indicating an environmental stress response.

Neurophysiology

Brainstem auditory-evoked responses

Prolonged transmission of information may be linked to dysfunctions of information-processing, and perceptual, particularly auditory, abnormalities in autism. Yet the evidence from these neurophysiological studies in autism is not conclusive.

In his review of 10 studies published in the previous 25 years reporting interpeak latencies of auditory brainstem responses (ABRs) in autism, Klin (1993) criticized the results as being only suggestive of brainstem involvement in autism. The reports displayed prolonged brainstem transmission times in five studies, as well as shortening (one study) or no abnormalities (five studies) in central transmission latencies. Moreover, the studies revealed peripheral hearing impairment in some of the autistic individuals. Some investigations show congruent findings of prolonged transmission times. Thivierge *et al.* (1990) studied 20 autistic and 13 mentally retarded subjects and found prolonged interpeak latencies in 80% of the autistic subjects. In a controlled study, Wong and Wong (1991) found a longer brainstem transmission time that correlated with autistic features rather than with mental retardation, age, or sex. Sersen *et al.* (1990) observed longer latencies for middle and late components, contrary to probands with Down's syndrome (who displayed shorter absolute and interpeak latencies for early components). Unfortunately, an effect of sedation could not be ruled out.

Event-related potentials

Event-related potentials (ERP) studies deal with orienting responses to novel information, modulation of attention, maintaining selective attention, and the topographic distribution of ERP components. Studies of ERP in autism are relatively rare and do not support a strong and unique discriminant effect related to autism. Positive (P) and negative (N) ERP amplitudes are measured in milliseconds after stimulus onset (e.g. P300 or P3) and such amplitudes are derived through substraction methods (e.g. PN as ERP differences between target and a different nontarget stimulus; Nd as ERP difference between target stimulus and the same stimulus previously presented as a nontarget).

Oades *et al.* (1990) published ERP amplitudes (e.g. N1, P3, PN, Nd) that were reduced in autistic subjects compared to normals, but the components affected varied. Kemner *et al.* (1995) (see below) overlooked auditory "oddball" studies in autism and concluded that the findings were inconsistent with respect to P3 and N1.

In a carefully designed study, Kemner *et al.* (1995) could not replicate earlier studies of abnormal mismatch negativity (MMN, resulting from the subtraction of potentials to different nontargets) in children with autism. Abnormal lateralization of abnormal MMN could not be found. Unexpected occipital P3 to deviant stimuli was significantly larger in the active than passive condition. This and the one replication that could be observed, namely the smaller A/Pcz/300, led to the suggestion that auditory occipital task effect is related to understimulation of the occipital lobe by visual stimuli in children with autism. As the autistic subjects differed not only from the normal control group but also from those with ADHD and dyslexia, the effects were suggested as highly specific for autism. Kemner *et al.* (1994) also reported differences specific to children with autism on ERPs for visual and somatosensory stimuli. Only the autistic group displayed a task effect on the visual P2N2 (mismatch activity) and larger P3s to novel than to deviant stimuli, again compared with hyperactive and dyslexic children. Therefore abnormalities in the processing of proximal and distal stimuli were regarded as specific for autism. No abnormal lateralization was observed.

Some more recent studies revealed abnormalities associated with the primary and secondary auditory cortex when the N1 (which is generated in the primary and secondary auditory cortex) in both children with autism and with receptive developmental language disorder (but not in controls) did not increase with increasing stimuli (Lincoln *et al.*, 1995). Lincoln *et al.* (1993) found an abnormally small amplitude of the P3b that was seen as evidence for difficulties of children with autism in auditory information. P3b was significantly diminished in size under focused selective attention conditions in autistic subjects compared with normals, which suggests abnormalities in selective attention in autism (Ciesielski *et al.*, 1990). "Emotional sounds" appeared to be particularly effective in activating the neural substrate of the P3 generator system. Autistic subjects with normal IQ did not differ in this respect from normals (Erwin *et al.*, 1991). P1 auditory ERP abnormalities in high-functioning adult autistic individuals were studied by Buchwald *et al.* (1992), who suggested that the ascending reticular activating system and their thalamic target cells may be dysfunctional in autism.

A correlation of ERP with attempts to identify idiomatic phrases in high-functioning adult autistic probands was found by Strandburg *et al.* (1993) (greatly reduced N400 to idioms). Additionally, autistic subjects produced larger N1 amplitudes in all tasks, and larger P3s in the Idiom Recognition Task and Continuous Performance Task.

Martineau *et al.* (1992a, 1992b) observed a cognitive deficit in the ability to maintain cross-modal associations in autism, preceded by a more elementary perceptive abnormality in studying auditory evoked responses to simple and cross-modal (audiovisual) stimuli in a controlled study of autistic, mentally retarded, and normal children. This could be related to dysfunctions of attention, intention, association, and communication.

Overall, many of these psychophysiological studies describe different aspects of possible links to some key or associated features of autism. At present an integrative approach to understand the impairment in perceptual and information processing (Oades & Eggers, 1994) on a neurophysiological level is needed in further studies.

Other medical conditions

Gillberg (1992) listed a number of syndromes and diseases associated with autism in at least two studies (fragile X syndrome, other X-chromosomal anomalies, partial trisomy 15, other chromosome anomalies, tuberous sclerosis, neurofibromatosis, hypomelanosis, Goldenhar's syndrome, Rett's syndrome, Möbius' syndrome, PKU, lactic acidosis, hypothyroidism, rubella embryopathy, herpes encephalitis, cytomegalovirus infection, Williams' syndrome, and Duchenne muscular dystrophy). The list could be continued. Fernell *et al.* (1991) found that 23% of a population of children with infantile hydrocephalus scored high on the Aberrant Behavior Checklist. These children comprised the most brain damaged and mentally retarded group.

More anecdotal reports deal with autism and exposure in utero to valproic acid (Christianson *et al.*, 1994), in fetal alcohol syndrome (Harris *et al.*, 1995), with lead exposure beyond the third year of life (and re-exposure) (Shannon & Graef, 1996), and thalidomide embryopathy (Stromland *et al.*, 1994). Also reported are syndromes such as Marfan-like disorder (and Asperger's syndrome; Tantam *et al.*, 1990), Sotos' syndrome (Morrow *et al.*, 1990), Brachmann–de Lange syndrome (Bay *et al.*, 1993), Joubert's syndrome (Holroyd *et al.*, 1991), and Noonan's syndrome (Ghaziuddin *et al.*, 1994). Other mixed causes have been studied, such as left temporal oligodenroglioma (Hoon & Reiss, 1992), herpes encephalitis at age 31 years (Gillberg, 1991), congenital hypothyreoidism (Gillberg *et al.*, 1992), Tourette's syndrome (Comings & Comings, 1991; Sverd, 1991), mutation in adenylsuccinate lyase (Stone *et al.*, 1992), PKU (Miladi *et al.*, 1992), gangliosides (Lekman *et al.*, 1995), high levels of glial fibril acidic protein (Ahlsen *et al.*, 1993; Rosengren *et al.*, 1992), and congenitally blind children (Goodman & Minne, 1995). Congenital rubella has been ruled out since the early reports by Chess (1977). Chess argued, that neither visual nor hearing impairments nor severity of mental retardation was of importance for autism; it does appear that "autistic features" become less striking in these individuals over time.

Chromosomal aberrations have also been associated with autistic symptoms. These include a de-novo translocation t(3;12) (p26.3;q23.3) of tuberous sclerosis and autistic behavior in a child (Fahsold *et al.*, 1991), deletion of chromosome 5 (Barber *et al.*, 1994), inv dup(15) (pter–q13) (Schinzel, 1990), 15q12 deletion (Kerbeshian *et al.*, 1990), tetrasomy 15 (Hotopf & Bolton, 1995), duplication of the 15q11–13 region (Bundey *et al.*, 1994), a partial 16p trisomy with autistic disorder and Tourette's syndrome (Hebebrand *et al.*, 1994), deletion of 17 (p11.2 p11.2), Asperger's syndrome in a balanced t(17;19)(p13.3;p11) translocation (Anneren *et al.*, 1995), trisomy 17 (Shaffer *et al.*, 1996), 18q-chromosomal abnormality (Ghaziuddin *et al.*, 1993; Seshadri *et al.*, 1992), Y chromosome (Blackman *et al.*, 1991), Xp duplication (Rao *et al.*, 1994), and 46,X,t(X;8) (p22.13;q22.1) duplication (Bolton *et al.*, 1995), revealing a mixed picture of locations.

Autism is relatively rarely to be seen in children with Down's syndrome. In anecdotal case reports an overlap between these two conditions has been observed (Ghaziuddin *et al.*, 1992; Howlin *et al.*, 1995). Bolton *et al.* (1994) reported a lesser variant of autism in 1.6% to 3.2% of the siblings of Down's syndrome cases.

Links to autoimmune disorders, C4 deficiency and autism, were proposed by Warren *et al.* (1991, 1994, 1995); antibodies to myelin basic protein have also been reported (Singh *et al.*, 1993). Daniels *et al.* (1995) suggested that one or more genes of the major histocompatibility complex are involved in the development of same cases of autism. α-Interferonemia, which contributes to allergies and autoimmune phenomena, was found to be increased in children with autism in a very preliminary study (Stubbs, 1995). Cook *et al.* (1993b) did not find that autoantibodies to serotonin receptors (5HT1A and 5HT2), α_2-adrenergic, D1 and D2 receptors and/or associated membrane proteins are of importance in children with autism.

Exposure to influenza epidemics during gestation was not found to be associated with autism in the study by Dassa *et al.* (1995). In addition, several studies were performed to investigate the existence of excesses of births of children with autism in certain seasons (speculations range from exposure to infections to nutrition or other effects). Gillberg found an excess for March births, as did Mouridsen *et al.* (1994) and Barak *et al.* (1995) for March and August births. Bolton *et al.* (1992) could not replicate earlier findings of any seasonal birth effects.

There are a few known medical conditions with some importance to autism, namely Rett's syndrome, fragile X syndrome, and tuberous scleroses.

Girls with Rett's syndrome exhibit autistic-like symptomatology, but they also show differences after the preschool years (Olsson & Rett, 1990).

Several reports initially indicated an association of the fragile X chromosomal anomaly with autism (Watson *et al.*, 1984; Blomquist *et al.*, 1985; Cohen *et al.*, 1991; Bailey *et al.*, 1993a), whereas others did not support this finding (Venter *et al.*, 1984; Einfeld *et al.*, 1989). With knowledge of the FMR-1 gene responsible for fragile X syndrome (Oberlé *et al.*, 1991; Verkerk *et al.*, 1991; Yu *et al.*, 1991) and the possibility of a more exact molecular genetic analysis, the lack of association of fragile X and autism was confirmed (Hallmayer *et al.*, 1994). Discrepancies between the various studies appear to be due to differences in ascertainment strategy, diagnostic criteria for autism, and varying thresholds for the cytogenetic diagnosis of fragile X at Xq27.3. Klauck *et al.* (1996) performed Southern blot analysis with a FMR-1 specific probe. No significant changes were found in 139 patients (99%) from 122 families other than the normal variations in the population. In the case of one multiplex family with three children showing no dysmorphic features of fragile X syndrome (one male meeting three out of four ADI-algorithm criteria, one normal male with slight learning disability but negative ADI-R testing, and one fully autistic female) FRAXA full mutation-specific CCG repeat expansion in the genotype was not consequently correlated with the autism phenotype. Further analysis revealed a mosaic pattern of methylation at the FMR-1 gene locus in the two sons of the family, indicating at least a partly functional gene. Therefore an association of autism with fragile X at Xq27.3 does not exist and excludes this location as a candidate gene region for autism.

According to prevalence studies of Hunt and Shepherd (1993) and Gillberg *et al.* (1994) tuberous sclerosis and autism are suggested to be strongly associated. Smalley *et al.* (1992) reported significantly more frequent seizures and more severe mental retardation in children with tuberous sclerosis and autism, compared with tuberous sclerosis without autism. Despite an equal ratio of males to females with tuberous sclerosis, those with both conditions were predominantly males.

There are two contrasting views about the etiology of autism (Bailey, 1993), which have wide implications for neurobiological research and interpretation.

Gillberg and Coleman (1992) on the one hand are convinced that autism is not a homogeneous disease but one with several different pathogenic pathways analogous to some other disorders with a stable course, such as cerebral palsy. Different syndromes are associated with autism (37% of cases with autism after intensive neurobiological investigation; Gillberg, 1992), and the significant psychopathology of autism or severity of mental retardation are not different from idiopathic cases. The search for autism-specific causes is therefore misleading in their view, but assessment requires neuropsychiatric assessment, including laboratory examination with lumbar punctures and CFS protein electrophoresis to rule out progressive encephalopathy and other more common clinical problems.

On the other hand, Rutter et al. (1994) reviewed the literature on the relationship between autism and different medical conditions and concluded that the rate of such underlying known conditions in autism is around 10% depending on the severity of the mental retardation; they are much more common in cases with profound mental retardation.

Furthermore the strength of association between autism and known medical conditions is seldom tested to compare the frequency of the association of autism with a certain condition versus the condition in relation to autism.

REFERENCES

Ahlsen, G., Rosengren, L., Belfrage, M. et al. (1993). Glial fibrillary acidic protein in the cerebrospinal fluid of children with autism and other neuropsychiatric disorders. *Biological Psychiatry*, **33**, 734–43.

Aylward, E. H., Minshew, N. J., Field, K., Sparks, B. F., and Singh, N. (2002). Effects of age on brain volume and head circumference in autism. *Neurology*, **59**(2), 175–83.

Aman, M. G., van Bourgondien, M. E., Wolford, P. L., and Sarphare, G. (1995). Psychotropic and anticonvulsant drugs in subjects with autism: prevalence and patterns of use. *Journal of the American Academy of Child and Adolescent Psychiatry*, **34**, 1672–81.

Anderson. G. M., Freedman, D. X., Cohen, D. J. et al. (1987). Whole blood serotonin in autistic and normal subjects. *Journal of Child Psychology and Psychiatry*, **28**, 885–900.

Anderson, G. M., Ross, D. L., Klykylo, W., Feibel, F. C., and Cohen, D. J. (1988). Cerebrospinal fluid indoleacetic acid in autistic subjects. *Journal of Autism and Developmental Disorders*, **18**, 259–62.

Anneren, G., Dahl, N., Uddenfeldt, U., and Janols, L. O. (1995). Asperger's syndrome in a boy with a balanced de novo translocation: t(17;19)(p13. 3;p11). *American Journal of Medical Genetics*, **56**, 330–1.

Arrieta, M. I., Martinez, B., Criado, B. *et al.* (1990). Dermatoglyphic analysis of autistic Basque children. *American Journal of Medical Genetics*, **35**, 1–9.

Bailey, A. J. (1993). The biology of autism [editorial] *Psychological Medicine*, **23**, 7–11.

Bailey, A., Bolton, P., Butler, L. *et al.* (1993a). Prevalence of the fragile X anomaly amongst autistic twins and singletons. *Journal of Child Psychology and Psychiatry*, **34**, 673–88.

Bailey, A., Luthert, P., Bolton, P. *et al.* (1993b). Autism and megalencephaly. *Lancet*, **341**(854), 1225–6.

Bailey, A., Luthert, P., Dean, A. *et al.* (1998). A clinicopathological study of autism. *Brain*, **121**, 189–905.

Barak, Y., Ring, A., Sulkes, J., Gabbay, U., and Elizur, A. (1995). Season of birth and autistic disorder in Israel. *American Journal of Psychiatry*, **152**, 798–800.

Barber, J. C., Ellis, K. H., Bowles, L. V. *et al.* (1994). Adenomatous polyposis coli and a cytogenetic deletion of chromosome 5 resulting from a maternal intrachromosomal insertion. *Journal of Medical Genetics*, **31**, 312–16.

Baron-Cohen, S., Ring, H., Moriarty, J. *et al.* (1994). Recognition of mental state terms. Clinical findings in autistic children and a functional neuroimaging study of normal adults. *British Journal of Psychiatry*, **165**, 640–9.

Baron-Cohen, S., Ring, H. A., Wheelwright, S. *et al.* (1999). Social intelligence in the normal and autistic brain: an fMRI study. *European Journal of Neuroscience*, **11**(6), 1891–8.

Barthelemy, C., Bruneau, N., Cottet-Eymard, J. M. *et al.* (1988). Urinary free and conjugated catecholamines and metabolites in autistic children. *Journal of Autism and Developmental Disorders*, **18**, 583–91.

Bauman, M. L. (1991). Microscopic neuroanatomic abnormalities in autism. *Pediatrics*, **87**, 791–6.

Bauman, M. and Kemper, T. L. (1985). Histoanatomic observations of the brain in early infantile autism. *Neurology*, **35**, 866–74.

Bauman, M. L. and Kemper, T. L. (1994). Neuroanatomical observations of the brain in autism. In M. L. Bauman and T. L. Kemper, eds., *The Neurobiology of Autism*. Baltimore: Johns Hopkins University Press, pp.119–45.

Bay, C, Mauk, J., Radcliffe, J., and Kaplan, P. (1993). Mild Brachmann–de Lange syndrome. Delineation of the clinical phenotype, and characteristic behaviors in a six-year-old boy. *American Journal of Medical Genetics*, **47**, 965–8.

Bieber-Martig, B., Werner, K., and Poustka, F. (1996). Die Rolle von prä- und perinatalen Faktoren in der Ätiologie des Autismus und neurologische Dysfunktion. *Zeitschift für Kinder- und Jugendpsychiatrie.*

Blackman, J. A., Selzer, S. C., Patil, S., and van Dyke, D. C. (1991). Autistic disorder associated with an iso-dicentric Y chromosome. *Developmental Medicine and Child Neurology*, **33**, 162–6.

Blomquist, H. K., Bohman, M., Edvinsson, S. O. *et al.* (1985). Frequency of the fragile X syndrome in infantile autism. *Clinical Genetics*, **27**, 113–17.

Boddaert, N. and Zilbovicius, M. (2002). Functional neuroimaging and childhood autism. *Pediatric Radiology*, **32**(1), 1–7.

Bolton, P., Pickles, A., Harrington, R., Macdonald, H., and Rutter, M. (1992). Season of birth: issues, approaches and findings for autism. *Journal of Child Psychology and Psychiatry*, **33**, 509–30.

Bolton, P., Murphy, M., Sim, L. *et al.* (1993). Obstetrical complications in autism: consequences rather than causes of the disorder? Paper presented at the 3rd World Congress of Psychiatric Genetics, New Orleans, October 25, 1993. *Psychiatric Genetics*, **3**, 178.

Bolton, P., Macdonald, H., Pickles, A. *et al.* (1994). A case-control family history study of autism. *Journal of Child Psychology and Psychiatry*, **35**, 877–900.

Bolton, P., Powell, J., Rutter, M. *et al.* (1995). Autism, mental retardation, multiple exostoses and short stature in a female with 46,X,t(X;8)(p22. 13;q22. 1). *Psychiatric Genetics*, **5**, 51–5.

Bolton, P. F., Murphy, M., Macdonald, H., Whitlock, B., Pickles, A., and Rutter, M. (1997). Obstetric complications in autism: consequences or causes of the condition? *Journal of the American Academy of Child and Adolescent Psychiatry*, **36**(2), 272–81.

Boucher, J., Lewis, V., and Collis, G. (1990). Hand dominance of parents and other relatives of autsitic children. *Developmental Medicine and Child Neurology*, **32**, 304–13.

Brambilla, P., Hardan, A., di Nemi, S. U., Perez, J., Soares, J. C., and Barale, F. (2003). Brain anatomy and development in autism: review of structural MRI studies. *Brain Research Bulletin*, **61**(6), 557–69.

Bryson, S. E., Smith, I. M., and Eastwood, D. (1988). Obstetrical suboptimality in autistic children. *Journal of the American Academy of Child and Adolescent Psychiatry*, **27**, 418–22.

Buchwald, J. S., Erwin, R., van Lancker, D. *et al.* (1992). Midlatency auditory evoked responses: PI abnormalities in adult autistic subjects. *Electroencephalography and Clinical Neurophysiology*, **84**, 164–71.

Buckle, V. J., Fujita, N., Bateson, A. N., Darlison, M. G., and Barnard, E. A. (1989). Localization of the human GABA-A3 receptor subunit gene to Xq28: a candidate gene for X-linked mental depression. *Cytogenetics and Cell Genetics*, **51**, 972.

Bundey, S., Hardy, C., Vickers, S., Kilpatrick, M. W., and Corbett, J. A. (1994). Duplication of the 15q 11–13 region in a patient with autism, epilepsy and ataxia. *Developmental Medicine and Child Neurology*, **36**, 736–42.

Burd, L., Severud, R., Kerbeshian, J., and Klug, M. G. (1999). Prenatal and perinatal risk factors for autism. *Journal of Perinatal Medicine*, **27**(6), 441–50.

Buznikov, G. A. (1984). The action of neurotransmitters and related substances on early embryo-genesis. *Pharmacology and Therapeutics*, **25**, 23–59.

Carod, F. J., Prats, J. M., Garaizar, C., and Zuazo, E. (1995). Clinical–radiological evaluation of infantile autism and epileptic syndromes associated with autism. *Revue Neurologique*, **23**, 1203–7.

Casanova, M. F., Buxhoeveden, D. P., Switala, A. E., and Roy, E. (2002). Minicolumnar pathology in autism. *Neurology*, **58**(3), 428–32.

Chakrabarti, S. and Fombonne, E. (2001). Pervasive developmental disorders in preschool children. *Journal of the American Medical Association*, **285**(24), 3093–9.

Chess, S. (1977). Follow-up report on autism in congenital rubella. *Journal of Autism and Childhood Schizophrenia*, **7**, 68–81.

Chiron, C, Leboyer, M., Leon, F. *et al.* (1995). SPECT of the brain in childhood autism: evidence for a lack of normal hemispheric asymmetry. *Developmental Medicine and Child Neurology*, **37**, 849–60.

Christianson, A. L., Chesler, N., and Kromberg, J. G. (1994). Fetal valproate syndrome: clinical and neuro-developmental features in two sibling pairs. *Developmental Medicine and Child Neurology*, **36**, 361–9.

Chugani, D. C., Muzik, O., Behen, M. *et al.* (1999). Developmental changes in brain serotonin synthesis capacity in autistic and nonautistic children. *Annals of Neurology*, **45**(3), 287–95.

Ciesielski, K. T. and Knight, J. E. (1994). Cerebellar abnormality in autism: a nonspecific effect of early brain damage? *Acta Neurobiologiae Experimental Warszawa*, **54**, 151–4.

Ciesielski, K. T., Courchesne, E., and Elmasian, R. (1990). Effects of focused selective attention tasks on event-related potentials in autistic and normal individuals. *Electroencephalography and Clinical Neurophysiology*, **75**, 207–20.

Cody, H., Pelphrey, K., and Piven, J. (2002). Structural and functional magnetic resonance imaging of autism. *International Journal of Developmental Neuroscience*, **20**(3–5), 421–38.

Cohen, I. L., Sudhalter, V., Pfadt, A. *et al.* (1991). Why are autism and the fragile-X-syndrome associated? Conceptual and methodological issues. *American Journal of Human Genetics*, **48**, 195–202.

Comings, D. E. and Comings, B. G. (1991). Clinical and genetic relationships between autism-pervasive developmental disorder and Tourette syndrome: a study of 19 cases. *American Journal of Medical Genetics*, **39**, 180–91.

Cook, E. H. (1990). Autism: review of neurochemical investigation. *Synapse*, **6**, 292–308.

Cook, E. H. Jr., Leventhal, B. L., Heller, W. *et al.* (1990). Autistic children and their first-degree relatives: relationships between serotonin and norepinephrine levels and intelligence. *Journal of Neuropsychiatry Clinical Neurosciences*, **2**, 268–74.

Cook, E. H. Jr., Arora, R. C., Anderson, G. M. *et al.* (1993a). Platelet serotonin studies in hyper-serotonemic relatives of children with autistic disorder. *Life Sciences*, **52**, 2005–15.

Cook, E. H. Jr., Perry, B. D., Dawson, G., Wainwright, M. S., and Leventhal, B. L. (1993b). Receptor inhibition by immunoglobulins: specific inhibition by autistic children, their relatives, and control subjects. *Journal of Autism and Developmental Disorders*, **23**, 67–78.

Cook, E. H. Jr., Charak, D. A., Arida, J. *et al.* (1994). Depressive and obsessive-compulsive symptoms in hyperserotonemic parents of children with autistic disorder. *Psychiatry Research*, **52**, 25–33.

Courchesne, E. (1991). Neuroanatomic imaging in autism. *Pediatrics*, **87**, 781–90.

Courchesne, E., Yeung-Courchesne, R., Press, G. A., Hesslink, J. R., and Jernigan, T. L. (1988). Hypoplasia of cerebellar vermal lobules VI and VII in autism. *New England Journal of Medicine*, **318**, 1349–54.

Courchesne, E., Press, G. A., and Yeung-Courchesne, R. (1993). Parietal lobe abnormalities detected with MR in patients with infantile autism. *American Journal of Roentgenology*, **160**, 387–93.

Courchesne, E., Townsend, J., and Saitoh, O. (1994a). The brain in infantile autism: posterior fossa structures are abnormal. *Neurology*, **44**, 214–23.

Courchesne, E., Saitoh, O., Yeung-Courchesne, R. *et al.* (1994b). Abnormality of cerebellar vermian lobules VI and VII in patients with infantile autism: identification of hypoplastic and hyperplastic subgroups with MR imaging. *American Journal of Roentgenology*, **162**, 123–30.

Courchesne, E., Townsend, J., Akshoomoff, N. A. *et al.* (1994c). Impairment in shifting attention in autistic and cerebellar patients. *Behavioural Neuroscience*, **108**, 848–65.

Courchesne, E., Karns, C., Davis, H. *et al.* (2001). Unusual brain growth patterns in early life in patients with autistic disorder: An MRI study. *Neurology*, **57**(2), 245–54.

Critchley, H. D., Daly, E. M., Bullmore, E. T. *et al.* (2000). The functional neuroanatomy of social behaviour: changes in cerebral blood flow when people with autistic disorder process facial expressions. *Brain*, **123**(11), 2203–12.

Croonenberghs, J., Delmeire, L., Verkerk, R. *et al.* (2000). Peripheral markers of serotonergic and noradrenergic function in post-pubertal, caucasian males with autistic disorder. *Neuropsychopharmacology*, **22**(3), 275–83.

Cuccaro, M. L., Wright, H. H., Abramson, R. K., Marsteller, F. A., and Valentine, J. (1993). Whole-blood serotonin and cognitive functioning in autistic individuals and their first-degree relatives. *Journal of Neuropsychiatry Clinical Neuroscience*, **5**, 94–101.

Daniels, W. W., Warren, R. P., Odell, J. D. *et al.* (1995). Increased frequency of the extended or ancestral haplotype B44-SC30-DR4 in autism. *Neuropsychobiology*, **32**, 120–3.

Dapretto, M., Davies, M. S., Pfeifer, J. H. *et al.* (2006). Understanding emotions in others: mirror neuron dysfunction in children with autism spectrum disorders. *Natural Neuroscience*, **9**(1), 28–30.

Dassa, D., Takei, N., Sham, P. C., and Murray, R. M. (1995). No association between prenatal exposure to influenza and autism. *Acta Psychiatrica Scandinavica*, **92**, 145–9.

Dawson, G., Klinger, L. G., Panagiotides, H., Lewy, A., and Castelloe, P. (1995). Subgroups of autistic children based on social behavior display distinct patterns of brain activity. *Journal of Abnormal Child Psychology*, **23**, 569–83.

DeLong, R. and Nohria, C. (1994). Psychiatric family history and neurological disease in autistic spectrum disorders. *Developmental Medicine and Child Neurology*, **36**, 441–8.

Derry, J. M. and Barnard, P. J. (1991). Mapping of the glycine receptor alpha 2-subunit gene and the GABAA alpha 3-subunit gene on the mouse X chromosome. *Genomics*, **10**, 593–7.

D'Eufemia, P., Finocchiaro, R., Celli, M. *et al.* (1995). Low serum tryptophan to large neutral amino acids ratio in idiopathic infantile autism. *Biomedical Pharmacotherapeutics*, **49**, 288–92.

Deutsch, C. K. and Joseph, R. M. (2003). Brief report: cognitive correlates of enlarged head circumference in children with autism. *Journal of Autism and Developmental Disorders*, **33**(2), 209–15.

Deykin, E. Y. and MacMahon, B. (1979). The incidence of seizures among children with autistic symptoms. *American Journal of Psychiatry*, **126**, 1310–12.

Deykin, E. Y. and MacMahon, B. (1980). Pregnancy, delivery, and neonatal complications among autistic children. *American Journal of Diseased Children*, **134**, 860–4.

Eaves, R. C. and Milner, B. (1993). The criterion-related validity of the Childhood Autism Rating Scale and the Autism Behavior Checklist. *Journal of Abnormal Child Psychology*, **21**, 481–91.

Egaas, B., Courchesne, E., and Saitoh, O. (1995). Reduced size of corpus callosum in autism. *Archives of Neurology*, **52**, 794–801.

Einfeld, S., Moloney, H., and Hall, W. (1989). Autism is not associated with the fragile X syndrome. *American Journal of Medical Genetics*, **34**, 187–93.

Ekman, G., de Chateau, P., Marions, O. *et al.* (1991). Low field magnetic resonance imaging of the central nervous system in 15 children with autistic disorder. *Acta Paediatrica Scandinavica*, **80**, 243–7.

Elia, M., Musumeci, S. A., Ferri, R., and Bergonzi, P. (1995). Clinical and neurophysiological aspects of epilepsy in subjects with autism and mental retardation. *American Journal of Mental Retardation*, **100**, 6–16.

Erdmann, J., Shimron-Abarbanell, D., Cichon, S. *et al.* (1995). Systematic screening for mutations in the promoter and the coding region of the 5-HT1A gene. *American Journal of Medical Genetics*, **60**, 393–9.

Fahsold, R., Rott, H. D., Claussen, U., and Schmalenberger, B. (1991). Tuberous sclerosis in a child with de novo translocation t(3.,12) (p26. 3.,q23. 3). *Clinical Genetics*, **40**, 326–8.

Fernell, E., Gillberg, C., and von Wendt, L. (1991). Autistic symptoms in children with infantile hydrocephalus. *Acta Paediatrica Scandinavica*, **80**, 451–7.

Folstein, S. and Rutter, M. (1977). Infantile autism: a genetic study of 21 twin pairs. *Journal of Child Psychology and Psychiatry*, **18**, 297–321.

Fombonne, E. (1992). Diagnostic assessment in a sample of autistic and developmentally impaired adolescents. *Journal of Autism and Developmental Disorders*, **22**, 563–81.

Garnier, C, Comoy, E., Barthelemy, C. *et al.* (1986). Dopamine-beta-hydroxylase (DBH) and homovanillic acid (HVA) in autistic children. *Journal of Autism and Developmental Disorders*, **16**, 23–9.

Garreau, B., Barthelemy, C., Jouve, J. *et al.* (1988). Urinary homovanillic acid levels of autistic children. *Developmental Medicine and Child Neurology*, **30**, 93–8.

George, M. S., Costa, D. C., Kouris, K., Ring, H. A., and Ell, P. J. (1992). Cerebral blood low abnormalities in adults with infantile autism. *Journal of Nervous and Mental Disease*, **180**, 413–17.

Gepner, B., Mestre, D., Masson, G., and de Schonen, S. (1995). Postural effects of motion vision in young autistic children. *Neuroreports*, **6**, 1211–14.

Ghaziuddin, M., Tsai, L. Y., and Ghaziuddin, N. (1992). Autism in Down's syndrome: presentation and diagnosis. *Journal of Intellectual Disability Research*, **36**, 449–56.

Ghaziuddin, M., Sheldon, S., Tsai, L. Y., and Alessi, N. (1993). Abnormalities of chromosome 18 in a girl with mental retardation and autistic disorder. *Journal of Intellectual Disability Research*, **37**, 313–17.

Ghaziuddin, M., Bolyard, B., and Alessi, N. (1994a). Autistic disorder in Noonan syndrome. *Journal of Intellectual Disability Research*, **38**, 67–72.

Ghaziuddin, M., Butler, E., Tsai, L., and Ghaziuddin, N. (1994b). Is clumsiness a marker for Asperger syndrome? *Journal of Intellectual Disability Research*, **38**, 519–27.

Gillberg, C. (1992). The Emanuel Miller Memorial Lecture 1991. Autism and autistic-like condi-
    tions. Subclasses among disorders of empathy. *Journal of Child Psychology and Psychiatry*, **33**,
    813–42.

Gillberg, C. (1995). Endogenous opioids and opiate antagonists in autism: brief review of empirical
    findings and implications for clinicians. *Developmental Medicine and Child Neurology*, **37**, 239–45.

Gillberg, C. and Coleman, M. (1992). *The Biology of the Autistic Syndromes*. Oxford: Blackwell
    Scientific.

Gillberg, C. and Gillberg, I. C. (1983). Infantile autism: a total population study of reduced opti-
    mality in the pre-, peri-, and neonatal period. *Journal of Autism and Developmental Disorders*,
    13, 153–66.

Gillberg, I. C. (1991). Autistic syndrome with onset at age 31 years: herpes encephalitis as a possible
    model for childhood autism. *Developmental Medicine and Child Neurology*, **33**, 920–4.

Gillberg, I. C., Gillberg, C., and Kopp, S. (1992). Hypothyroidism and autism spectrum disorders.
    Journal of Child Psychology and Psychiatry, **33**, 531–42.

Gillberg, I. C, Bjure, J., Uvebrant, P., Vestergren, E., and Gillberg, C. (1993). SPECT (single photon
    emission computed tomography) in 31 children and adolescents with autism and autism-like
    conditions. *European Child and Adolescent Psychiatry*, **2**, 50–9.

Gillberg, I. C., Gillberg, C., and Ahlsen, G. (1994). Autistic behaviour and attention deficits in
    tuberous sclerosis: a population-based study. *Developmental Medicine and Child Neurology*, **36**,
    50–6.

Goa, J. H., Parsons, L. M., Bower, J. M. *et al.* (1996). Cerebellum implicated in sensory acquisition
    and discrimination rather than motor control. *Science*, **272**, 545–7.

Goodman, R. (1990). Technical note: are perinatal complications causes or consequences of autism?
    Journal of Child Psychology and Psychiatry, **31**, 809–12.

Goodman, R. and Minne, C. (1995). Questionnaire screening for comorbid pervasive developmen-
    tal disorders in congenitally blind children: a pilot study. *Journal of Autism and Developmental
    Disorders*, **25**, 195–203.

Hallett, M., Lebiedowska, M. K., Thomas, S. L. *et al.* (1993). Locomotion of autistic adults. *Archives
    Neurology*, **50**, 1304–8.

Hallmayer, J., Pintado, E., Lotspeich, L. *et al.* (1994). Molecular analysis and test of linkage between
    the FMR-1 gene and infantile autism in multiplex families. *American Journal of Human Genetics*,
    55, 951–9.

Harris, S. R., MacKay, L. L., and Osborn, J. A. (1995). Autistic behaviors in offspring of mothers
    abusing alcohol and other drugs: a series of case reports. *Alcohol Clinics and Experimental
    Research*, **19**, 660–5.

Hashimoto, T., Tayama, M., Miyazaki, M. *et al.* (1991). Reduced midbrain and pons size in autistic
    children. *Tokushima Journal of Experimental Medicine*, **38**, 15–18.

Hashimoto, T., Murakawa, K., Miyazaki, M., Tayama, M., and Kuroda, Y. (1992a). Magnetic
    resonance imaging of the brain structures in the posterior fossa in retarded autistic children.
    Acta Paediatrica, **81**, 1030–4.

Hashimoto, T., Tayama, M., Miyazaki, M. *et al.* (1992b). Reduced brainstem size in autistic children. *Brain Development*, **14**, 94–7.

Hashimoto, T., Tayama, M., Miyazaki, M. *et al.* (1993). Brainstem involvement in high-functioning autistic children. *Acta Neurologica Scandinavica*, **88**, 123–8.

Hashimoto, T., Tayama, M., Murakawa, K. *et al.* (1995). Development of the brainstem and cerebellum in patients with autism. *Journal of Autism and Developmental Disorders*, **25**, 1–18.

Heath, M. J. S. and Hen, R. (1995). Genetic insights into serotonin function. *Current Biology*, **5**, 997–9.

Hebebrand, J., Martin, M., Korner, J. *et al.* (1994). Partial trisomy 16p in an adolescent with autistic disorder and Tourette's syndrome. *American Journal of Medical Genetics*, **54**, 268–70.

Holroyd, S., Reiss, A. L., and Bryan, R. N. (1991). Autistic features in Joubert syndrome: a genetic disorder with agenesis of the cerebellar vermis [see comments]. *Biological Psychiatry*, **29**(3), 287–94.

Holttum, J. R., Minshew, N. J., Sanders, R. S., and Phillips, N. E. (1992). Magnetic resonance imaging of the posterior fossa in autism. *Biological Psychiatry*, **32**, 1091–101.

Hoon, A. H. Jr., and Reiss, A. L. (1992). The mesial-temporal lobe and autism: case report and review. *Developmental Medicine and Child Neurology*, **34**, 252–9.

Hotopf, M. and Bolton, P. (1995). A case of autism associated with partial tetrasomy 15. *Journal of Autism and Developmental Disorders*, **25**, 41–9.

Howlin, P., Wing, L., and Gould, J. (1995). The recognition of autism in children with Down's syndrome: implications for intervention and some speculations about pathology. *Developmental Medicine and Child Neurology*, **37**, 406–14.

Hsu, M., Yeung-Courchesne, R., Courchesne, E., and Press, G. A. (1991). Absence of magnetic resonance imaging evidence of pontine abnormality in infantile autism. *Archives of Neurology*, **48**, 1160–3.

Hubl, D., Bolte, S., Feineis-Matthews, S. *et al.* (2003). Functional imbalance of visual pathways indicates alternative face processing strategies in autism. *Neurology*, **61**(9), 1232–7.

Hultman, C. M., Sparen, P., and Cnattingius, S. (2002). Perinatal risk factors for infantile autism. *Epidemiology*, **13**(4), 417–23.

Hunt, A. and Shepherd, C. (1993). A prevalence study of autism in tuberous sclerosis. *Journal of Autism and Developmental Disorders*, **23**, 323–39.

Jorde, L. B., Hasstedt, S. J., Ritvo, E. R. *et al.* (1991). Complex segregation analysis of autism. *American Journal of Human Genetics*, **49**, 932–8.

Juul-Dam, N., Townsend, J., and Courchesne, E. (2001). Prenatal, perinatal, and neonatal factors in autism, pervasive developmental disorder-not otherwise specified, and the general population. *Pediatrics*, **107**(4), E63.

Kates, W. R., Burnette, C. P., Eliez, S. *et al.* (2004). Neuroanatomic variation in monozygotic twin pairs discordant for the narrow phenotype for autism. *American Journal of Psychiatry*, **161**(3), 539–46.

Kemner, C., Verbaten, M. N., Cuperus, J. M., Camfferman, G., and van Engeland, H. (1994). Visual and somatosensory event-related brain potentials in autistic children and three different control groups. *Electroencephalography and Clinical Neurophysiology*, **92**, 225–37.

Kemner, C., Verbaten, M. N., Cuperus, J. M., Camfferman, G., and van Engeland, H. (1995). Auditory event-related brain potentials in autistic children and three different control groups. *Biological Psychiatry*, **38**, 150–65.

Kemper, T. L. and Bauman, M. L. (1992). Neuropathology of infantile autism. In H. Naruse and E. M. Ornitz, eds., *Neurobiology of Infantile Autism*. Amsterdam: Elsevier Science, pp. 43–57.

Kerbeshian, J., Burd, L., Randall, T., Martsolf, J., and Jalal, S. (1990). Autism, profound mental retardation and atypical bipolar disorder in a 33-year-old female with a deletion of 15ql2. *Journal of Mental Deficiency Research*, **34**, 205–10.

Klauck, S. M., Münstermann, E., Bieber-Martig, B. *et al.* (1997). Molecular genetic analysis of the FMR-1 gene in a large collection of patients with autism. *Human Genetics*, **100**, 224–9.

Kleiman, M. D., Neff, S., and Rosman, N. P. (1992). The brain in infantile autism: are posterior fossa structures abnormal? *Neurology*, **42**, 753–60.

Klin, A. (1993). Auditory brainstem responses in autism: brainstem dysfunction or peripheral hearing loss? *Journal of Autism and Developmental Disorders*, **23**, 15–35.

Knobloch, H. and Pasamanick, B. (1975). Some etiologic and prognostic factors in early infantile autism and psychosis. *Pediatrics*, **55**, 182–91.

Kohen-Raz, R. (1991). Application of tetra-ataxiametric posturography in clinical and developmental diagnosis. *Perception and Motor Skills*, **73**, 635–56.

Kohen-Raz, R., Volkmar, F. R., and Cohen, D. J. (1992). Postural control in autistic children. *Journal of Autism and Developmental Disorders*, **22**, 419–32.

Kokubun, M., Haishi, K., Okuzumi, H., and Hosobuchi, T. (1995). Factors affecting age of walking by children with mental retardation. *Perception and Motor Skills*, **80**, 547–52.

Lappalainen, J., Zhang, L., Dean, M. *et al.* (1995). Identification, expression, and pharmacology of a Cys23-Ser23 subsitution in the human 5-HT2C receptor gene (HTR2C). *Genomica*, **27**, 287–94.

Launay, J. M., Bursztejn, C, Ferrari, P. *et al.* (1987). Catecholamines metabolism in infantile autism: a controlled study of 22 autistic children. *Journal of Autism and Developmental Disorders*, **17**, 333–47.

Leboyer, M., Philippe, A., Bouvard, M. *et al.* (1999). Whole blood serotonin and plasma beta-endorphin in autistic probands and their first-degree relatives. *Biological Psychiatry*, **45**(2), 158–63.

Lekman, A., Skjeldal, O., Sponheim, E., and Svennerholm, L. (1995). Gangliosides in autistic children. *Acta Paediatrica*, **84**, 787–90.

Lensing, P., Klinger, D., Panksepp, J. *et al.* (1992). Opiathypothese zur Genese des fruhkindlichen Autismus und Folgerungen zur Psychopharmakotherapie. [Opiate hypothesis of the origin of early childhood autism and sequelae for psychopharmacotherapy] *Z-Kinder-Jugenpsychiatry*, **20**, 185–96.

Leventhal, B. L., Cook, E. H. Jr., Morford, M., Ravitz, A., and Freedman, D. X. (1990). Relationships of whole blood serotonin and plasma norepinephrine within families. *Journal of Autism and Developmental Disorders*, **20**, 499–511.

Levy, S., Zoltak, B., and Saelens, T. (1988). A comparison of obstetrical records of autistic and nonautistic referrals for psychoeducational evaluations. *Journal of Autism and Developmental Disorders*, **18**, 573–81.

Lincoln, A. J., Courchesne, E., Harms, L., and Allen, M. (1993). Contextual probability evaluation in autistic, receptive developmental language disorder, and control children: event-related brain potential evidence. *Journal of Autism and Developmental Disorders*, **23**, 37–58.

Lincoln, A. J., Courchesne, E., Harms, L., and Allen, M. (1995). Sensory modulation of auditory stimuli in autistic children and receptive developmental language disorder: event-related brain potential evidence. *Journal of Autism and Developmental Disorders*, **25**, 521–39.

Lisch, S., Ruhl, D., Sacher, A. *et al.* (1993). Beziehungen zwischen autistischem Syndrom und dem FraX-Syndrom. In P. Baumann, ed., *Biologische Psychiatrie der Gegenwart*. Vienna: Springer Verlag, pp. 390–8.

Lobascher, M. E., Kingerlee, P. E., and Gubbay, S. S. (1970). Childhood autism: an investigation of aetiological factors in twenty-five cases. *British Journal of Psychiatry*, **117**, 525–9.

Martineau, J., Barthelemy, C., Jouve, J., Muh, J. P., and Lelord, G. (1992a). Monoamines (serotonin and catecholamines) and their derivatives in infantile autism: age-related changes and drug effects. *Developmental Medicine and Child Neurology*, **34**, 593–603.

Martineau, J., Roux, S., Adrien, J. L. *et al.* (1992b). Electrophysiological evidence of different abilities to form cross-modal associations in children with autistic behavior. *Electroencephalography and Clinical Neurophysiology*, **82**, 60–6.

McBride, P. A., Anderson, G. M., Hertzig, M. E. *et al.* (1989). Serotonergic responsivity in male young adults with autistic disorder. Results of a pilot study. *Archives of General Psychiatry*, **46**, 213–321.

McDougle, C. J., Naylor, S. T., Cohen, D. J. *et al.* (1996). Effects of tryptophan depletion in drug-free adults with autistic disorder. *Archives of General Psychiatry*, **53**, 993–1000.

McKelvey, J. R., Lambert, R., Mottron, L., and Shevell, M. I. (1995). Right-hemisphere dysfunction in Asperger's syndrome. *Journal of Child Neurology*, **10**, 310–14.

Miladi, N., Larnaout, A., Kaabachi, N., Helayem, M., and Ben-Hamida, M. (1992). Phenylketonuria: an underlying etiology of autistic syndrome. A case report. *Journal of Child Neurology*, **7**, 22–3.

Miller, G. (1989). Minor congenital anomalies and ataxic cerebral palsy. *Archives of Disease in Childhood*, **64**, 557–62.

Minderaa, R. B., Anderson, G. M., Volkmar, F. R., Akkerhuis, G. W., and Cohen, D. J. (1987). Urinary 5-hydroxyindoleacetic acid and whole blood serotonin and tryptophan in autistic and normal subjects. *Biological Psychiatry*, **22**, 933–40.

Minderaa, R. B., Anderson, G. M., Volkmar, F. R., Akkerhuis, G. W., and Cohen, D. J. (1994). Noradrenergic and adrenergic functioning in autism. *Biological Psychiatry*, **36**, 237–41.

Minshew, N. J. (1991). Indices of neural function in autism: clinical and biologic implications. *Pediatrics*, **87**(5 pt.2), 774–80.

Minshew, N. J. and Dombrowski, S. M. (1994). In vivo neuroanatomy of autism: neuroimaging studies. In M. L. Bauman and T. L. Kemper, eds., *The Neurobiology of Autism*. Baltimore: Johns Hopkins University Press, pp. 66–85.

Minshew, N. J., Goldstein, G., Dombrowski, S. M., Panchalingam, K., and Pettegrew, J. W. (1993). A preliminary 31P MRS study of autism: evidence for undersynthesis and increased degradation of brain membranes. *Biological Psychiatry*, **33**, 762–73.

Morrow, J. D., Whitman, B. Y., and Accardo, P. J. (1990). Autistic disorder in Sotos' syndrome: a case report. *European Journal of Pediatrics*, **149**, 567–9.

Mouridsen, S. E., Nielsen, S., Rich, B., and Isager, T. (1994). Season of birth in infantile autism and other types of childhood psychoses. *Child Psychiatry and Human Development*, **25**, 31–43.

Murphy, D. G., Critchley, H. D., Schmitz, N. *et al.* (2002). Asperger syndrome: a proton magnetic resonance spectroscopy study of brain. *Archives of General Psychiatry*, **59**(10), 885–91.

Myrianthopoulos, N. C. and Melnick, M. (1977). Malformations in monozygotic twins: a possible example of environmental influence on the developmental genetic clock. In E. Inouye and H. Nishimura, eds., *Gene Environment Interaction in Common Diseases*. Tokyo: University of Tokyo Press, pp. 206–20.

Naffah-Mazzacoratti, M. G., Rosenberg, R., Fernandes, M. J. *et al.* (1993). Serum serotonin levels of normal and autistic children. *Brazilian Journal of Medical and Biological Research*, **26**, 309–17.

Nagamitsu, S. (1993). CSF beta-endorphin levels in pediatric neurologic disorders. *Kurume Medical Journal*, **40**, 233–41.

Narayan, M., Srinath, S., Anderson, G. M., and Meundi, D. B. (1993). Cerebrospinal fluid levels of homovanillic acid and 5-hydroxyindoleacetic acid in autism. *Biological Psychiatry*, **33**, 630–5.

Nelson, K. B. (1991). Prenatal and perinatal factors in the etiology of autism. *Pediatrics*, **87**(5 Pt. 2), 761–6.

Nelson, K. B. and Ellenberg, J. H. (1986). Antecedents of cerebral palsy: multivariate analysis of risk. *New England Journal of Medicine*, **315**, 81–6.

Nicole, J., Rinehart, M., Bellgrove, B., Tonge, A., Brereton, D., Bradshaw, J. (2006). An examination of movement kinematics in young people with high-functioning autism and asperger's disorder: further evidence for a motor planning deficit. *Journal of Autism and Developmental Disorders*, **36**(6), 757–67.

Nowell, M. A., Hackney, D. B., Muraki, A. S., and Coleman, M. (1990). Varied MR appearance of autism: fifty-three pediatric patients having the full autistic syndrome. *Magnetic Resonance Imaging*, **8**, 811–16.

Oades, R. D. and Eggers, C. (1994). Childhood autism: an appeal for an integrative and psychobiological approach. *European Child and Adolescent Psychiatry*, **3**, 159–75.

Oades, R. D., Stern, L. M., Walker, M. K., Clark, C. R., and Kapoor, V. (1990). Event-related potentials and monoamines in autistic children on a clinical trial of fenfluramine. *International Journal of Psychophysiology*, **8**, 197–212.

Oberlé, I., Rousseau, F., Heitz, D. *et al.* (1991). Instability of a 550-base pair DNA segment and abnormal methylation in fragile X syndrome. *Science*, **252**, 1097–102.

Ogdie, M. N., Macphie, I. L., Minassian, S. L. *et al.* (2003). A genomewide scan for attention-deficit/hyperactivity disorder in an extended sample: suggestive linkage on 17p11. *American Journal of Human Genetics*, **72**(5), 1268–79.

Olsson, B. and Rett, A. (1990). A review of the Rett syndrome with a theory of autism. *Brain and Development*, **12**, 11–15.

Ornitz, E. M. (1978). Biological homogeneity or heterogeneity. In M. Rutter and E. Schopler, eds., *Autism: A Reappraisal of Concepts and Treatments*. New York: Plenum Press, pp. 243–50.

Perry, B. D., Cook, E. H. Jr., Leventhal, B. L., Wainwright, M. S., and Freedman, D. X. (1991). Platelet 5-HT2 serotonin receptor binding sites in autistic children and their first-degree relatives. *Biological Psychiatry*, **30**, 121–30.

Peterson, B. S. (1995). Neuroimaging in child and adolescent neuropsychiatric disorders. *Journal of the American Academy of Child and Adolescent Psychiatry*, **34**, 1560–76.

Pierce, K., Muller, R. A., Ambrose, J., Allen, G., and Courchesne, E. (2001). Face processing occurs outside the fusiform "face area" in autism: evidence from functional MRI. *Brain*, **124**(10), 2059–73.

Piven, J., Berthier, M. L., Starkstein, S. E. *et al.* (1990). Magnetic resonance imaging evidence for a defect of cerebral cortical development in autism. *American Journal of Psychiatry*, **147**, 734–9.

Piven, J., Tsai, G. C, Nehme, E. *et al.* (1991). Platelet serotonin: a possible marker for familial autism. *Journal of Autism and Developmental Disorders*, **21**, 51–9.

Piven, J., Nehme, E., Simon, J. *et al.* (1992). Magnetic resonance imaging in autism: measurement of the cerebellum, pons, and fourth ventricle. *Biological Psychiatry*, **31**, 491–504.

Piven, J., Arndt, S., Bailey, J. *et al.* (1995). An MRI study of brain size in autism. *American Journal of Psychiatry*, **152**, 1145–9.

Prechtl, H. F. R. (1980). The optimality concept [editorial]. *Early Human Development*, **4**, 201–5.

Rantakallio, P. and von Wendt, L. (1985). Risk factors for mental retardation. *Archives of Disease in Childhood*, **60**, 946–52.

Rao, P. N., Klinepeter, K., Stewart, W. *et al.* (1994). Molecular cytogenetic analysis of a duplication Xp in a male: further delineation of a possible sex-influencing region on the X chromosome. *Human Genetics*, **94**, 149–53.

Raymond, G. V., Bauman, M. L., and Kemper, T. L. (1989). Hippocampus in autism: Golgi analysis. *Annals of Neurology*, **26**, 483–4.

Realmuto, G. M., Jensen, J. B., Reeve, E., and Garfinkel, B. D. (1990). Growth hormone response to L-dopa and clonidine in autistic children. *Journal of Autism and Developmental Disorders*, **20**, 455–65.

Reiss, A. L., Patel, S., Kumar, A. J., and Freund, L. (1988). Preliminary communication: neuroanatomical variations of the posterior fossa in men with the fragile X (Martin Bell) syndrome. *American Journal of Medical Genetics*, **31**, 407–14.

Reiss, A. L., Aylward, E., Freund, L., Joshi, P. K., and Bryan, R. N. (1991). Neuroanatomy in fragile X syndrome: the posterior fossa. *Annals of Neurology*, **29**, 26–32.

Richdale, A. L. and Prior, M. R. (1992). Urinary cortisol circadian rhythm in a group of high-functioning autistic children. *Journal of Autism and Developmental Disorders*, **22**, 433–47.

Ritvo, E. R., Freeman, B. J., Scheibel, A. B. *et al.* (1986). Lower Purkinje cell counts in the cerebella of four autistic subjects: initial findings of the UCLA–NSAC autopsy research report. *American Journal of Psychiatry*, **143**, 862–6.

Ritvo, E. R., Ritvo, R., Yuwiler, A. *et al.* (1993). Elevated daytime melatonin concentrations in autism: a pilot study. *European Child and Adolescent Psychiatry*, **2**, 75–8.

Rolf, L. H., Haarmann, F. Y., Grotemeyer, K. H., and Kehrer, H. (1993). Serotonin and amino acid content in platelets of autistic children. *Acta Psychiatrica Scandinavica*, **87**, 312–16.

Root-Bernstein, R. S. and Westall, F. C. (1990). Serotonin binding sites. II. Muramyl dipeptide binds to serotonin binding sites on myelin basic protein, LHRH, and MSH-ACTH 4–10. *Brain Research Bulletin*, **25**, 827–41.

Rosengren, L. E., Ahlsen, G., Belfrage, M. *et al.* (1992). A sensitive ELISA for glial fibrillary acidic protein: application in CSF of children. *Journal of Neuroscience Methods*, **44**, 113–19.

Rossi, P. G., Parmeggiani, A., Bach, V., Santucci, M., and Visconti, P. (1995). EEG features and epilepsy in patients with autism. *Brain and Development*, **17**, 169–74.

Ruhl, D., Bolte, S., and Poustka, F. (2001). [Speech development and intelligence in autism. How uniform is Asperger syndrome?]. *Nervenarzt*, **72**(7), 535–40.

Rutter, M. (1984). Autistic children growing up. *Developmental Medicine and Child Neurology*, **26**, 122–9.

Rutter, M. (1988). Biological basis to autism: implications for intervention. In F. J. Menolascino and J. A. Stark, eds., *Preventive and Curative Interventions in Mental Retardation*. Baltimore: Brookes Publishing, pp. 265–94.

Rutter, M. and Redshaw, J. (1991). Annotation: growing up as a twin. Twin-singleton differences in psychological development. *Journal of Child Psychology and Psychiatry*, **32**, 885–95.

Rutter, M., Bailey, A., Bolton, P., and Le Couteur, A. (1994). Autism and known medical conditions: myth and substance. *Journal of Child Psychology and Psychiatry*, **35**, 311–22.

Saitoh, O., Courchesne, E., Egaas, B., Lincoln, A. J., and Schreibman, L. (1995). Cross-sectional area of the posterior hippocampus in patients with autism with cerebellar and corpus callosum abnormalities. *Neurology*, **45**, 317–24.

Sameroff, A. J., Seifer, R., and Zax, M. (1982). Early development of children at risk for emotional disorder. *Monographs of the Society for Research in Child Development*, **47**, 1–82.

Schaefer, G. B., Thompson, J. N., Bodensteiner, J. B. *et al.* (1996). Hypoplasia of the cerebellar vermis in neurogenetic syndromes. *Annals of Neurology*, **39**, 382–5.

Schain, R. J. and Freedman, D. X. (1961). Studies on 5-hydroxyindole metabolism in autistic and mentally retarded children. *Journal of Pediatrics*, **58**, 315–20.

Schifter, T., Hoffman, J. M., Hatten, H. P. Jr. *et al.* (1994). Neuroimaging in infantile autism. *Journal of Child Neurology*, **9**, 155–61.

Schinzel, A. (1990). Autistic disorder and additional inv dup(15)(pter–q13) chromosome. *American Journal of Medical Genetics*, **35**, 447–8.

Schmamann, J. D. (1991). An emerging concept. The cerebellar contribution to higher function. *Archives of Neurology*, **271**, 153–84.

Schultz, R. T., Gauthier, I., Klin, A. *et al.* (2000). Abnormal ventral temporal cortical activity during face discrimination among individuals with autism and Asperger syndrome. *Archives of General Psychiatry*, **57**(4), 331–40.

Schultz, R. T., Grelotti, D. J., Klin, A. *et al.* (2003). The role of the fusiform face area in social cognition: implications for the pathobiology of autism. *Philosophical Transactions of the Royal Society of London – Series B: Biological Sciences*, **358**(1430), 415–27.

Sersen, E. A., Heaney, G., Clausen, J., Belser, R., and Rainbow, S. (1990). Brainstem auditory-evoked responses with and without sedation in autism and Down's syndrome. *Biological Psychiatry*, **15**, 834–40.

Seshadri, K., Wallerstein, R., and Burack, G. (1992). 18q-chromosomal abnormality in a phenotypically normal $2\frac{1}{2}$-year-old male with autism. *Developmental Medicine and Child Neurology*, **34**, 1005–9.

Shaffer, L. G., McCaskill, C., Hersh, J. H., Greenberg, F., and Lupski, J. R. (1996). A clinical and molecular study of mosaicism for trisomy 17. *Human Genetics*, **97**, 69–72.

Shannon, M. and Graef, J. W. (1996). Lead intoxication in children with pervasive developmental disorders. *Journal of Toxicology and Clinical Toxicology*, **34**, 177–81.

Siegel, B. V. Jr., Asarnow, R., Tanguay, P. *et al.* (1992). Regional cerebral glucose metabolism and attention in adults with a history of childhood autism. *Journal of Neuropsychiatry Clinical Neuroscience*, **4**, 406–14.

Siegel, B. V. Jr., Nuechterlein, K. H., Abel, L., Wu, J. C., and Buchsbaum, M. S. (1995). Glucose metabolic correlates of continuous performance test performance in adults with a history of infantile autism, schizophrenics, and controls. *Schizophrenia Research*, **17**, 85–94.

Singh, V. K., Warren, R. P., and Singh, E. A. (1990). Binding of [3H]serotonin to lymphocytes in patients with neuropsychiatric disorders. *Molecular Chemistry and Neuropathology*, **13**, 167–73.

Singh, V. K., Warren, R. P., Odell, J. D., and Cole, P. (1993). Changes of soluble interleukin-2, interleukin-2 receptor, T8 antigen, and interleukin-1 in the serum of autistic children. *Clinical Immunology and Immunopathology*, **61**, 448–55.

Skjeldal, O. H., Sponheim, E., Ganes, T., Jellum, E., and Bakke, S. (1998). Childhood autism: the need for physical investigations. *Brain and Development*, **20**(4), 227–33.

Smalley, S. L., Tanguay, P. E., Smith, M., and Gutierrez, G. (1992). Autism and tuberous sclerosis. *Journal of Autism and Developmental Disorders*, **22**, 339–55.

Sparks, B. F., Friedman, S. D., Shaw, D. W. *et al.* (2002). Brain structural abnormalities in young children with autism spectrum disorder. *Neurology*, **59**(2), 184–92.

Steffenburg, S., Gillberg, C., Hellgren, L. *et al.* (1989). A twin study of autism in Denmark, Finland, Iceland, Norway and Sweden. *Journal of Child Psychology and Psychiatry*, **30**, 405–16.

Steffenburg, S., Gillberg, C., and Steffenburg, U. (1996). Psychiatric disorders in children and adolescents with mental retardation and active epilepsy. *Archives of Neurology*, **53**, 904–12.

Stone, R. L., Aimi, J., Barshop, B. A. *et al.* (1992). A mutation in adenylosuccinate lyase associated with mental retardation and autistic features. *Nature Genetics*, **1**, 59–63.

Strandburg, R. J., Marsh, J. T., Brown, W. S. *et al.* (1993). Event-related potentials in high-functioning adult autistics: linguistic and nonlinguistic visual information processing tasks. *Neuropsychologia*, **31**, 413–34.

Stromland, K., Nordin, V., Miller, M., Akerstrom, B., and Gillberg, C. (1994). Autism in thalidomide embryopathy: a population study. *Developmental Medicine and Child Neurology*, **36**, 351–6.

Stubbs, G. (1995). Interferonemia and autism. *Journal of Autism and Developmental Disorders*, **25**, 71–3.

Sturm, H., Fernell, E., and Gillberg, C. (2004). Autism spectrum disorders in children with normal intellectual levels: associated impairments and subgroups. *Developmental Medicine and Child Neurology*, **46**(7), 444–7.

Sverd, J. (1991). Tourette syndrome and autistic disorder: a significant relationship. *American Journal of Medical Genetics*, **39**, 173–9.

Tantam, D., Evered, C., and Hersov, L. (1990). Asperger's syndrome and ligamentous laxity. *Journal of the American Academy of Child and Adolescent Psychiatry*, **29**, 892–6.

Thivierge, J., Bedard, C., Cote, R., and Maziade, M. (1990). Brainstem auditory evoked response and subcortical abnormalities in autism. *American Journal of Psychiatry*, **147**, 1609–13.

Todd, R. D., Hickok, J. M., Anderson, G. M., and Cohen, D. J. (1988). Antibrain antibodies in infantile autism. *Biological Psychiatry*, **23**, 644–7.

Tordjman, S., Anderson, G. M., McBride, P. A. *et al.* (1995). Plasma androgens in autism. *Journal of Autism and Developmental Disorders*, **25**, 295–304.

Tsai, L. Y. and Stewart, M. A. (1983). Etiological implication of maternal age and birth order in infantile autism. *Journal of Autism and Developmental Disorders*, **13**, 57–65.

Tsai, L. Y., Tsai, M. C., and August, G. J. (1985). Brief report: implication of EEG diagnoses in the subclassification of infantile autism. *Journal of Autism and Developmental Disorders*, **15**, 339–44.

Tuchman, R. and Rapin, I. (2002). Epilepsy in autism. *Lancet Neurology*, **1**(6), 352–8.

Tuchman, R. F., Rapin, I., and Shinnar, S. (1991). Autistic and dysphasic children. II. Epilepsy. *Pediatrics*, **88**, 1219–25.

Venter, P. A., Op't Hof, J., Coetzee, D. J., van der Walt, C., and Retief, A. E. (1984). No marker (X) syndrome in autistic children. *Human Genetics*, **67**, 107.

Verkerk, A. J. M. H., Pieretti, M., Sutclifle, J. S. *et al.* (1991). Identification of a gene (FMR-l) containing a CGG repeat coincident with a breakpoint cluster region exhibiting length variation in fragile X syndrome. *Cell*, **65**, 905–14.

Volkmar, F. R. and Cohen, D. J. (1988). Diagnosis of pervasive developmental disorders. In B. Lahey and A. Kazdin, eds., *Advances in Clinical Child Psychology*. New York: Plenum Press, pp. 249–84.

Volkmar, F. R. and Nelson, D. S. (1990). Seizure disorders in autism. *Journal of the American Academy of Child and Adolescent Psychiatry*, **29**, 127–9.

Volkmar, F. R., Cicchetti, D. V., Bregman, J., and Cohen, D. J. (1992). Three diagnostic systems for autism: DSM-III, DSM-III-R, and ICD-10. *Journal of Autism and Developmental Disorders*, **22**, 483–92.

Volkmar, F. R., Klin, A., Siegel, B. *et al.*, and Members of the DSM-IV Autism/PDD Field Trial Group. DSM-IV Autism/Pervasive Developmental Disorders Field Trial (1994). *American Journal of Psychiatry*, **151**, 1361–7.

Warren, R. P., Singh, V. K., Cole, P. *et al.* (1991). Increased frequency of the null allele at the complement C4b locus in autism. *Clinical and Experimental Immunology*, **83**, 438–40.

Warren, R. P., Burger, R. A., Odell, D., Torres, A. R., and Warren, W. L. (1994). Decreased plasma concentrations of the C4B complement protein in autism. *Archives of Pediatric and Adolescent Medicine*, **148**, 180–3.

Warren, R. P., Yonk, J., Burger, R. W., Odell, D., and Warren, W. L. (1995). DR-positive T cells in autism: association with decreased plasma levels of the complement C4B protein. *Neuropsychobiology*, **31**, 53–7.

Watson, M. S., Leckman, J. F., Annex, B. *et al.* (1984). Fragile X in a survey of 75 autistic males. *New England Journal of Medicine*, **310**, 1462.

Wilcox, J., Tsuang, M. T., Ledger, E., Algeo, J., and Schnurr, T. (2002). Brain perfusion in autism varies with age. *Neuropsychobiology*, **46**(1), 13–6.

Willemsen-Swinkels, S. H., Buitelaar, J. K, Nijhof, G. J., and van Engeland, H. (1995). Failure of naltrexone hydrochloride to reduce self-injurious and autistic behavior in mentally retarded adults. Double-blind placebo-controlled studies. *Archives of General Psychiatry*, **52**, 766–73.

Williams, R. S., Mauser, S. L., Purpura, D. P., Delong, G. R., and Swisher, C. W. (1980). Autism and mental retardation. *Archives of Neurology*, **37**, 749–53.

Wolman, S. R., Campbell, M, Marchi, M. L., Deutsch, S. I., and Gershon, T. D. (1990). Dermatoglyphic study in autistic children and controls. *Journal of the American Academy of Child and Adolescent Psychiatry*, **29**, 878–84.

Wong, V. (1993). Epilepsy in children with autistic spectrum disorder. *Journal of Child Neurology*, **8**, 316–22.

Wong, V. and Wong, S. N. (1991). Brainstem auditory evoked potential study in children with autistic disorder. *Journal of Autism and Developmental Disorders*, **21**, 329–40.

Yu, S., Pritchard, M., Kremer, E. *et al.* (1991). Fragile X genotype characterized by an unstable region of DNA. *Science*, **252**, 1179–81.

Yuwiler, A., Shih, J. C, Chen, C. H. *et al.* (1992). Hyperserotoninemia and antiserotonin antibodies in autism and other disorders. *Journal of Autism and Developmental Disorders*, **22**, 33–45.

Zilbovicius, M., Garreau, B., Tzourio, N. *et al.*(1992). Regional cerebral blood flow in childhood autism: a SPECT study. *American Journal of Psychiatry*, **149**, 924–30.

Zilbovicius, M., Garreau, B., Samson, Y. *et al.* (1995). Delayed maturation of the frontal cortex in childhood autism. *American Journal of Psychiatry*, **152**, 248–52.

7

Psychopharmacology

Craig A. Erickson, Kimberly A. Stigler, David J. Posey, and
Christopher J. McDougle

Department of Psychiatry, Indiana University School of Medicine, and
Christian Sarkine Autism Treatment Center, James Whitcomb Riley Hospital for Children

Introduction

Research into the pharmacotherapy of individuals with pervasive developmental disorders (PDDs) has increased steadily over the last 20 years, and more rapidly over the last several years, as treatment successes have triggered more rigorous study. The use of drugs targeted to possible neurochemical systems involved in the pathophysiology of autistic disorder (autism) have been shown to often reduce aggression, self-injury, and interfering repetitive behavior in these patients (Cook, 1990). No pharmacotherapeutics have yet shown a consistent primary effect on the core social disability of autism. Combined with comprehensive individualized treatment programs, appropriate pharmacotherapy can enhance an autistic person's ability to benefit from educational and behavior modification techniques (McDougle et al., 1994). This chapter will comprehensively highlight significant research in the psychopharmacology of PDDs from the perspective of specific neurochemical systems.

Drug treatment studies focusing on subtypes of PDD, other than autism, have not yet been conducted (McDougle, 2002). Many trials thus far have used heterogeneous samples, including individuals with autism, Asperger's disorder, and PDD not otherwise specified (PDD-NOS). As appropriate, differences in drug response among patients with different PDD subtypes will be highlighted. Because of their rarity, little systematic pharmacologic research has occurred in subjects with Rett's disorder or childhood disintegrative disorder.

Drugs affecting dopamine function

Evidence from clinical neurobiological studies and drug treatment response data suggest that dopamine (DA) function may be increased in some patients with

Autism and Pervasive Developmental Disorders, 2nd edn., ed. Fred R. Volkmar.
Published by Cambridge University Press. © Cambridge University Press 2007.

autism. Gillberg *et al.* (1983) found cerebrospinal fluid (CSF) concentrations of homovanillic acid – the primary metabolite of brain DA – to be elevated in 13 medication-free autistic children compared to matched controls. In addition, the indirect DA receptor agonist amphetamine has been shown to exacerbate stereotypic motor symptoms and hyperactivity in some autistic children.

Haloperidol

The potent DA (D_2) receptor antagonist haloperidol has been studied extensively in patients with autism. Campbell and colleagues have published several large, well-designed, controlled studies of the efficacy of this agent in young children with autism (Anderson *et al.*, 1984; Anderson *et al.*, 1989; Campbell *et al.*, 1978; Cohen *et al.*, 1980; Perry *et al.*, 1989). In these studies, the authors reported haloperidol (doses 1–2 mg/day) to be efficacious in young children (ages 2–8 years) for the treatment of severe symptoms associated with autism including stereotypies, aggression, withdrawal, hyperactivity, and irritability. Some studies showed a positive treatment effect on learning, and in one study older children responded better than younger children. Sedation and acute dystonic reactions were the most frequent short-term adverse effects. Dyskinesias were also frequent, occurring especially upon medication withdrawal.

Due to the frequency of dyskinesias associated with haloperidol use in children with autism, Campbell *et al.* (1997) prospectively studied these side-effects in 118 autistic children (ages 2.3–8.2 years) who had no history of seizure disorder or pre-existing dyskinesias. Forty (33.9%) children developed dyskinesias during this six-month study of haloperidol treatment followed by four weeks of placebo. The majority of dyskinesias were associated with medication withdrawal and were reversible. In a subgroup of ten children receiving a higher cumulative dose of haloperidol, nine developed dyskinesias. Since haloperidol is associated with a high incidence of dyskinesias, its use is reserved for severe treatment-refractory symptoms associated with autism.

Psychostimulants

Psychostimulant medications, such as dextroamphetamine and methylphenidate, affect a number of neurotransmitter systems, although their most potent effect is to enhance DA neurotransmission. Early reports of stimulants in patients with PDDs showed little benefit, but more recent studies suggest a modest effect.

Quintana *et al.* (1995) conducted a double-blind, crossover study of methylphenidate (10 or 20 mg twice a day for two weeks) in ten children aged 7 to 11 years with autism. Irritability and hyperactivity showed significant improvement as determined by the Aberrant Behavior Checklist (ABC) and Connors Teacher Questionnaire. In general, though, the authors considered the overall treatment effect to be modest.

A more recent double-blind, placebo-controlled study of stimulants in autistic children with symptoms of hyperactivity conducted by Handen *et al.* (2000) treated 13 children (aged 5 to 11 years) with methylphenidate (0.3 or 0.6 mg/kg per dose) and found that the medication was associated with a 50% decrease on the Connors Hyperactivity Index in 8 (62%) of the children studied. Adverse effects, which were more common with the higher dose, included social withdrawal and irritability.

The National Institute of Mental Health (NIMH)-funded Research Units on Pediatric Psychopharmacology (RUPP) Autism Network recently completed a large controlled investigation of methylphenidate that may help to elucidate the role of stimulants in the treatment of symptoms of hyperactivity, inattention, and impulsivity associated with PDDs.

Atypical antipsychotic agents

Atypical antipsychotics have the potential to attenuate the maladaptive symptoms of patients with PDDs, and potentially target core socialization deficits. This potential is derived from initial studies that have indicated that in schizophrenia, these agents were shown to improve both "positive" (hallucinations and delusions) and "negative" (blunted affect, social withdrawal, lack of interest in relationships, difficulty with spontaneous conversation, and stereotyped thinking) symptoms (McDougle, 2002). Numerous investigators have suggested that the negative symptoms of schizophrenia are similar to those deficits that compose the social deficit associated with autism. The indication from work in schizophrenia that these agents are better tolerated than conventional antipsychotics, with a lower risk of acute and tardive dyskinesias, has also led to their increased standing in addressing severe behavior issues associated with PDDs.

Risperidone

Risperidone is a highly potent serotonin $(5\text{-HT})_{2A}/D_2$ antagonist that has been found effective in controlled trials in treating the positive and negative symptoms of schizophrenia. It has been the most widely studied atypical antipsychotic in patients with PDDs. Several open-label and controlled studies have shown positive benefits of risperidone in moderating maladaptive behaviors in children and adults with autism.

Masi *et al.* (2001) conducted a 16-week, open-label trial of risperidone (optimal dose 0.5 mg/day) in 24 children (aged 3 to 6 years) with PDDs, including 19 subjects with autism and 5 subjects with PDD-NOS. Thirteen patients (54%) were judged treatment responders based on Clinical Global Impression (CGI) global improvement item (CGI-I) ratings of "much improved" or "very much improved" and a 25% decrease in Children's Psychiatric Rating Scale (CPRS) scores. Two subjects left the study because of sedation and tachycardia. No severe side-effects were noted in this analysis; the most common adverse effect was increased appetite in six subjects (25%).

Masi and colleagues (2003) published the results of a larger open-label evaluation of risperidone usage (optimal dose 0.55 ± 0.22 mg/day) in 45 boys and 8 girls (aged 3–6 years) with autism or PDD-NOS. The patients participated in the trial for an average of 7.9 ± 6.8 months. Using the same definition of patient response as in their previous study, the authors judged 22 (46.8%) of the subjects to be responders to the medication. After the study, 28 children (52.8%) stopped taking the medication because of side-effects. The most frequent side-effects included an asymptomatic increase in prolactin levels – 24 (65%) children of 37 tested – and increased appetite – 8 (15%) of 53 children participating.

An attempt to evaluate the long-term safety and effectiveness of risperidone in children was conducted by Malone *et al.* in 2002. Twenty-two children (mean age 7.1 years) with autism were treated with risperidone (mean dose 1.2 mg/day) during a one-month, short-term phase, and 13 of the children continued into a 6-month, long-term treatment phase. At the conclusion of the long-term phase of this open-label trial, the medication was discontinued to evaluate withdrawal effects. At the end of the one-month treatment period, the children's mean CPRS score had significantly declined and 17 (77.3%) of the patients were defined as "much improved" or "very much improved" on the CGI-I. During the long-term treatment phase, the authors had data on 11 of the 13 children who began this phase and of these participants 10 (77% of those entering phase two) had improved CGI-I scores. The most common side-effect noted during the one-month phase was sedation in 15 (68.1%) of the participants. Increased appetite was noted in 7 (32%) of the subjects in the one-month trial, and this side-effect continued to be prevalent in the six-month phase with an average weight gain in those who completed both phases of 7.33 ± 3.7 pounds. Two (15.4%) of 13 children in the 6-month phase developed mild, reversible withdrawal dyskinesias upon medication discontinuation.

In addition to these open-label studies, two controlled investigations of the use of risperidone in patients with PDD have been conducted. McDougle *et al.* (1998a) conducted a 12-week, double-blind, placebo-controlled trial of risperidone, mean dose 2.9 mg/day, in 31 adults with autism (17 patients) or PDD-NOS (14 patients). Repetitive behavior, aggression, anxiety, irritability, depression, and general behavioral symptoms decreased in 8 of 14 patients, as measured by ratings of "much improved" or "very much improved" on the CGI-I scale. Sixteen subjects who received placebo showed no response. Objective improvement in social behavior or language did not occur with the treatment. Fifteen patients who received placebo during the study were subsequently given open-label risperidone for 12 weeks, and 9 (60%) of these patients were noted to be responders. Mild, transient sedation was the only noted side-effect. Generally, the authors reported the medication to be well tolerated without extrapyramidal, cardiac, or seizure effects.

The NIMH-sponsored RUPP Autism Network completed an eight-week, double-blind, placebo-controlled study of risperidone (mean dose 1.8 mg/day) in 101 children and adolescents (aged 5 to 17 years) with autism (RUPP Autism Network, 2002). At the completion of the study, 69% of the treatment participants as compared to only 12% of the placebo group were defined as responders. Response was defined by at least a 25% decrease on ABC Irritability subscale scores, and a rating of "much improved" or "very much improved" on the CGI-I. Risperidone was noted to be effective in treating aggression, agitation, hyperactivity, and repetitive behaviors. The medication was associated with a significantly greater weight gain than placebo (2.7 ± 2.9 kg vs. 0.8 ± 2.2 kg). Increased appetite, fatigue, drowsiness, dizziness, and drooling were also more common in the treatment group. However, no children were withdrawn from the study because of adverse effects. The authors commented that most side-effects were mild and self-limited. This study represents the largest controlled drug trial to date in patients with PDD. A follow-up report to this study found that in addition to the measures used in the primary analysis, risperidone was superior to placebo in reducing symptoms most concerning to the participating patients (Arnold et al., 2003).

Overall, risperidone has been shown in open-label and controlled studies to be efficacious in addressing maladaptive behaviors often associated with autism.

Olanzapine

Four open-label studies have described the use of the atypical antipsychotic olanzapine in subjects with PDD. No placebo-controlled studies of olanzapine in patients with PDD have been published to date.

Potenza et al. (1999) reported that six (86%) of seven children, adolescents and adults with autism or another PDD (mean age 20.9 ± 11.7 years) who completed a 12-week, open-label trial of olanzapine (mean dose 7.8 ± 4.7 mg/day) were medication responders based on the CGI-I. Significant improvement was noted on many symptoms, including aggression, anxiety, and social relatedness. An average weight gain of 18.44 lb (8.4 kg) per patient was noted during this trial.

Seven male patients (aged 8 to 52 years) with PDD (five with autism, two with PDD-NOS) were evaluated for a mean duration of 17.7 months while on olanzapine therapy (5–10 mg/day) in addition to their current medication regimens (five patients on concurrent psychoactive medications) (Stavrakaki et al., 2004). All patients showed improvement based on CGI and Global Assessment of Function scores. Few side-effects were noted by the authors, with dose-related sedation being the most common in four (57%) of the patients.

Kemner et al. (2002) conducted a three-month, open-label trial of olanzapine (mean dose 10.7 mg/day) in 25 children (aged 6–16 years) with autism or PDD-NOS. Twenty-three children who completed the study showed improvement on the Irritability, Hyperactivity, and Inappropriate Speech subscales of the ABC, but only three (12%) of those who started the study were noted to have improvement on the CGI. The most common side-effect noted was weight gain with increased appetite. Three children (12%) developed extrapyramidal side-effects that disappeared after the dose was lowered.

Olanzapine was compared to haloperidol treatment in 12 children with autism (mean age 7.8 ± 2.1 years) during a six-week, open-label treatment study (Malone et al., 2001). The mean final dose of olanzapine was 7.9 ± 2.5 mg/day. Both treatment groups showed symptom reduction, with five (83%) children in the olanazpine group and three (50%) children in the haloperidol treatment group showing an improved CGI score. The most common side-effects noted included sedation and weight gain.

Quetiapine

Only one report to date has evaluated the usage of the atypical antipsychotic quetiapine in patients with PDD. Martin et al. (1999) conducted an open-label, 16-week trial of quetiapine (1.6–5.2 mg/kg per day) in six children and adolescents with autism. Only two patients completed the trial, both of whom were noted to be "much improved" or "very much improved" on the CGI-I. Overall, the group showed no statistically significant behavior improvement on rating scale measures. One subject dropped out because of a possible seizure, and two others left the study because of sedation or a lack of treatment effect.

Ziprasidone

Two open-label trials of the atypical antipsychotic ziprasidone have been published in patients with PDD.

McDougle *et al.* (2002) conducted a naturalistic, open-label study of ziprasidone, 20–120 mg/day (mean dose 59.2 mg/day), in 12 patients aged 8–20 years. Nine of the patients were diagnosed with autism and three with PDD-NOS. Six patients (50%) were noted to be responders over the 14-week trial, with response being defined by a rating of "much improved" or "very much improved" on the CGI-I. Transient sedation was the most common side-effect, and no cardiovascular effects were reported.

Cohen *et al.* (2004) reported on a retrospective study of ten autistic adults (mean age 43.8 years) switched to ziprasidone (mean dose 128 ± 41 mg/day) from other atypical antipsychotics. The study covered six months of treatment after the patients were switched, and all patients continued with ziprasidone at the end of this review. Primarily, patients switched antipsychotics because of weight gain, but other reasons, including increased cholesterol, maladaptive behaviors, and depression were noted. Seven patients (70%) were noted to have improvement or no worsening in their maladaptive behaviors on ziprasidone. No significant adverse effects were noted with ziprasidone, and eight patients (80%) lost weight after the medication switch.

Clozapine

The atypical antipsychotic clozapine's mechanism of action is proposed to be blockage of the $5\text{-}HT_{2A}$, $5\text{-}HT_{2C}$, $5\text{-}HT_3$, and dopamine $D_1\text{-}D_4$ receptors. Only small case reports of the usage of clozapine in patients with PDD exist in the literature.

Zuddas *et al.* (1996) treated three children with autism and hyperactivity and aggression refractory to typical antipsychotics with clozapine. After three months of treatment (up to 200 mg/day), all three children were noted to have improvement in their target symptoms. Gobbi and Pulvirenti (2001) reported one case of a 32-year-old man with autism receiving clozapine (300 mg/day) with clinical improvement noted on the CGI, including improved socialization and decreased ritualistic behavior. No side-effects were reported in either case report.

The scarcity of reports of clozapine usage in patients with PDD may be due, in part, to the concern regarding agranulocytosis or seizures that have been associated with administering the drug. In particular, patients with PDD have been reported to have a higher prevalence of seizure disorders. Furthermore, the frequent blood draws necessary for clozapine administration are not ideal for children, particularly those with autism.

Drugs affecting serotonin function

While little is definitively known regarding the pathophysiology of autism, abnormalities of the 5-HT neurotransmitter system have been identified in a subset of patients. Schain and Freedman (1961) first reported on elevated levels of whole-blood 5-HT in the peripheral vascular system of autistic children compared to normal controls. Others have replicated this finding in groups of children compared to normal controls (Anderson *et al.*, 1987). Conflicting data do exist, however, with one controlled study reporting low whole-blood and high urinary 5-HT levels in autistic children (Herault *et al.*, 1996).

Research into the genetic basis of 5-HT dysfunction in individuals with autism has yielded mixed results. Several studies have looked for polymorphisms in the 5-HT transporter gene specific to individuals with autism. Four studies have shown nominally significant excess transmission of alleles of the transporter gene, while three studies have reported no excess transmission (Conroy *et al.*, 2004).

Finally, acute dietary depletion of the 5-HT precursor tryptophan has been associated with an exacerbation of behavioral symptoms in drug-free autistic adults (McDougle *et al.*, 1996a). Based upon the large amount of evidence pointing to 5-HT dysregulation in patients with autism, drugs that affect this system have been extensively studied.

Fenfluramine

Early reports of elevated levels of whole-blood 5-HT in subjects with autism, combined with information that the indirect 5-HT agonist fenfluramine decreased brain and blood 5-HT levels in animals, led to this drug receiving extensive investigations in autism.

Despite early enthusiasm generated by reports of treatment success in open-label settings, most controlled studies have shown no significant benefits when using fenfluramine to treat symptoms associated with autism (Campbell *et al.*, 1988; Stern *et al.*, 1990). Problems with poor drug tolerability over time were also noted during a 2-year follow-up of six children with autism (Varley & Holm, 1990). Furthermore, increasing evidence of possible neurotoxic effects of the drug on 5-HT neurons in animals and the association of fenfluramine with primary pulmonary hypertension and (in combination with phentermine) valvular heart disease have eliminated its use as a safe agent in treating children with maladaptive behaviors.

Clomipramine

Clomipramine is a nonselective tricyclic agent that has been shown in double-blind, placebo-controlled trials to be efficacious in the treatment of depression and obsessive–compulsive disorder (OCD) (Greist *et al.*, 1995). Although clomipramine affects norepinephrine (NE) and DA neuronal uptake, its most potent action is to inhibit 5-HT uptake.

The impact of clomipramine on the treatment of compulsions associated with OCD and the resemblance, in part, of these behaviors to repetitive and stereotyped behavior in autism, have led some researchers to assess the benefit of the drug in patients with PDD. Gordon *et al.* (1993) published the first controlled study of clomipramine in patients with autism. The authors found clomipramine (152 ± 56 mg/day) to be superior to the relatively selective NE uptake inhibitor desipramine (127 ± 52 mg/day) and placebo in a ten-week (five weeks each on drug or placebo), randomized, crossover study in children with autism (mean age 9.6 years). In comparison to placebo, improvement from clomipramine was noted with regard to anger, hyperactivity and obsessive–compulsive symptoms. As compared to desipramine, patients taking clomipramine had significantly less anger and obsessive–compulsive symptoms. Adverse effects from clomipramine included prolongation of the cardiac QT interval, tachycardia, and *grand mal* seizure.

Brodkin *et al.* (1997) completed a 12-week, open-label trial of clomipramine (139.4 ± 50.4 mg/day) in 35 adults (mean age 30.2 years) who met DSM-IV criteria for PDD (autism $n = 15$; Asperger's disorder $n = 8$; PDD-NOS $n = 12$). Of the 33 patients who completed the trial, 18 (55%) were noted to be responders based on the CGI-I. Improvement was seen in aggression, self-injurious behavior, interfering repetitive thoughts and behavior, and social relatedness. Thirteen (39%) of the 33 patients had significant side-effects including seizures (three patients, two with pre-existing seizure disorder previously controlled on medications), weight gain, constipation, sedation, agitation, and anorgasmia.

Similar concerns regarding the tolerability of clomipramine in individuals with PDD were mentioned in a seven-week, double-blind, placebo-controlled trial of clomipramine (mean dose 128 mg/day), haloperidol (mean dose 1.3 mg/day), and placebo in 36 autistic patients (aged 10 to 36 years) (Remington *et al.*, 2001). Among the patients who completed the trial, clomipramine and haloperidol were similarly effective in reducing overall autistic symptoms, irritability, and stereotypy. The authors noted, though, that significantly fewer individuals receiving clomipramine versus haloperidol were able to complete the trial (37.5% vs. 69.7%). Reasons noted for those leaving the trial during clomipramine treatment included lack of efficacy, side-effects, or behavior problems. Among the side-effects noted, fatigue and tremor were the most prevalent.

Fluvoxamine

Selective serotonin reuptake inhibitors (SSRIs), such as fluvoxamine, are also potent inhibitors of 5-HT uptake. Because of their better side-effect profile than clomipramine, SSRIs have been receiving increased attention as a treatment for the symptoms of autism.

To date, only one controlled trial of fluvoxamine in patients with PDD has been published. Fluvoxamine (mean dose 276.7 mg/day) or placebo was given to 30 adults with autism for 12 weeks (McDougle et al., 1996b). Eight patients (53%) in the treatment group were categorized a "much improved" or "very much improved" on the CGI-I (compared to none of the placebo-treated patients). Fluvoxamine was significantly better than placebo at reducing repetitive thoughts and aggression. In addition, fluvoxamine increased the communicative use of language as measured by the Ritvo–Freeman Real Life Rating Scale. Adverse effects from the treatment included sedation and nausea, which were minimal and self-limited.

Less encouraging data on the use of fluvoxamine in children and adolescents with PDD were generated by McDougle and colleagues (unpublished data). A 12-week, double-blind, placebo-controlled study of 34 patients (mean age 9.5 years) with PDD (12 with autism, 8 with Asperger's disorder, 14 with PDD-NOS) found no significant treatment difference between groups for any target symptoms. The average dose of fluvoxamine in the treatment group was 106.9 mg/day (range 25–250 mg/day). Only 1 of 18 children in the treatment group showed a significant clinical improvement. Adverse effects were noted in 14 (78%) patients in the fluvoxamine group. The most common adverse effects included insomnia, motor hyperactivity, agitation, and aggression.

The markedly lower efficacy and tolerability of fluvoxamine in children and adolescents with PDD from this preliminary study underscores the importance of a developmental approach to pharmacotherapy in autistic patients.

Paroxetine

Only a few reports, none of them controlled, have been published on the use of the SSRI paroxetine in individuals with PDD.

Two case reports of the effective use of paroxetine in individuals with autism exist. Paroxetine (20 mg/day) decreased self-injury in a 15-year-old boy with high-functioning autism (Snead et al., 1994). In the second report, paroxetine resulted in a reduction of irritability, tantrums, and interfering preoccupations in a 7-year-old boy with autism (Posey et al., 1999).

Davanzo et al. (1998) conducted a 4-month, open-label study of 15 adults with severe and profound mental retardation (seven with PDD) who were treated with paroxetine (20–50 mg/day). The treatment was noted to be successful in reducing aggression at 1 month, but not at the 4-month follow-up. The authors hypothesized that adaptive changes may have occurred in 5-HT receptor density and sensitivity, thus leading to the decreased response.

In a retrospective study of both fluoxetine (20–80 mg/day) and paroxetine (20–40 mg/day), Branford et al. (1998) noted that 3 (25%) of 12 adults with "intellectual disability" and autistic traits (mean age 39 years) treated with paroxetine (mean duration of treatment 13 months) were rated as "much improved" or "very much improved" on the CGI-I.

Fluoxetine

The SSRI fluoxetine has been evaluated in two open-label trials and one small controlled study in patients with PDD.

Fatemi et al. (1998) conducted a longitudinal open-label trial of seven autistic patients (aged 9 to 20 years) given fluoxetine 20–80 mg/day (mean dose 37.1 mg/day) for 1–32 months (mean duration 18 ± 10.4 months). As measured by the ABC, irritability, lethargy, and stereotypy improved during the trial. Adverse effects noted included increased hyperactivity and transient appetite suppression.

A second open-label trial enrolled 129 children (aged 2 to 8 years) with autism (DeLong et al., 2002). The patients received fluoxetine (0.15 to 0.5 mg/kg per day) for 5–76 months (mean 34 months). The investigators rated the medication response as "excellent" in 22 children (17%), "good" in 67 (52%), and "fair/poor" in 40 (31%). The authors reported that medication response correlated strongly with a familial history of major affective disorder, unusual intellectual achievement, and hyperlexia. Aggression was the most prevalent side-effect noted in this trial.

Buchsbaum et al. (2001) conducted a 16-week, placebo-controlled, crossover trial of fluoxetine in six adult patients with PDD (five with autism, one with Asperger's disorder). Patients also received positron emission tomography and magnetic resonance imaging at baseline and at the end of fluoxetine administration. A significant treatment effect was noted with decreased obsessions subscale scores on the Yale–Brown Obsessive–Compulsive Scale. Three of the patients (50%) were noted to have scores of "much improved" on the CGI-I. The results of the imaging studies showed that patients with higher metabolic rates in the medial and frontal region and anterior cingulate gyrus at baseline were more likely to respond to the medication.

Sertraline

To date only open-label trials of the SSRI sertraline exist in patients with PDD.

Steingard *et al.* (1997) conducted an open-label trial of sertraline (25–50 mg/day for 2–8 weeks) in nine autistic children aged 6 to 12 years. Eight of the children (88%) were noted to show clinical improvement during the trial. Improvement was observed in irritability, transition-associated anxiety, and the need for sameness.

Over the course of a 12-week, open-label study, McDougle *et al.* (1998b) evaluated 42 adults with PDD (autism, Asperger's disorder, or PDD-NOS) taking sertraline (mean dose 122 mg/day). The authors reported the drug to be effective in improving aggression and interfering repetitive behavior, without any improvement in social relatedness. As determined by a CGI-I score of "much improved" or "very much improved," 15 (68%) of 22 subjects with autism, none of 6 with Asperger's disorder, and 9 (64%) of 14 with PDD-NOS were judged responders. Those subjects with autism or PDD-NOS showed significantly more improvement than those with Asperger's disorder. The authors hypothesized that this difference may have been because those diagnosed with Asperger's disorder were less symptomatic at baseline. Three (7%) of the 42 subjects in the study dropped out due to intolerable agitation and anxiety.

Citalopram

Only retrospective chart review studies are available regarding the use of the SSRI citalopram in patients with PDD.

Couturier and Nicolson (2002) first evaluated the use of citalopram in a retrospective case series of 17 children and adolescents (age range 4–15 years) with PDD (14 with autism, 3 with Asperger's disorder). Treatment was for a minimum of two months with an average treatment duration of 7.4 ± 5.3 months and a mean final dose of 19.7 ± 7.8 mg/day. Ten (58%) of 17 patients were reported to be "much improved" or "very much improved" on the CGI. Core symptoms of PDD, including social interaction and communication, showed no improvement. Four patients discontinued the medication because of adverse effects that included two patients with increased agitation, one with possible tic development and one with severe insomnia.

A second retrospective case series involving the use of citalopram in children and adolescents with PDDs was conducted by Namerow *et al.* in 2003. This investigation reviewed the charts of 15 children and adolescents with PDDs (aged 6–16 years). Six patients met criteria for Asperger's disorder, 2 for autism, and 7 for PDD-NOS. The average final dose of citalopram was 16.9 ± 12.1 mg/day for an average duration of 218.8 ± 167.2 days. Analysis of CGI improvement found that 11 (73%) of the 15 patients were rated as "much improved" or "very much improved." This improvement was observed for all patients with Asperger's disorder, 1 of 2 patients with autism, and 4 of 7 with PDD-NOS. According to symptom domain, 10 patients (66%) showed improved repetitive and/or stereotyped behaviors and 7 patients (47%) showed improved mood profile, including decreased aggression and/or irritability. Also, of the patients who responded, 9 out of 10 were reported to have previously been nonresponsive to other SSRIs. Five patients (33%) in this study reported side-effects that included headaches, sedation, agitation, and lip dyskinesias; two patients stopped the medication because of these side-effects.

Buspirone

Buspirone is a 5-HT$_{1A}$ receptor partial agonist approved by the Food and Drug Administration (FDA) for the treatment of generalized anxiety disorder.

Several case reports and small open-label studies have reported on the effectiveness of buspirone in the treatment of patients with autism (reviewed in Posey & McDougle, 2000). Larger prospective studies have generated mixed results.

King and Davanzo (1996) in a prospective, open-label study of buspirone (30–60 mg/day daily for 28–413 days) found the drug to be ineffective in treating the target symptoms of aggression and self-injury in 26 adults with severe to profound mental retardation, including 9 patients with PDDs.

In another open-label study, Buitelaar et al. (1998) treated 22 children and adolescents with PDD with buspirone (15–45 mg/day) for 6–8 weeks. Nine subjects (40%) showed marked improvement on the CGI. Improvement was noted in the target symptoms of anxiety and irritability. In cases of treatment response, patients were followed for 1 year and benefits were sustained in all cases. After 10 months of treatment, one patient developed an orofacial–lingual dyskinesia, which remitted after discontinuation of treatment.

No controlled studies of buspirone in patients with PDD have been published.

Mirtazapine

The antidepressant mirtazapine (a medication with both serotonergic and noradrenergic properties) has been evaluated in one open-label trial in patients with PDD.

Posey et al. (2001) treated 26 patients, aged 2 to 23, diagnosed with a PDD (20 with autism, 1 with Asperger's disorder, 1 with Rett's disorder, and 4 with PDD-NOS) with mirtazapine (7.5–45 mg/day, duration of treatment 150 ± 103 days). Nine patients (34%) were reported to have decreased aggression, self-injury, irritability, hyperactivity, anxiety, depression, and insomnia with ratings of "much improved" or "very much improved" on the CGI-I. Mirtazapine was not reported to have an impact on social or communication impairment. Side-effects were noted to be mild, including increased appetite, irritability, and sedation.

Tianeptine

Tianeptine is a newer antidepressant with a novel neurochemical profile. It is not currently available in the United States. The drug decreases brain 5-HT uptake and reduces stress-induced atrophy of neuronal dendrites (Wagstaff *et al.*, 2001).

Niederhofer *et al.* (2003) conducted the only trial to date of tianeptine in patients with PDD. This double-blind, placebo-controlled, 12-week, crossover trial enrolled 12 male children (aged 4–15) with autism. The dosage was 37.5 mg/day and outcome measures included ABC scores as reported by patients' teachers and clinician ratings of videotaped sessions using the behavior checklist and CGI scores. The study had mixed results with teachers reporting improved irritability, stereotyped behavior and, inappropriate speech, while clinicians' ratings showed no significant difference on any measure.

Inositol

Inositol is a precursor of the second messenger for some 5-HT receptors. Clinical trials have indicated it may be an effective treatment for patients with depression, panic disorder, or OCD (Einat & Belmaker, 2001).

Only one trial of inositol in patients with PDDs has been conducted. Levin *et al.* (1997) conducted an 8-week, double-blind, placebo-controlled, crossover study of inositol (200 mg/kg per day) in ten children (aged 3–8) with autism. No significant benefit was noted on any behavioral measure. No side-effects were reported during the inositol treatment.

Venlafaxine

The antidepressant venlafaxine is a dual 5-HT and NE uptake inhibitor. Its use in patients with PDD is limited to a single case report and one retrospective chart analysis.

Marshall *et al.* (2003) reported a case of venlafaxine (37.5–75 mg/day) being associated with increased aggressive behavior in an autistic teenager on maintainance olanzapine (10 mg/day) whose treatment goals included decreased anxiety, aggression, and severe self-injurious behavior.

The cases of ten individuals with autism spectrum disorders being treated with venlafaxine (6.25–50 mg/day) were analyzed retrospectively to assess the impact of the medication on all domains of autistic impairment including socialization, repetitive behaviors, and communication (Hollander *et al.*, 2000). Six of the patients reviewed (60%) were noted to be "much improved" or "very much improved" on the CGI-I. The authors reported that improvement occurred in repetitive behaviors, socialization, communication, inattention, and hyperactivity. The medication was reported to have been well tolerated by all participants.

Drugs affecting norepinephrine function

Studies investigating NE function and the response to drugs affecting this system suggest that this neurochemical may not be significantly involved in the pathophysiology of autism (Minderaa *et al.*, 1994). This is despite an early report by Lake *et al.* (1977) which found elevated levels of plasma NE in autistic patients compared to age-matched controls. Not all of these patients were drug-free at the time of the study. Later work investigated levels of the principal metabolite of NE, 3-methoxy-4-hydroxyphenethylene glycol (MHPG), in the plasma (Young *et al.*, 1981) and CSF (Gillberg *et al.*, 1983) of patients with autism compared to control subjects. No difference was found in MHPG levels in either the plasma or CSF in these investigations.

Despite this lack of positive evidence for a correlation between NE dysregulation and autism, several noradrenergic agents have been evaluated in controlling the maladaptive symptoms of autism.

Beta-adrenergic blockers

Beta-adrenergic blockers are drugs that block NE receptors and reduce overall NE neurotransmission.

Ratey *et al.* (1987a,b) described a reduction in aggressive, impulsive, and self-injurious behavior and an improvement in speech and socialization in eight hospitalized adults with autism treated with open-label propranolol or nadolol. Patients were started on propranolol or nadolol (40 mg/day) and the dose was increased weekly or biweekly in 40-mg increments until a positive effect occurred, or hypotension developed. The final mean dose was 225 mg/day and the average duration of treatment was 14.2 months. All eight patients showed moderate or markedly reduced aggression, six (75%) showed improved social skills, and four (50%) developed improved speech during the treatment period. Seven of the participants were on concomitant neuroleptic treatment during this trial, and of these patients, five were able to decrease their neuroleptic dosage and one was able to discontinue neuroleptic treatment. The authors felt that the improvement noted was due to the beta-blockers decreasing patients' chronic hyperarousal.

Clonidine

The α_2-adrenergic agonist clonidine has been evaluated in two controlled trials involving patients with autism.

Jaselskis *et al.* (1992) conducted a double-blind, placebo-controlled trial of clonidine in eight autistic boys (mean age 8.1 years) who demonstrated symptoms of inattention, impulsivity, and hyperactivity. Clonidine (0.004–0.01 mg/kg per day) or placebo was given during a six-week period, followed by a one-week washout, and finally the administration of the alternative treatment for six weeks. Teacher and parent ratings showed statistically significant improvement with regard to hyperactivity and irritability, but clinician ratings of videotaped sessions showed no drug–placebo differences. Adverse effects included hypotension, sedation, and irritability.

Transdermal clonidine (0.005 mg/kg per day) was evaluated in a double-blind, placebo-controlled, crossover study (four weeks in each treatment phase) involving nine males (aged 5 to 33 years) with autism (Fankhauser *et al.*, 1992). Significant improvement was noted on the CGI, and specifically hyperactivity and anxiety were reduced. The most common adverse effects noted were sedation and fatigue.

Guanfacine

Guanfacine, also an α_2-adrenergic agonist, has been evaluated retrospectively in one report involving 80 children and adolescents, aged 3 to 18 years, with PDDs (Posey *et al.*, 2004a). The mean dosage was 2.6 mg/day and 19 subjects (23.8%) were noted to have improved hyperactivity, inattention, and tics along with being rated as "much improved" or "very much improved" on the CGI-I. Sedation was the most commonly reported side-effect.

Lofexidine

The α_2-adrenergic agonist lofexidine, which is not currently available in the United States, has been the subject of one small controlled trial in individuals with PDD.

Niederhofer *et al.* (2002) conducted a double-blind, placebo-controlled, crossover trial of lofexidine (final dose 0.8–1.2 mg/day) in 12 male children (aged 5–13) with autism. Treatment periods lasted six weeks and outcome measures included weekly parent and teacher behavior checklist reports and clinician ratings of three taped behavior examples. The authors reported significant improvement with lofexidine noted by parents and teachers, with the greatest change noted in hyperactivity. None of the clinician ratings showed significant differences between placebo and lofexidine. The only side-effect reported was hypotension in three subjects (25%) whose medication doses needed to be blindly tapered down to alleviate this effect.

Drugs affecting glutamate function

The N-methyl D-aspartate (NMDA) subtype of glutamate receptor is central to neurodevelopmental processes including neuronal migration, plasticity, and differentiation (Coyle 1996). As such, disturbances in this system, via reduced neurotropic effects or excessive neurotoxicity, could substantially alter neurodevelopment (Krystal et al., 1999). These ideas have led to hypotheses of glutamatergic dysfunction in patients with PDD (Carlsson, 1998). Such theories have laid the groundwork for investigation of drugs affecting glutamate in patients with PDD.

Lamotrigine

Lamotrigine is an anticonvulsant of the phenyltriazine class. The drug attenuates some forms of cortical glutamate release via inhibition of sodium channels, P- and N-type calcium channels, and potassium channels.

In a subgroup of 50 children given lamotrigine (mean maintanance dose 4.5 mg/kg per day; mean duration 14 months) for intractable epilepsy, Uvebrandt and Bauziene (1994) treated 13 children with autism (aged 3–13 years). The authors reported eight (62%) of the autistic patients showed a decrease in "autistic symptoms." Adverse effects were noted in 42% of all study participants, with sleep disturbance and rash being the most common reactions.

Belsito et al. (2001) conducted a four-week, double-blind, placebo-controlled, trial of lamotrigine (5.0 mg/kg per day) in 14 children (aged 3–11 years) with autism. Lamotrigine and placebo showed no difference in effect as measured by the ABC, Vineland scales, Childhood Autism Rating Scale (CARS), and PreLinguistic Autism Diagnostic Observation Scale. Insomnia and hyperactivity were the most common side-effects reported.

Two case reports of successful use of lamotrigine in patients with Rett's syndrome have been reported (Kumandas et al., 2001). Two girls, aged 2.5 and 4.5 years, were treated with lamotrigine (3.0 mg/kg per day) for six months. The authors reported that after lamotrigine therapy, their convulsions were controlled, and stereotyped hand movements and autistic behaviors were markedly decreased.

Amantadine

Amantadine is a noncompetitive NMDA antagonist routinely used for the treatment of influenza, herpes zoster, and Parkinson's disease.

King *et al.* (2001) conducted a double-blind, placebo-controlled study of amantadine in 39 subjects with autism (aged 5–19 years). The design included a one-
week, single-blind, placebo lead-in, followed by a single daily dose of amantadine
(2.5 mg/kg per day) or placebo for the following week, then twice daily dosing
for the subsequent three weeks. No significant difference was found between
drug and placebo on parent ratings, although clinician-rated measures of hyperactivity and inappropriate speech showed statistically significant improvement.
The authors reported that the medication was well tolerated.

D-Cycloserine

D-Cycloserine is an NMDA partial agonist which has been shown in adults to
reduce the negative symptoms associated with schizophrenia (Goff *et al.*, 1999).
To date, one study has looked at the use of D-cycloserine in children with autism.

Posey *et al.* (2004b) conducted an eight-week trial of D-Cycloserine (0.7, 1.4,
and 2.8 mg/kg per day, each for two weeks) that began with a two-week placebo
lead-in phase. Twelve drug-free children with autism (mean age 10.0 ± 7.7 years)
were enrolled in the trial, and ten participants completed the study. Two patients
left the study after the placebo lead-in phase. D-Cycloserine was associated with a
statistically significant improvement on the CGI-severity item and the ABC Social
Withdrawal subscale. Overall, the medium and high doses of the medication
were associated with significant change from baseline. Four patients (40%) who
finished the study were considered responders based on CGI-I ratings of "much
improved." Two subjects in this study (20%) experienced adverse effects at the
highest dose. These included a transient motor tic and increased echolalia.

Mood stabilizers

Divalproex sodium

Divalproex sodium is approved by the FDA for the treatment of epilepsy and
manic episodes associated with bipolar illness.

A single, open-label trial has investigated the use of divalproex sodium in
patients with PDD. Hollander *et al.* (2001) conducted an open-label trial of
divalproex sodium (125–2500 mg/day; mean dose 768 mg/day; mean blood
level 75.8 mcg/ml) in 14 subjects aged 5–40, with PDDs (10 with autism, 2
with Asperger's disorder, 2 with PDD-NOS). Treatment lasted an average of
10.7 ± 12.3 months (range 0.5–43 months). Affective instability, repetitive behavior, impulsivity, and aggression improved in 10 patients (71%) as measured by
CGI-I ratings of "much improved" or "very much improved." Adverse effects

reported included sedation, weight gain, hair loss, elevated liver enzymes, and behavioral activation. Two subjects left the trial within the first two weeks because of severe behavioral activation.

Lithium

Three case reports of the use of the mood stabilizer lithium in patients with PDDs have been published.

Two reports exist of lithium decreasing manic symptoms in individuals with autism and a family history of bipolar disorder (Kerbeshian *et al.*, 1987; Steingard & Biederman, 1987). A single report of lithium augmentation of fluvoxamine treatment in an adult with autism noted improved aggression and impulsivity after two weeks of treatment as measured by the CGI, Brown Aggression Scale, and Vineland Adaptive Behavior Scale (Epperson *et al.*, 1994).

Other therapeutic agents

Carnosine

The dipeptide carnosine is thought to possess some neuroprotective or anti-convulsant effects by having a chelating effect on zinc and copper in the brain (Horning *et al.*, 2000), perhaps acting to modulate the impact of these metals at GABA receptor sites (Chez *et al.*, 2002).

A single study has assessed the use of carnosine in treating patients with PDD. Chez *et al.* (2002) conducted a double-blind, placebo-controlled, eight-week crossover study of L-carnosine (800 mg/day) in 31 children (aged 3–12 years) with either autism or PDD-NOS. Thirteen of the participants (42%) had a previously abnormal EEG, and thirteen subjects were on maintenance val-proic acid treatment during the trial. This trial generated mixed results with significant treatment changes noted on the Receptive One-Word Picture Vocab-ulary Test and all domains of the Gilliam Autism Rating Scale, but no significant changes were reported on the CGI, CARS, or the Expressive One-Word Picture Vocabulary test. No children had to leave the study because of medication side-effects. The authors reported only sporadic hyperactivity with the medication that resolved by decreasing the dosage.

Dimethylglycine

The dietary supplement dimethylglycine has been shown to decrease seizure activity in humans (Freed, 1984) and activate immune systems in animal studies (Reap & Lawson, 1990).

Bolman and Richmond (1999) investigated the use of dimethylglycine in males with autism in a double-blind, placebo-controlled, crossover pilot study. Eight males (aged 4–30 years) received either one, two, or three 125 mg medication tablets (depending on their weight) over a four-week period. No statistically significant difference was found between treatment and placebo on any measure employed including the Campbell–NIMH rating scale, an experimental rating scale, and an individualized scale created for each child. The medication was reportedly well tolerated.

In a second study, Kern *et al.* (2001) conducted a four-week, double-blind, placebo-controlled study of dimethylglycine (125 mg, 1–5 tablets per day depending on weight) in 18 children (aged 3–11 years) with autism or another PDD. Improvement on all behavioral measures, including Vineland scales and the ABC, were found for both placebo and treatment groups. No statistically significant difference was found between groups.

Donepezil

The cholinesterase inhibitor donepezil has been evaluated in two open-label investigations in patients with PDDs.

Chez *et al.* (2000) conducted a 12-week, open-label trial of donepezil (2.5 or 5 mg/day) in 25 boys (mean age 6.59 years) with PDDs. Significant improvement was observed in speech production as measured by the Expressive and Receptive One-Word Picture Vocabulary Tests. Autistic features, as measured by the CARS, did not show statistically significant improvement. Adverse effects noted included aggression, irritability, lethargy, and sleep disturbances.

A smaller, retrospective, open-label review of donepezil given to children with autism reported that half of the children showed a significant response to the medication (Harden & Handen, 2002). Eight children (aged 7–19 years), each on additional psychoactive medications during the review, were given donepezil (mean dose 9.37 ± 1.76 mg) over a two-month period. After treatment, four (50%) children had CGI-I scores of either "much improved" or "very much improved." Among all subjects, ABC Irritability and Hyperactivity subscale scores decreased, without any changes on the Inappropriate Speech, Lethargy, or Stereotypies subscale scores being noted. Side-effects were reported as limited, with one patient developing nausea and vomiting and one patient reporting mild irritability while taking the drug.

Levetiracetam

Levetiracetam is a novel anticonvulsant with an unknown mechanism of action currently approved to treat adult partial seizures in the United States.

Rugino and Samsock (2002) conducted an open-label study of levetiracetam (925 ± 307 mg/day) in ten males (age range 4–10 years) with autism or PDD-NOS. Patient evaluation was carried out at the beginning of the trial and again after taking the drug for an average of 4.1 weeks. Patient data were grouped and the authors reported a significant improvement in mood instability as measured by the Conners Global Index (Emotional Lability Scale and Global Scale). Improvement in hyperactivity, impulsivity, and inattention was found using the Conners ADHD Index scale and Achenbach Attention scale; no significant difference was noted with regard to aggression as measured by the Achenbach Aggression scale. The authors noted that this was due to worsening aggression in those children weaned off medications targeting aggression before the trial. Side-effects were mild with the exception of one patient who developed a diffuse rash that resolved with medication discontinuation.

No controlled trials of levetiracetam in PDD have been published to date.

Naltrexone

The opiate receptor antagonist naltrexone has been evaluated in four controlled studies in patients with autism. This research was stimulated by past investigations which have implicated the opioid system in the pathophysiology of autism. Controlled studies have found increased endorphin levels in the blood (Weizman et al., 1984) and CSF (Gillberg et al., 1985; Ross et al., 1987) of individuals with autism.

In a small, double-blind, placebo-controlled trial, Leboyer et al. (1992) studied naltrexone (0.5–2.0 mg/kg per day) given for one week in four autistic children (aged 4–19 years). Three of the children had high blood endorphin levels at baseline, and all children demonstrated significant symptom improvement on the medication; the patient with normal blood endorphin levels showed no improvement. Positive changes noted in those with elevated blood endorphin levels included improved eye contact, increased socialization, verbalization, and attentiveness, and decreased restlessness and self-injurious behavior.

A larger, double-blind, placebo-controlled study of 41 children with autism found naltrexone useful only for symptoms of hyperactivity, with no positive gains noted with regard to ability to learn (Campbell et al., 1993). Side-effects in this study were noted to be mild and transient.

Two double-blind, placebo-controlled studies of naltrexone in individuals with autism have shown no positive effects from medication usage. Willemsen-Swinkels et al. (1995) conducted a four-week trial of naltrexone (50 mg/day or 150 mg/day) versus placebo in 16 adults with autism. Naltrexone was noted to have no therapueitic effect on autistic symptoms or self-injurious behavior, and the medication was noted to cause an increase in stereotyped behavior. Feldman *et al.* (1999) evaluated 24 children with autism (aged 3–8.3 years) who were treated with naltrexone (1 mg/kg per day) or placebo for two weeks. No differences were found between naltrexone and placebo for any measures of communication. In summary, most controlled studies suggest that the core symptoms of autism and maladaptive behavior are not significantly affected by naltrexone.

Percy *et al.* (1994) conducted a four-month, double-blind, placebo-controlled trial of naltrexone in 25 patients with Rett's syndrome (aged 2–15.7 years). Positive treatment effect on respiratory disturbance was noted. Overall, the authors suggested that the treatment had a deleterious effect, with declines in motor function and a more rapid progression of the disorder noted in the treatment group.

Oxytocin

Oxytocin is a neurohypophyseal peptide that has an established role in milk ejection and uterine contraction during labor. Oxytocin's role in social development has been supported in animal studies (Carter *et al.*, 1992; Insel & Hulihan, 1995; Popik & van Ree, 1992; Witt *et al.*, 1992). Animals administered oxytocin have also been noted to develop repetitive behaviors (Drago *et al.*, 1986; Insel & Winslow, 1991; Nelson & Alberts, 1997). Modahl *et al.* (1998) found lower plasma oxytocin levels in 29 prepubertal autistic children compared to age-matched normally developing controls. These findings have supported the investigation of oxytocin as a treatment option for individuals with PDD.

Hollander *et al.* (2003) conducted a double-blind, placebo-controlled study of oxytocin (continuous four-hour infusion) in 15 high-functioning (IQ $= 90 \pm 9.90$) adults with PDD (6 with autism and 9 with Asperger's disorder). A significant difference was noted in the number and severity of repetitive behaviors as measured during the infusion. Side-effects were reportedly mild and those with autism and Asperger's disorder responded similarly.

No multidose or long-term follow up studies of oxytocin have been published in patients with PDD.

Secretin

Secretin is a polypeptide hormone secreted primarily by the endocrine cells of the upper gastrointestinal (GI) tract that are involved in regulating pancreatic exocrine secretion. Horvath *et al.* (1998) reported on three children with autism who showed marked improvement in language and social behavior after receiving secretin during a routine workup for GI complaints. Since this time, a wave of excitement and optimism was generated regarding secretin as a potential "cure" for autism. In response, a large number of well-designed controlled trials have been conducted testing this hypothesis.

Nine single-dose, double-blind, placebo-controlled trials of synthetic (four trials) or porcine (five trials) secretin in a total of 433 children with autism all reported no significant improvements on any parameter tested, including measures of language, socialization, and maladaptive behavior (Carey *et al.*, 2002; Coniglio *et al.*, 2001; Corbett *et al.*, 2001; Dunn-Geier *et al.*, 2000; Kern *et al.*, 2002; Malloy *et al.*, 2002; Owley *et al.*, 2001; Sandler *et al.*, 1999; Unis *et al.*, 2002).

Two studies have evaluated multiple doses of secretin in patients with autism. Roberts *et al.* (2001) conducted a double-blind, placebo-controlled trial using two doses of secretin given six weeks apart to 64 autistic children. No significant treatment effects were found in this investigation. A much smaller study was carried out with six children in a crossover design used three doses of secretin (Sponheim *et al.*, 2002). Again, this study found no significant differences between secretin and placebo.

Based on the results of these 11 systematic investigations, secretin is not currently recommended as a treatment for target symptoms associated with autism.

Conclusion

Significant progress in the pharmacotherapy of PDD has been made in recent years. This progress is best exemplified by the development of the RUPP Autism Network and the large multisite controlled study of risperidone already conducted by this group. As these advances continue, one can anticipate a continuous flow of open-label reports with successful reports followed by rigorous controlled studies. Ongoing work is necessary to further begin to tease out medication effects on specific subtypes of PDD. As the most recognized and prevalent PDD, autism has garnered the most research attention. It will be important to continue to address the difference in medication response between all subtypes of PDD whenever possible. It will also be necessary to continue to follow children and adults with PDD on psychopharmacologic agents over a long period to determine both the impact of development on drug response and assess for long-term side-effects.

The recent increase of available data has allowed for the development of symptom-based algorithms for the psychopharmacologic management of autism (Stigler *et al.*, 2003). This is important in that it gives emphasis to the importance of specific target symptoms while recognizing that to date there is no one drug designed to alleviate all possible maladaptive behaviors associated with PDDs. These published algorithms address hyperactivity/inattention, anxiety, repetitive behaviors, and aggression. In addition to behavior therapy being recommended as a first-line approach to most symptoms, α_2-adrenergic agonists followed by atypical antipsychotics (if no response) are recommended for treatment of hyperactivity or inattention. In this report, anxiety is recommended to be approached with mirtazapine first followed by low-dose SSRI, and then α_2-adrenergic agonists, if necessary. Repetitive behaviors are referred to a trial of low-dose SSRI followed by an atypical antipsychotic if no response is seen with the SSRI. Aggressive behavior is divided in this analysis between mild and severe degrees, with mild cases referred to an α_2-adrenergic agonist, followed by an atypical antipsychotic and then a mood stabilizer, if necessary. Severe cases follow a similar progression with the exception that treatment is recommended to begin with an atypical antipsychotic. The fact that such algorithms have been developed is a testament to the continued growth and maturation of the research surrounding autism and psychopharmacology. These proposals will be able to be adjusted and refined as new information becomes available and over time, after adequate testing, such protocols could even possibly be adopted by governing bodies of professionals as official recommendations.

While it is recognized that medications work to assist patients with severe behaviors to gain from nonpharmacologic treatment modalities, research that investigates drug treatment in combination with certain educational and behavioral therapies should be pursued. This would help to determine in which areas medications specifically enhance learning experiences for individuals with PDD. A future goal will be giving practitioners information about which drugs offer the greatest efficacy to address a specific behavioral deficit, which may be limiting a participant's progress in a particular area of education or behavioral treatment.

Pharmacogenetics (the study of the genetic basis of treatment response or lack thereof) will continue to be important in the research of PDD psychopharmacology. Examples thus far are the numerous studies looking at the 5-HT transporter gene in autistic individuals. The fields of genetics and psychopharmacology will continue to be best served by working together to understand the basis of treatment response, always with an eye toward linking treatment effects to possible etiologic factors of PDDs.

The advancement of neuroimaging to look at both functional and structural entities should serve psychopharmacologic research well as treatment response can be viewed in both behavioral manifestations and at the level of altered brain activity. This combination, again like that with genetics, can also point toward potential pathophysiologic causes of the impairments associated with PDD.

Finally, the scientific community will need to continue to be cognizant of reputed autism "cures" and the impact such reports have on the families of patients with PDDs. It will be necessary for such claims to be continually evaluated in a scientifically rigorous manner.

Acknowledgments

This work was supported in part by a Daniel X. Freedman Psychiatric Research Fellowship Award (Dr. Posey), a National Alliance for Research in Schizophrenia and Depression (NARSAD) Young Investigator Award (Dr. Posey), a Research Units on Pediatric Psychopharmacology Grant (U10-MH66766-02) from the National Institute of Mental Health (NIMH) to Indiana University (Drs. McDougle, Stigler, and Posey), a Research Career Development Award (K23-MH068627-01) from the NIMH (Dr. Posey), a National Institutes of Health Clinical Research Center Grant to Indiana University (M01-RR00750), and a Department of Housing and Urban Development (HUD) Grant No. B-01-SP-IN-0200 (Dr. McDougle).

REFERENCES

Anderson, G. M., Freedman, D. X., Cohen, D. J. et al. (1987). Whole blood serotonin in autistic and normal subjects. *Journal of Child Psychology and Psychiatry*, **28**, 885–900.

Anderson L. T., Campbell, M., Grega, D. M. et al. (1984). Haloperidol in the treatment of infantile autism: effects on learning and behavioral symptoms. *American Journal of Psychiatry*, **141**, 1195–202.

Anderson L. T., Campbell, M., Adams, P. et al. (1989). The effects of haloperidol on discrimination learning and behavioral symptoms in autistic children. *Journal of Autism and Developmental Disorders*, **19**, 227–39.

Arnold, L. E., Vitiello, B., McDougle, C. et al. (2003). Parent-defined target symptoms respond to risperidone in RUPP autism study: customer approach to clinical trials. *Journal of the American Academy of Child and Adolescent Psychiatry*, **42**, 1443–50.

Belsito, K. M., Law, P. A., Kirk, K. S., Landa, R. J., and Zimmerman, A.W. (2001). Lamotrigine therapy for autistic disorder: a randomized, double-blind, placebo-controlled trial. *Journal of Autism and Developmental Disorders*, **31**, 175–81.

Bolman, W. M. and Richmond, J. A. (1999). A double-blind placebo controlled, crossover pilot trial of low dose dimethylglycine in patients with autistic disorder. *Journal of Autism and Developmental Disorders*, **29**, 191–4.

Branford, D., Bhaumik, S., and Naik, B. (1998). Selective serotonin re-uptake inhibitors for the treatment of pervasive and maladaptive behaviors of people with intellectual disability. *Journal of Intellectual Disability Research*, **42**, 301–6.

Brodkin, E. S., McDougle, C. J., Naylor, S. T., Cohen, D. J., and Price L. H. (1997). Clomipramine in adults with pervasive developmental disorders: a prospective open-label investigation. *Journal of Child and Adolescent Psychopharmacology*, **7**, 109–21.

Buchsbaum, M. S., Hollander, E., Hazendar, M. M. *et al.* (2001). Effects of fluoxetine on regional cerebral metabolism in autistic spectrum disorder: a pilot study. *International Journal of Neuropsychopharmacology*, **4**, 119–25.

Buitelaar, J. K., van der Gaag, R. J., and van der Hoeven, J. (1998). Buspirone in the management of anxiety and irritability in children with pervasive developmental disorders: results of an open-label trial. *Journal of Clinical Psychiatry*, **59**, 56–9.

Campbell, M., Anderson, L. T., Meier, M. *et al.* (1978). A comparison of haloperidol and behavior therapy and their interaction in autistic children. *Journal of the American Academy of Child and Adolescent Psychiatry*, **17**, 640–55.

Campbell, M., Adams, P., Small, A. M. *et al.* (1988). Efficacy and safety of fenfluramine in autistic children. *Journal of the American Academy of Child and Adolescent Psychiatry*, **27**, 434–9.

Campbell, M., Anderson, L. T., Small, A. M. *et al.* (1993). Naltrexone in autistic children: behavioral symptoms and attentional learning. *Journal of the American Academy of Child and Adolescent Psychiatry*, **32**, 1283–91.

Campbell, M., Armenteros, J. L., Malone, R. P. *et al.* (1997). Neuroleptic-related dyskinesias in autistic children: a prospective, longitudinal study. *Journal of the American Academy of Child and Adolescent Psychiatry*, **36**, 835–43.

Carey, T., Ratliff-Schaub, K., Funk, J. *et al.* (2002). Double-blind placebo-controlled trial of secretin: effects on aberrant behavior in children with autism. *Journal of Autism and Developmental Disorders*, **32**, 161–7.

Carlsson, M. L. (1998). Hypothesis: is infantile autism a hypoglutamatergic disorder? Relevance of glutamate–serotonin interactions for pharmacotherapy. *Journal of Neural Transmission*, **105**, 525–35.

Carter, C. S., Williams, J. R., Witt, D. M., and Insel T. R. (1992). Oxytocin and social bonding. *Annals of the New York Academy of Science*, **652**, 204–11.

Chez, M. G., Nowinski, C. V., Buchanan, C. P., and Jones, C. (2000). Donepezil use in children with autistic spectrum disorders. *American Neurological Association Annual Meeting* [abstract].

Chez, M. G., Buchanan, C. P., Aimonovitch, M. C. *et al.* (2002). Double-blind, placebo-controlled study of L-carnosine supplementation in children with autistic spectrum disorders. *Journal of Child Neorology*, **17**, 833–7.

Cohen, I. L., Campbell, M., Posner, D. *et al.* (1980). Behavioral effects of haloperidol in young autistic children. *Journal of the American Academy of Child and Adolescent Psychiatry*, **19**, 665–77.

Cohen, S. A., Fitzgerald, B. J., Khan, S. R., and Khan, A. (2004). The effect of a switch to ziprasidone in an adult population with autistic disorder: chart review of naturalistic, open-label treatment. *Journal of Clinical Psychiatry*, **65**, 110–13.

Coniglio, S. J., Lewis, J. D., Lang, C., and Burns, T. G. (2001). A randomized, double-blind, placebo-controlled trial of single-dose intravenous secretin as a treatment for children with autism. *Journal of Pediatrics*, **138**, 649–55.

Conroy, J., Meally, E., Kearney, G. *et al.* (2004). Serotonin transporter gene and autism: a haplotype analysis in an Irish autistic population. *Molecular Psychiatry*, **9**, 587–93.

Cook, E. H. (1990). Autism: review of neurochemical investigation. *Synapse*, **6**, 292–308.

Corbett, B., Khan, K., Czapansky-Beilman, D., and Brady, N. (2001). A double-blind, placebo-controlled crossover study investigating the effect of porcine secretin in children with autism. *Clinical Pediatrics*, **40**, 327–31.

Couturier, J. L. and Nicolson, R. (2002). A retrospective assessment of citalopram in children and adolescents with pervasive developmental disorders. *Journal of Child and Adolescent Psychopharmacology*, **12**, 243–8.

Coyle, J. T. (1996). The glutaminergic dysfunction hypothesis for schizophrenia. *Harvard Review of Psychiatryy*, **3**, 241–53.

Davanzo, P. A., Belin, T. R., Widawski, M. H., and King, B. H. (1998). Paroxetine treatment of aggression and self-injury in persons with mental retardation. *American Journal of Mental Retardation*, **102**, 427–37.

DeLong, G. R., Ritch, C. R., and Burch, S. (2002). Fluoxetine response in children with autistic spectrum disorders, correlation with familial major affective disorder and intellectual achievement. *Developmental Medicine and Child Neurology*, **44**, 652–9.

Drago, F., Pedersen, C. A., Caldwell, J. D., and Prange, A. J. Jr. (1986). Oxytocin potently enhances novelty-induced grooming behavior in the rat. *Brain Research*, **368**, 287–95.

Dunn-Geier, J. Ho, H. H., Auersperg, E., and Coyle, D. (2000). Effect of secretin on children with autism: a randomized controlled trial. *Developmental Medicine and Child Neurology*, **42**, 796–802.

Einat, H. and Belmaker, R. H. (2001). The effects of inositol treatment in animal models of psychiatric disorders. *Journal of Affective Disorders*, **62**, 113–21.

Epperson, C. N., McDougle, C. J., and Anand, A. (1994). Lithium augmentation of fluvoxamine in autistic disorder: a case report. *Journal of Child and Adolescent Psychopharmacology*, **4**, 201–7.

Fankhauser, M. P., Karumanchi, V. C., German, M. L., Yates, A., and Karumanchi, S. D. (1992). A double-blind, placebo-controlled study of the efficacy of transdermal clonidine in autism. *Journal of Clinical Psychiatry*, **53**, 77–82.

Fatemi, S. H., Realmuto, G. M., Khan, L., and Thuras, P. (1998). Fluoxetine in treatment of adolescent patients with autism: a longitudinal open trial. *Journal of Autism and Developmental Disorders*, **28**, 303–7.

Feldman, H. M., Kolman, B. K., and Gonzaga, A. M. (1999). Naltexone and communication skills in young children with autism. *Journal of the American Academy of Child and Adolescent Psychiatry*, **38**, 587–93.

Freed, W. J. (1984). *N,N*-Dimethylglycine, betaine, and seizures. *Archives of Neurology*, **41**, 1129–30.

Gillberg, C., Terenius, L., and Lonnerholm, G. (1985). Endorphin activity in childhood psychosis. *Archives of General Psychiatry*, **42**, 780–3.

Gillberg, C. Svennerholm, L., and Hamilton-Hellberg, C. (1983). Childhood psychosis and monoamine metabolites in spinal fluid. *Journal of Autism and Developmental Disorders*, **13**, 383–96.

Gobbi, G. and Pulvirenti, L. (2001). Long-term treatment with clozapine in an adult with autistic disorder accompanied by aggressive behavior. *Journal of Psychiatry and Neuroscience*, **26**, 340–1.

Goff, D. C., Tsai, G., Levitt, J. *et al.* (1999). A placebo-controlled trial of D-cycloserine added to conventional neuroleptics in patients with schizophrenia. *Archives of General Psychiatry*, **56**, 21–7.

Gordon, C. T., State, R. C., Nelson, J. E., Hamburger, S. D., and Rapoport, J. L. (1993). A double-blind comparison of clomipramine, desipramine, and placebo in the treatment of autistic disorder. *Archives of General Psychiatry*, **50**, 441–7.

Greist, J. H., Jefferson, J. W., Kobak, K. A., Katzelnick, D. J., and Serlin R. C. (1995). Efficacy and tolerability of serotonin transport inhibitors in obsessive–compulsive disorder. A meta-analysis. *Archives of General Psychiatry*, **52**, 53–60.

Handen, B. L., Johnson, C. R., and Lubetsky, M. (2000). Efficacy of methylphenidate among children with autism and symptoms of attention-deficit hyperactivity disorder. *Journal of Autism and Developmental Disorders*, **30**, 245–55.

Harden, A. Y. and Handen, B. L. (2002). A retrospective open trial of adjunctive donepezil in children and adolescents with autistic disorder. *Journal of Child and Adolescent Psychopharmacology*, **12**, 237–41.

Herault, J., Petit, E., Martineau, J. *et al.* (1996). Serotonin and autism: biochemical and molecular biology features. *Psychiatry Research*, **65**, 33–43.

Hollander, E., Kaplan, A., Cartwright, C., and Reichman, D. (2000). Venlafaxine in children, adolescents and young adults with autism spectrum disorders: an open retrospective clinical report. *Journal of Child Neurology*, **15**, 132–5.

Hollander, E., Dolgoff-Kaspar, R., Cartwright, C., Rawitt, R., and Novotny, S. (2001). An open trial of divalproex sodium in autism spectrum disorders. *Journal of Clinical Psychiatry*, **62**, 530–4.

Hollander, E., Novotny, S., Hanratty, M. *et al.* (2003). Oxytocin infusion reduces repetitive behaviors in adults with autistic and Asperger's disorders. *Neuropsychopharmacology*, **28**, 193–8.

Horning, M. S., Blakemore, L. J., and Trombley, P. Q. (2000). Endogenous mechanisms of neuroprotection: role of zinc, copper, and carnosine. *Brain Research*, **852**, 56–61.

Horvath, K., Stefanatos, G., Sokolski, K. N. *et al.* (1998). Improved social and language skills after secretin administration in patients with autistic spectrum disorder. *Journal of the American Association for Academic Minority Physicians*, **9**, 9–15.

Insel, T. R. and Hulihan, T. J. (1995). A gender-specific mechanism for pair bonding: oxytocin and partner preference formation in monogamous voles. *Behavioral Neuroscience*, **109**, 782–9.

Insel T. R. and Winslow J. T. (1991). Central administration of oxytocin modulates the infant rat's response to social isolation. *European Journal of Pharmacology*, **203**, 149–52.

Jaselskis, C. A., Cook, E. H. Jr., Fletcher, K. E., and Levanthal, B. L. (1992). Clonidine treatment of hyperactive and impulsive children with autistic disorder. *Journal of Clinical Psychopharmacology*, **12**, 322–7.

Kemner, C., Willemsen-Swinkels, S. H., de Jonge, M., Tuynman-Qua, H., and van Engeland, H. (2002). Open-label study of olanzapine in children with pervasive developmental disorder. *Journal of Clinical Psychopharmacology*, **22**, 455–60.

Kerbeshian, J., Burd, L., and Fisher, W. (1987). Lithium carbonate in the treatment of two patients with infantile autism and atypical bipolar symptomology. *Journal of Clinical Psychopharmacology*, **7**, 401–5.

Kern, J. K., Miller, V. S., Cauller, L. *et al.* (2001). Effectiveness of *N,N*-dimethylglycine in autism and pervasive developmental disorder. *Journal of Child Neurology*, **16**, 169–73.

Kern, J. K., Miller, V. S., Evans, P. A., and Trivendi, M. H. (2002). Efficacy of porcine secretin in children with autism and pervasive developmental disorder. *Journal of Autism and Developmental Disorder*, **32**, 153–60.

King, B. H. and Davanzo, P. (1996). Buspirone treatment of aggression self-injury in autistic and nonautistic persons with severe mental retardation. *Developmental Brain Dysfuntion*, **9**, 22–31.

King, B. H., Wright, D. M., Handen, B. L. *et al.* (2001). Double-blind placebo-controlled study of amantadine hydrochloride in the treatment of children with autistic disorder. *Journal of the American Academy of Child and Adolescent Psychiatry*, **40**, 658–65.

Krystal, J. H., Belger, A., and D'Souza, D. C. (1999). Therapeutic implications of the hyperglutaminergic effects of NMDA antagonists. *Neuropsychopharmacology*, **22**, S143–S157.

Kumandas, S., Caksen, H., Ciftci, A., Ozturk, M., and Per, H. (2001). Lamotrigine in two cases of Rett syndrome. *Brain and Development*, **23**, 240–2.

Lake, C. R., Ziegler, M. G., and Murphy, D. L. (1977). Increased norepinephrine levels and decreased dopamine-β-hydroxylase activity in primary autism. *Archives of General Psychiatry*, **34**, 553–6.

Leboyer, M., Bouvard, M. P., Launay, J. M. *et al.* (1992). Brief report: a double-blind study of naltrexone in infantile autism. *Journal of Autism and Developmental Disorders*, **22**, 309–19.

Levin, J., Aviram, A., Holan, A. *et al.* (1997). Inositol treatment of autism. *Journal of Neural Transmission*, **104**, 307–10.

Malloy, C. A., Manning-Courtney, P., Swayne, S. *et al.* (2002). Lack of benefit of intravenous synthetic human secretin in the treatment of autism. *Journal of Autism and Developmental Disorders*, **32**, 545–51.

Malone, R. P., Cater, J., Sheikh, R. M., Choudhury, M. S., and Delaney, M. A. (2001). Olanazapine versus haloperidol in children with autistic disorder: an open label pilot study. *Journal of the American Academy of Child and Adolescent Psychiatry*, **40**, 887–94.

Malone, R. P., Maislin, G., Choudhury, M. S., Gifford, C., and Delaney, M. A. (2002). Risperidone treatment in children and adolescents with autism: short- and long-term safety and effectiveness. *Journal of the American Academy of Child and Adolescent Psychiatry*, **41**, 140–7.

Marshall, B. L., Napolitano, D. A., McAdam, D. B. *et al.* (2003). Venlafaxine and increased aggression in a female with autism. *Journal of the American Academy of Child and Adolescent Psychiatry*, **42**, 383–4.

Martin, A., Koenig, K., Scahill, L., and Bregman, J. (1999). Open-label quetiapine in the treatment of children and adolescents with autistic disorder. *Journal of Child and Adolescent Psychopharmacology*, **9**, 99–107.

Masi, G., Cosenza, A., Mucci, M., and Brovedani, P. (2001). Open trial of risperidone in 24 young children with pervasive developmental disorders. *Journal of the American Academy of Child and Adolescent Psychiatry*, **40**, 1206–14.

Masi, G., Cosenza, A., Mucci, M., and Brovedani, P. (2003). A 3-year naturalistic study of 53 preschool children with pervasive developmental disorders treated with risperidone. *Journal of Clinical Psychiatry*, **64**, 1039–47.

McDougle, C. J. (2002). Current and emerging therapeutics of autistic disorder and related pervasive developmental disorders. In David, K. L., Charney, D., Coyle, J. T., and Nemeroff, C., eds., *Neuropsychopharmacology: The Fifth Generation of Progress*. Philadelphia: Lippincott, Williams & Wilkins, pp. 565–76.

McDougle, C. J., Price, L. H., and Volkmar, F. R. (1994). Recent advances in the pharmacotherapy of autism and related conditions. In F. R. Volkmar, ed., *Child and Adolescent Psychiatric Clinics of North America*. Vol. 3. *Psychoses and Pervasive Developmental Disorders*. Philadelphia: W. B. Saunders, pp. 71–89.

McDougle, C. J., Naylor, S. T., Cohen, D. J. *et al.* (1996a). Effects of typtophan depletion in drug-free adults with autism. *Archives of General Psychiatry*, **53**, 993–1000.

McDougle, C. J., Naylor, S. T., Cohen, D. J. *et al.* (1996b). A double-blind, placebo-controlled study of fluvoxamine in adults with autistic disorder. *Archives of General Psychiatry*, **53**, 1001–8.

McDougle, C. J., Holmes, J. P., Carlson, D. C. *et al.* (1998a). A double-blind placebo-controlled study of risperidone in adults with autistic disorder and other pervasive developmental disorders. *Archives of General Psychiatry*, **55**, 633–41.

McDougle, C. J., Brodkin, E. S., Naylor, S. T. *et al.* (1998b). Sertraline in adults with pervasive developmental disorders: a prospective open-label investigation. *Journal of Clinical Psychopharmacology*, **18**, 62–6.

McDougle, C. J., Kem, D. L., and Posey, D. J. (2002). Case series: use of ziprasidone for maladaptive symptoms in youths with autism. *Journal of the American Academy of Child and Adolescent Psychiatry*, **41**, 921–7.

Minderaa, R. B. Anderson, G. M., Volkmar, F. R., Akkerhuis, G. W., and Cohen, D. J. (1994). Noradrenergic and adrenergic functioning in autism. *Biological Psychiatry*, **36**, 237–41.

Modahl, C., Green, L., Fein, D. *et al.* (1998). Plasma oxytocin levels in autistic children. *Biologic Psychiatry*, **43**, 270–7.

Namerow, L. B., Thomas, P., Bostic, J. Q., Prince, J., and Montuteaux, M. C. (2003). Use of citalopram in pervasive developmental disorders. *Developmental and Behavioral Pediatrics*, **24**, 104–8.

Nelson E. and Alberts J. R. (1997). Oxytocin-induced paw sucking in infant rats. *Annals of the New York Academy of Science*, **807**, 543–5.

Niederhofer, H., Staffen, W., and Mair, A. (2002). Lofexidine in hyperactive and impulsive children with autistic disorder. *Journal of the American Academy of Child and Adolescent Psychiatry*, **41**, 1396–7.

Niederhofer, H., Staffen, W., and Mair, A. (2003). Tianeptine: a novel strategy of psychopharmacological treatment of children with autistic disorder. *Human Psychopharmacology*, **18**, 389–93.

Owley, T., McMahon, W., Cook, E. H. *et al.* (2001). Multisite, double-blind, placebo-controlled trial of porcine secretin in autism. *Journal of the American Academy of Child and Adolescent Psychiatry*, **40**, 1293–9.

Percy, A. K., Glaze, D. G., Schultz, R. J. *et al.* (1994). Rett syndrome: controlled study of an oral opiate antagonist, naltrexone. *Annals of Neurology*, **35**, 464–70.

Perry, R., Campbell, M., Adams, P. *et al.* (1989). Long-term efficacy of haloperidol in autistic children: continuous versus discontinuous drug administration. *Journal of the American Academy of Child and Adolescent Psychiatry*, **28**, 87–92.

Popik, P. and van Ree, J. M. (1992). Long-term facilitation of social recognition in rats by vasopressin related peptides: a structure–activity study. *Life Science*, **50**, 567–72.

Posey, D. J. and McDougle, C. J. (2000). The pharmacotherapy of target symptoms associated with autistic disorder and other pervasive developmental disorders. *Harvard Review of Psychiatry*, **8**, 45–63.

Posey, D. J., Litwiller, M., Koburn, A., and McDougle, C. J. (1999). Paroxetine in autism. *Journal of the American Academy of Child and Adolescent Psychiatry*, **38**, 111–12.

Posey, D. J., Guenin, K. D., Kohn, A. E., Swiezy, N. B., and McDougle, C. J. (2001). A naturalistic open-label study of mirtazapine in autistic and other pervasive developmental disorders. *Journal of Child and Adolescent Psychopharmacology*, **11**, 267–77.

Posey, D. J., Puntney, J. I., Sasher, T. M. *et al.* (2004a). Guanfacine treatment of hyperactivity and inattention in autism: a retrospective analysis of 80 cases. *Journal of Child and Adolescent Psychopharmacology*, **14**, 233–41.

Posey, D. J., Kem, D. L., Swiezy, N. B. *et al.* (2004b). A pilot study of D-cycloserine in autistic disorder. *American Journal of Psychiatry*, **161**, 2115–17.

Potenza, M. N., Holmes, J. P., Kanes, S. J., and McDougle, C. J. (1999). Olanzapine treatment of children, adolescents, and adults with pervasive developmental disorders: an open-label pilot study. *Journal of Clinical Psychopharmacology*, **19**, 37–44.

Quintana, H., Birmaher, B., Stedge, D. *et al.* (1995). Use of methylphenidate in the treatment of children with autistic disorder. *Journal of Autism and Developmental Disorders*, **25**, 283–95.

Ratey, J. J., Bemporad, J., Sorgi, J. *et al.* (1987a). Brief report: open trial effects of beta-blockers on speech and social behaviors in 8 autistic adults. *Journal of Autism and Developmental Disorders*, **17**, 439–46.

Ratey, J. J., Mikkelsen, E., Sorgi, P. *et al.* (1987b). Autism: the treatment of aggressive behaviors. *Journal of Clinical Psychopharmacology*, **7**, 35–41.

Reap, E. and Lawson, J. (1990). Stimulation of the immune system by dimethylglycine, a nontoxic metabolite. *Journal of Laboratory and Clinical Medicine*, **115**, 481–6.

Remington, G., Sloman, L., Konstantareas, M., Parker, K., and Gow, R. (2001). Clomipramine versus haloperidol in the treatment of autistic disorder: a double-blind, placebo-controlled, crossover study. *Journal of Clinical Psychopharmacology*, **21**, 440–4.

Research Units on Pediatric Psychopharmacology Autism Network (2002). Risperidone in children with autism and serious behavior problems. *New England Journal of Medicine*, **347**, 314–21.

Roberts, W., Weaver, L., Brian, J., and Bryson, S. (2001). Repeated doses of porcine secretin in the treatment of autism: a randomized, placebo controlled trial. *Pediatrics*, **107**, E71.

Ross, D. L., Klykylo, W. M., and Hitzemann, R. (1987). Reduction of elevated CSF beta-endorphin by fenfluramine in infantile autism. *Pediatric Neurology*, **3**, 83–6.

Rugino, T. A. and Samsock, T. C. (2002). Levetiracetam in autistic children: an open-label study. *Developmental and Behavioral Pediatrics*, **23**, 225–30.

Sandler, A. D., Sutton, K. A., DeWeese, J. *et al.* (1999). Lack of benefit of single dose of synthetic human secretin in the treatment of autism and pervasive developmental disorder. *New England Journal of Medicine*, **341**, 1801–6.

Schain, R. J. and Freedman, D. X. (1961). Studies on 5-hydroxyindole metabolism in autistic and other mentally retarded children. *Journal of Pediatrics*, **58**, 315–20.

Snead, R. W., Boon, F., and Presberg, J. (1994). Paroxetine for self-injurious behavior. *Journal of the American Academy of Child and Adolescent Psychiatry*, **33**, 909–10.

Sponheim, E., Oftedal, G., and Helverschou, B. (2002). Multiple doses of secretin in the treatment of autism: a controlled study. *Acta Paediatrica*, **91**, 540–5.

Stavrakaki, C., Antochi, R., and Emery, P. C. (2004). Olanazpine in the treatment of pervasive developmental disorders: a case series analysis. *Journal of Psychiatry and Neuroscience*, **29**, 57–60.

Steingard, R. and Biederman, J. (1987). Lithium-responsive manic-like symptoms in two individuals with autism and mental retardation. *Journal of the American Academy of Child and Adolescent Psychiatry*, **26**, 932–5.

Steingard, R. J., Zimnitsky, B., DeMaso, D. R. Bauman, M. L., and Bucci, J. P. (1997). Sertraline treatment of transition-associated anxiety and agitation in children with autistic disorder. *Journal of Child and Adolescent Psychopharmacology*, **7**, 9–15.

Stern, L. M., Walker, M. K., Sawyer, M. G. *et al.* (1990). A controlled crossover trial of fenfluramine in autism. *Journal of Child Psychology and Psychiatry*, **31**, 569–85.

Stigler, K. A., Posey, D. J., and McDougle, C. J. (2003). Drug therapy algorithms target autism's problem behaviors. *Current Psychiatry*, **2**, 33–48.

Unis, I. S., Munson, J. A., Rogers, S. J. *et al.* (2002). A randomized, double-blind, placebo controlled trial of porcine versus synthetic secretin for reducing symptoms of autism. *Journal of the American Academy of Child and Adolescent Psychiatry*, **41**, 1315–21.

Uvebrant, P. and Bauziene, R. (1994). Intractable epilepsy in children. The efficacy of lamotrigine treatment, including non-seizure-related benefits. *Neuropediatrics*, **25**, 284–8.

Varley, C. K. and Holm, V. A. (1990). A two-year follow-up of autistic children treated with fenfluramine. *Journal of the American Academy of Child and Adolescent Psychiatry*, **29**, 137–40.

Wagstaff, A. J., Ormrod, D., and Spencer, C. M. (2001). Tianeptine: a review of its use in depressive disorders. *CNS Drugs*, **15**, 231–59.

Weizman, R., Weizman, A., Thano, S. *et al.* (1984). Humoral-endorphin blood levels in autistic, schizophrenic and healthy subjects. *Psychopharmacology*, **82**, 368–70.

Willemsen-Swinkels, S. H. N., Buitelaar, J. K, Nijhof, G. J., and van Engeland, H. (1995). Failure of naltrexone hydrochloride to reduce self-injurious and autistic behavior in mentally retarded adults: double-blind placebo-controlled studies. *Archives of General Psychiatry*, **52**, 766–73.

Witt, D. M., Winslow, J. T., and Insel, T. R. (1992). Enhanced social interactions in rats following chronic, centrally infused oxytocin. *Pharmacology, Biochemistry, and Behavior*, **43**, 855–61.

Young, J. G., Cohen, D. J., Kavanagh, M. E. *et al.* (1981). Cerobrospinal fluid, plasma, and urinary MHPG in children. *Life Sciences*, **28**, 2837–45.

Zuddas, A. Ledda, M. G., Fratta, A., Muglia, P., and Cianchetti, C. (1996). Clinical effects of clozapine on autistic disorder. *American Journal of Psychiatry*, **153**, 738.

8

Behavioral and educational approaches to the pervasive developmental disorders

Sandra L. Harris

Graduate School of Applied and Professional Psychology, Rutgers, The State University of New Jersey

Our understanding of the pervasive developmental disorders (PDDs) has radically altered in the past 40 years. The initial recognition that these are biologically based conditions (Rimland, 1964), and rejection of the psychoanalytic concept of parental blame as an explanatory mechanism (Bettelheim, 1967), created an intellectual context in which behavioral and educational interventions could take root. Beginning with demonstrations by Ferster (1961), Lovaas *et al.* (1966), and Bartak and Rutter (1971) that principles of learning influenced the behavior of these clients, there developed an appreciation of highly structured, carefully planned interventions to meet the needs of people with autistic disorder and related conditions. Since the mid 1960s the teaching technology for this population has grown increasingly sophisticated and effective.

This chapter reviews the state of the art in behavioral and educational treatments for people with PDDs. The focus is on assessment and treatment of skill deficits, especially language and social skills, and intervention with dangerous or disruptive behaviors, such as self-injury or aggression. The behavioral technology for early intervention is addressed, as are the controversial treatment approaches of facilitated communication and auditory integration therapy. Finally, the need to consider the family context in which treatment takes place is discussed.

This chapter is based on research with people diagnosed as exhibiting autistic disorder, Asperger's disorder, and pervasive developmental disorder not otherwise specified (PDD-NOS). In some cases they are described as "autistic" or demonstrating "autistic behaviors." These variations in language reflect the changing state of the diagnostic art as well as variation among client populations.

Autism and Pervasive Developmental Disorders, 2nd edn, ed. Fred R. Volkmar.
Published by Cambridge University Press. © Cambridge University Press 2007.

Behavioral assessment

Behavioral assessment is integral to applied behavior analysis. Van Houten and his colleagues (1988) call for an initial behavioral assessment and ongoing evaluation as every client's basic right. This assessment approaches each client as a unique person, and examines the learning history, biological factors, and current setting in which that person functions. The evaluator explores such questions as "What are the conditions under which the maladaptive behavior occurs?", "Is it possible to change environmental cues to reduce the likelihood of triggering a problem behavior?", or "What existing skills may be engaged to assist this client in learning a new skill?" It is important for this assessment to continue over time. Typically, one does an initial assessment, tries an intervention, and based on the outcome, either continues the treatment or changes it. Changes in treatment strategy should be data based.

Behavioral assessment also examines the generalization and maintenance of target behaviors. When we teach a new skill we intend that it be used in every appropriate setting (generalization) and that its use continues over time (maintenance). If a child speaks only to her teacher, or uses the word "ball" only for a single blue ball, the skill has limited generality. If the skill drops away over time, it has shown poor maintenance. Both generalization of skills to new persons, places, and objects, and maintenance of skills over time are vital if a behavior is to have adaptive value for the client.

Clients come for treatment presenting a variety of concerns. For example, if a child with autistic disorder has severe tantrums, is not toilet trained, and does not speak, one needs to decide where to begin treatment. The educator or clinician chooses from among several presenting problems those that merit immediate intervention and those to be addressed later. In their discussion of this decision-making process Mash and Terdal (1988) note that some behaviors, such as those that are physically dangerous, or keep the client from accessing naturally reinforcing environmental events, would be more urgent than behaviors that do not pose an immediate crisis, or isolate the client from the community. For example, treating self-injury is usually more urgent than toilet-training, although both are important to a client's long-term functioning. Developing an intervention hierarchy is typically done by the clinician in consultation with the client's family and teachers. Clients of normal intellectual functioning, such as the person with Asperger's disorder, may have their own treatment priorities.

A good behavioral assessment considers the developmental appropriateness of the targeted skill. Both chronological age and mental age should be considered in a treatment plan. Although a person may not be capable of fully mastering the skills being acquired by typically developing peers, it is important to bring that person as close as possible to that goal. An adolescent with autistic disorder and mental retardation may not "surf the net," but he or she can probably learn to play some video games.

Teaching new skills

Teaching new, adaptive skills to persons with PDDs is at the heart of the educational enterprise. There are repeated demonstrations that when properly taught, persons with autistic disorder, Asperger's disorder, and PDD-NOS can markedly improve their expressive and receptive language, social awareness, and performance on academic, life skills, and vocational tasks.

Language

Teaching language to people with PDDs was one of the earliest accomplishments of applied behavior analysts. Beginning with the demonstration by Lovaas *et al.* (1966) that previously mute children could acquire rudimentary speech, there has been continuing research on speech and language. Initially this work used behavioral techniques in artificial settings to teach specific grammatical forms including nouns (e.g. Guess *et al.*, 1968), prepositions (Frisch & Schumaker, 1974), and interrogative sentences (Twardosz & Baer, 1973). Gradually there was a shift toward teaching functional language in the natural world. This shift was motivated by the discovery that skills learned in a restrictive setting were not automatically generalized to the student's natural environment, and the observation that if skills were to be functional they had to be taught in ways that facilitate generalized use (Harris, 1975).

Teaching spontaneous functional language to people with PDDs has benefited considerably in recent years by research based on Skinner's (1957) writings about verbal behavior. This work has led to important advances in the sequencing of language instruction (e.g. Sundberg & Partington, 1998). For example, it is now widespread practice to begin by teaching children of limited verbal ability to request the things they want (mand training) rather than teaching them to name common objects (tacting) as used to be done. The logic behind this concerns the strong motivation and direct reinforcement for requesting desired items and thus the opportunity for the learner to experience speech (or Sign) as valuable. Tacting now comes later in training than does requesting. There is also an appreciation of the need to provide objects and experiences that are highly reinforcing for the child and to create conditions that heighten the child's interest in these items.

This process of capitalizing on a child's motivation is called creating or capturing an establishing operation (Michael, 1993). For example, one could give a child a can of favorite drink, but leave it sealed so she or he must ask her teacher to open it and thus use language functionally. Along with the focus on the sequence of teaching verbal behavior skills and the careful consideration of the learner's preferences for reinforcement, applied behavior analysts continue to rely on other more traditional techniques such as discrete trial instruction, prompting of responses, and shaping of new skills.

Although current technology enables many people to speak who would previously have been mute, there are still learners for whom limited speech remains a major barrier to community life. Increasingly, for these people, there is a reliance on augmentative communication methods (Harris, 1995). Sign language, the Picture Exchange Communication System (Bondy & Frost, 2001), a board with pictures or words to which a person can point, or a handheld electronic device which provides a printed message, or functions as a voice synthesizer can enhance communication in mute clients. The choice among these items requires a careful assessment of the individual's cognitive abilities, verbal and nonverbal imitative skills, and motor control.

Social skills

Deficits in social skills characterize the PDDs. These problems range from a profound lack of social engagement exhibited by some people with autistic disorder and co-occurring mental retardation, to a relatively subtle but nonetheless serious problem in empathic understanding exhibited by a highly intelligent person with Asperger's disorder. Social skills programs should be part of the treatment agenda for nearly every person in this diagnostic grouping. Interest in social skills deficits has stirred both theoretical research on "theory of mind" (e.g. Happe, 1995; Hobson, 1993; Leslie, 1987), and applied work on specific interventions to help persons with PDDs become more socially adept.

Countless social skills are necessary to be a competent adult in an industrialized society. For example, one needs to greet other people, keep an appropriate physical distance, make purchases in a store, and recognize emotions. To be an active member of the community many other skills are required such as participating in leisure activities, sharing resources, exchanging compliments, and so forth. Most of us learned these skills through informal lessons, but for the person with a PDD they must be painstakingly taught. Among the interventions for teaching social skills are programs for increasing proximity to peers during play (Hoch et al., 2002), increasing social initiations (Shabani et al., 2002), increasing social communication (Thiemann & Goldstein, 2001), showing appropriate affective behavior (Gena *et al.*, 1996), and engaging in symbolic (Stahmer, 1995) and sociodramatic play (Thorp *et al.*, 1995).

Peer modeling is a potent tool for teaching social skills. Research on the benefits of exposure to competent peers has been carried out primarily with preschool-aged children (e.g. Odom *et al.*, 1985; Odom & Strain, 1986), with a few studies looking at older children (e.g. Lord & Hopkins, 1986; Sasso & Rude, 1987) including junior high school youngsters (Haring & Breen, 1992). Initially the research in this area relied heavily on adult intervention (e.g. Strain & Timm, 1974; Strain *et al.*, 1976) while later work taught typically developing peers how to engage the child with a PDD (e.g. McGee *et al.*, 1992; Pierce & Schreibman, 1995). Another promising line of work teaches the child with autism to initiate social interactions (e.g. Belchic & Harris, 1994; Zanolli *et al.*, 1996). In clinical practice one is not confined to a single intervention; the teacher may prompt behavior as needed, peers may be taught skills for initiating play, and the child with autism may learn to initiate and respond to social bids. Several studies have demonstrated that classwide interventions involving peer tutoring and cooperative learning groups can improve the academic progress of an entire class, including children with autistic disorder (e.g. Dugan *et al.*, 1995; Kamps *et al.*, 1994).

Decreasing maladaptive behavior

Well-trained applied behavior analysts makes relatively little use of punishment and a great deal of use of positive reinforcement in bringing maladaptive behavior under control. Although some strategies such as ignoring inappropriate behavior (extinction) or the use of a punishment such as time out from positive reinforcement may be part of a treatment plan, the heart of each plan should be teaching new adaptive behaviors to replace those that are inappropriate. One key to the shift from the field's historic use of aversive procedures to the current emphasis on nonaversive techniques has been the increased effectiveness of methods for assessing the functions of maladaptive responding (Pelios *et al.*, 1999). The research shows that if one does a careful functional assessment, teaches the client alternative ways to communicate needs, and alters controlling environmental variables, it is possible to reduce the frequency of many intrusive behaviors such as aggression, self-injury, and stereotyped behavior (Durand & Carr, 1991). However, it is essential that this assessment be tailored to each client's needs. For example, Kennedy *et al.* (2000) identified multiple functions for the stereotypic behavior of young people with autism with some instances of stereotypic (i.e. "self-stimulatory") behavior being reinforced by escape or avoidance of work rather than the automatic reinforcement that has traditionally been assumed to underlie all repetitive behavior. One cannot make assumptions about the motivating factors in disruptive behavior, but instead must carry out a careful assessment to determine what is maintaining the behavior for each individual learner.

Many of the studies examining the relationship between environmental or contextual events and maladaptive behavior have focused on two patterns: escape-motivated behavior and attention-seeking behavior (Durand & Carr, 1987). These two variables account for many of the disruptive behaviors emitted by people with PDDs. Among other environmental factors that may influence maladaptive behaviors are such diverse events as the noise of another child crying (Tang et al., 2002), variations in meal schedule (Wacker et al., 1996), certain kinds of verbal reprimands (Fisher et al., 1996), brief breaks from work (Zarcone et al., 1996), and giving warnings before changing activities (Tustin, 1995). Physical factors such as middle-ear infections, allergies, and sleep disruption must also be considered in a comprehensive assessment (O'Neill et al., 1997). It may be important to carry out an assessment in more than a single setting. Haring and Kennedy (1990) reported that disruptive behavior in an instructional setting was controlled by different factors than that same behavior during leisure time.

The most powerful way to identify the factors controlling a maladaptive behavior is through a functional analysis in which variables such as teacher attention, work demands, and other potentially important factors can be systemically manipulated in brief, highly controlled analogs of the client's usual routines. Once a functional analysis is performed, and the controlling variables have been identified, it is often possible to provide functional communication training to teach the client an alternative response. For example, a person whose self-injury results in work avoidance may be taught to ask for a break (e.g. Lalli et al., 1995), and in this way work activities may be modified.

Early intervention

Early intervention with children who have PDDs can, in some cases, markedly alter their developmental trajectory. Some of these children can enter a regular kindergarten or first grade following an intensive preschool experience. Lovaas's (1987) very influential demonstration of the benefits of early intervention reported that nearly half of his young participants with autistic disorder achieved normal intellectual and educational functioning by first grade. A number of subsequent studies have likewise reported significant gains for very young children exposed to intensive treatment (e.g. Birnbrauer & Leach, 1993; Harris et al., 1991; Howard et al., 2005; Sallows & Graupner, 2005). However, in the only study using randomized assigment, Smith *et al.* (2000) – while finding that the children who received intensive treatment were superior to a comparison group on such factors as post-treatment IQ – visuospatial skills, language, academic skills, and school placement, did not find as great a benefit as did Lovaas (1987). A number of differences between the two studies in such factors as total hours of instruction and initial functioning level of the children may have influenced the outcome. For example, children who are younger and have higher IQs appear to benefit more than those who are older or have lower IQs (Harris & Handleman, 2000). Much research remains to be performed to determine who benefits in what ways from these intensive methods.

A number of factors characterize some of the most effective early intervention programs (Handleman & Harris, 2001). One feature is individualized, comprehensive programming. As noted above, one of the things behavioral technology does well is to study each child, and identify the specific strengths and deficits of that child, as well as the contextual variables that influence the child's behavior. This assessment, when linked to a comprehensive curriculum that meets a range of needs, serves children with PDDs well. The highly effective treatment programs also emphasize identifying children as early as possible, and working with them in a very favorable teacher-to-child ratio, often one-to-one in the early stages. Most effective programs also have a highly systematic approach to helping children with autistic disorder and related conditions learn to interact with peers, and function in the natural environment of childhood. As discussed above, peers can play an integral role in this treatment.

Controversial treatments

Perhaps because we do not fully understand the etiologies of the PDDs, and are not effective at treating every person with these disorders, there continue to be reports of controversial treatments. Were the PDDs as minor as the common cold, or as responsive to treatment as many bacterial infections, few parents or professionals would adopt alternative treatments without rigorous supporting data. One must be cautious of uncontrolled case reports of dramatic changes in people with PDDs. Skepticism is especially in order when these reports make no sense on theoretical grounds, or in terms of our knowledge of PDDs, or when disinterested scientists cannot replicate the finding. Those principles are part of the "common sense" of science, but are still brushed aside by some.

Facilitated communication

One controversial treatment that has passed its peak of popularity, but is still used by some, is facilitated communication (Biklen, 1990). Following a great deal of attention in the media, extensive empirical effort was directed toward facilitated communication, a method that provides the nonverbal person with autism an opportunity to communicate through graduated physical guidance at a keyboard or other communication device (Jacobson *et al.*, 1995). Initial public response to this method was enthusiastic. For example, based on the sophisticated communications that arose using facilitated communication, children with autistic disorder who had been assumed to have co-occurring mental retardation, were moved from specialized to regular classes, and a normative curriculum, through the support of their facilitator.

A major review by Jacobson and his colleagues (1995), and a more recent follow-up by Mostert (2001), note that scores of well-controlled studies in independent laboratories failed to find that the communications that arise during facilitated communication can be attributed to the person with a PDD. Equally of concern is the repeated finding that it is the facilitator, and not the client, who controls the communication (e.g. Montee *et al.*, 1995). Thus there is reason to question whether children are benefiting from their new educational placements, and whether, in fact, they are being denied the opportunity to learn essential skills for later life.

Based on their research Montee and her colleagues (1995) recommend that facilitated communication not be used. They suggest that if individuals are committed to the continuing use of this approach, in spite of the lack of validation, it is essential that ". . . every communication produced through facilitated communication should be verified through another means . . ." (p. 198), and that informed consent be required when facilitated communication is attempted. Smith (1996) urges that service providers who rely on facilitated communication be avoided. Given the lack of supporting data, and the potential danger of failing to provide an appropriate education, a rigorous assessment of the benefits of facilitated communication for any individual client should be routine if a parent or educator insists upon applying the techniques. The experimental literature has countless models for such an assessment.

Auditory integration training

Auditory integration training (AIT) was initially based on the idea that hypersensitive hearing causes some of the maladaptive behaviors of people with PDDs. It was argued that decreasing this sensitivity by systematic exposure to problematic sound frequencies led to improved behavior (Stehli, 1991). However, it is no longer clear whether hypersensitivity plays a major role in predicting response to this treatment (Rimland & Edelson, 1994). During AIT people listen to music electronically modulated, and sometimes filtered, to create what are believed to be therapeutic sounds. Interestingly, questions have been raised about whether filtered sounds are required for beneficial effects (Bettison, 1996; Rimland & Edelson, 1994). At present this method is still experimental, and there are too few data to be certain whether the approach benefits people with PDDs. However, some of the people who advocate AIT are studying whether and when it might be helpful (e.g. Rimland & Edelson, 1995). In the absence of consistently demonstrated benefits it is essential that if AIT is used, data are collected to determine whether a client is benefiting. Unlike facilitated communication, there is no reason to believe that AIT interferes with effective education.

Role of the family

Once it was recognized that poor parenting did not cause a child to have a PDD, it became possible to think about parents as partners in a treatment process, rather than as part of the child's problem (Lovaas *et al.*, 1973; Schopler & Reichler, 1971). It was evident that family support was essential if a child's newly learned skills were to be maintained and generalized (Lovaas *et al.*, 1973). Recognition of the crucial role of parents led to research on the most effective ways to teach behavioral technology (e.g. Harris, 1983, 1989; Koegel *et al.*, 1984). That work shows that parents can master essentially any behavioral skill, and that their application of these skills can be highly effective, especially when the family is provided with ongoing programming support (Harris, 1986).

Every family that includes a child with a PDD should learn behavioral teaching strategies to support their child's education. However, it is also important to recognize that being the parent of a child with a PDD is inherently stressful. As a result, parents may require considerable formal and informal support in dealing with the demands imposed on them by their child's unusual needs (National Research Council, 2001).

Conclusion

In the past 40 years there have been major advances in our ability to meet the needs of people with PDDs. Early intervention is especially potent for many young children, but older children, adolescents, and adults can also experience a markedly improved quality of life through behavioral technology. One of the challenges facing the field is disseminating this technology as widely as possible to ensure that every young child who requires early intervention, and every older child and adult who needs longer-term education and training, has those resources available. Education dollars spent early in the life of a person with a PDD can yield major benefits in both human and economic terms over a lifetime.

REFERENCES

Bartak, L. and Rutter, M. (1971). Educational treatment of autistic children. In M. L. Rutter, ed., *Infantile Autism: Concepts, Characteristics and Treatment*. Baltimore: Williams & Wilkins, pp. 258–88.

Belchic, J. K. and Harris, S. L. (1994). The use of multiple peer exemplars to enhance the generalization of play skills to the siblings of children with autism. *Child and Family Behavior Therapy*, **16**, 1–25.

Bettelheim, B. (1967). *The Empty Fortress*. New York: The Free Press.

Bettison, S. (1996). The long-term effects of auditory training on children with autism. *Journal of Autism and Developmental Disorders*, **26**, 361–74.

Biklen, D. (1990). Communication unbound: autism and praxis. *Harvard Educational Review*, **62**, 291–314.

Birnbrauer, J. S. and Leach, D. J. (1993). The Murdoch early intervention program after 2 years. *Behaviour Change*, **10**, 63–74.

Bondy, A. and Frost, L. (2001). *A Picture's Worth. PECS and Other Visual Communication Strategies in Autism*. Bethesda, MD: Woodbine House.

Dugan, E., Kamps, D., Leonard, B. *et al.* (1995). Effects of cooperative learning groups during social studies for students with autism and fourth-grade peers. *Journal of Applied Behavior Analysis*, **28**, 175–88.

Durand, V. M. and Carr, E. G. (1987). Social influences on "self-stimulatory" behavior: analysis and treatment application. *Journal of Applied Behavior Analysis*, **20**, 119–32.

Durand, V. M. and Carr, E. G. (1991). Functional communication training to reduce challenging behavior: maintenance and application in new settings. *Journal of Applied Behavior Analysis*, **24**, 251–64.

Ferster, C. B. (1961). Positive reinforcement and behavioral deficits of autistic children. *Child Development*, **32**, 437–56.

Fisher, W. W., Ninness, H. A. C., Piazza, C. C., and Owen-DeSchryver, J. S. (1996). On the reinforcing effects of the content of verbal attention. *Journal of Applied Behavior Analysis*, **29**, 235–8.

Frisch, S. A. and Schumaker, J. B. (1974). Training generalized receptive prepositions in retarded children. *Journal of Applied Behavior Analysis*, **7**, 611–21.

Gena, A., Krantz, P. J., McClannahan, L. E., and Poulson, C. L. (1996). Training and generalization of affective behavior displayed by youths with autism. *Journal of Applied Behavior Analysis*, **29**, 291–304.

Guess, D., Sailor, W., Rutherford, G., and Baer, D. M. (1968). An experimental analysis of linguistic development: the productive use of the plural morpheme. *Journal of Applied Behavior Analysis*, **1**, 297–306.

Handleman, J. S. and Harris, S. L., eds. (2001). *Preschool Education Programs for Children with Autism*, 2nd edn. Austin, TX: Pro-Ed.

Happe, F. (1995). *Autism: An Introduction to Psychological Theory.* Cambridge, MA: Harvard University Press.

Haring, T. G. and Breen, C. G. (1992). A peer-mediated social network intervention to enhance the social integration of persons with moderate and severe disabilities. *Journal of Applied Behavior Analysis,* **25**, 319–33.

Haring T. G. and Kennedy, C. H. (1990). Contextual control of problem behaviors in students with severe disabilities. *Journal of Applied Behavior Analysis,* **23**, 235–43.

Harris, S. L. (1975). Teaching language to nonverbal children – with emphasis on problems of generalization. *Psychological Bulletin,* **82**, 564–80.

Harris, S. L. (1983). *Families of the Developmentally Disabled: A Guide to Behavioral Intervention.* Elmsford, NY: Pergamon Press.

Harris, S. L. (1986). Parents as teachers: a four- to seven-year follow-up of parents of children with autism. *Child and Family Behavior Therapy,* **8**, 39–47.

Harris, S. L. (1989). Training parents of children with autism: an update on models. *The Behavior Therapist,* **12**, 219–21.

Harris, S. L. (1995). Educational strategies in autism. In E. Schopler and G. B. Mesibov, eds., *Learning and Cognition in Autism.* New York: Plenum, pp. 293–309.

Harris, S. L. and Handleman, J. S. (2000). Age and IQ at intake as predictors of placement for young children with autism: a four- to six-year follow-up. *Journal of Autism and Developmental Disorders,* **30**, 137–142.

Harris, S. L., Handleman, J. S., Gordon, R., Kristoff, B., and Fuentes, F. (1991). Changes in cognitive and language functioning of preschool children with autism. *Journal of Autism and Developmental Disorders,* **21**, 281–90.

Hobson, P. (1993). *Autism and the Development of Mind.* Hillsdale, NJ: Lawrence Earlbaum.

Hoch, H., McComas, J. J., Johnson, L., Faranda, N., and Guenther, S. L. (2002). The effects of magnitude and quality of reinforcement on choice responding during play activities. *Journal of Applied Behavior Analysis,* **35**, 171–81.

Howard, J. S., Sparkman, C. R., Cohen, H. G., and Stanislaw, H. (2005). A comparison of intensive behavior analytic and eclectic treatments for young children with autism. *Research in Developmental Disabilities,* **26**, 359–83.

Jacobson, J. W., Mulick, J. A., and Schwartz, A. A. (1995). A history of facilitated communication. Science, pseudoscience, and antiscience. Science working group on facilitated communication. *American Psychologist,* **50**, 750–65.

Kamps, D. M., Barbetta, P. M., Leonard, B. R., and Delquadri, J. (1994). Classwide peer tutoring: an integration strategy to improve reading skills and promote peer interactions among students with autism and general education peers. *Journal of Applied Behavior Analysis,* **27**, 49–61.

Kennedy, C. H., Meyer, K. A., Knowles, T., and Shukla, S. (2000). Analyzing the multiple functions of stereotyped behavior for students with autism: implications for assessment and treatment. *Journal of Applied Behavior Analysis,* **33**, 559–71.

Koegel, R. L., Schreibman, L., Johnson, J., O'Neill, R. E., and Dunlap, G. (1984). Collateral effects of parent training on families of autistic children. In R. F. Dangel and R. A. Polster, eds., *Parent Training: Foundations of Research and Practice.* New York: Guilford Press, pp. 358–78.

Lalli, J. S., Casey, S., and Kates, K. (1995). Reducing escape behavior and increasing task completion with functional communication training, extinction, and response chaining. *Journal of Applied Behavior Analysis*, **28**, 261–8.

Leslie, A. M. (1987). Pretence and representation: the origins of "theory of mind." *Psychological Review*, **94**, 412–26.

Lord, C. and Hopkins, J. M. (1986). The social behavior of autistic children with younger and same-age nonhandicapped peers. *Journal of Autism and Developmental Disorders*, **16**, 249–62.

Lovaas, O. I. (1987). Behavioral treatment and normal educational and intellectual functioning in young autistic children. *Journal of Consulting and Clinical Psychology*, **55**, 3–9.

Lovaas, O. I., Berberich, J. P., Perloff, B. F., and Schaeffer, B. (1966). Acquisition of imitative speech by schizophrenic children. *Science*, **151**, 705–7.

Lovaas, O. I., Koegel, R. L., Simmons, J. Q., and Long, J. S. (1973). Some generalization and follow-up measures on autistic children in behavior therapy. *Journal of Applied Behavior Analysis*, **6**, 131–66.

Mash E. J. and Terdal L. G. (1988). Behavioral assessment of child and family disturbance. In E. J. Mash and L. G. Terdal, eds., *Behavioral Assessment of Childhood Disorders*, 2nd edn. New York, Guilford Press, pp. 3–65.

McGee, G. G., Almeida, M. C., Sulzer-Azaroff, B., and Feldman, R. S. (1992). Prompting reciprocal interactions via peer incidental teaching. *Journal of Applied Behavior Analysis*, **25**, 117–26.

Michael, J. (1993). Establishing operations. *The Behavior Analyst*, **16**, 191–206.

Montee, B. B., Miltenberger, R. G., and Wittrock, D. (1995). An experimental analysis of facilitated communication. *Journal of Applied Behavior Analysis*, **28**, 189–200.

Mostert, M. P. (2001). Facilitated communication since 1995: a review of published studies. *Journal of Autism and Developmental Disorders*, **31**, 287–313.

National Research Council (2001). *Educating Children with Autism*. Committee on educational interventions for children with autism. Division of Behavioral and Social Sciences. Washington, DC: National Academy Press.

Odom, S. L. and Strain, P. S. (1986). A comparison of peer-initiation and teacher–antecedent intervention for promoting reciprocal social interaction of autistic preschoolers. *Journal of Applied Behavior Analysis*, **19**, 59–71.

Odom, S. L., Hoyson, M., Jamieson, B., and Strain, P. S. (1985). Increasing handicapped preschoolers' peer social interactions: cross-setting and component analysis. *Journal of Applied Behavior Analysis*, **18**, 3–16.

O'Neill R. E., Horner, R. H., Albin, R. W. *et al*. (1997). *Functional Assessment and Program Development for Problem Behavior*, 2nd edn. Pacific Grove, CA: Brooks Cole.

Pelios, L., Morren, J., Tesch, D., and Axelrod, S. (1999). The impact of functional analysis methodology on treatment choices for self-injurious and aggressive behavior. *Journal of Applied Behavior Analysis*, **32**, 185–95.

Pierce, K. and Schreibman, L. (1995). Increasing complex social behaviors in children with autism: effects of peer-implemented pivotal response training. *Journal of Applied Behavior Analysis*, **28**, 285–95.

Rimland, B. (1964). *Infantile Autism*. New York: Appleton Century Crofts.

Rimland, B. and Edelson, S. M. (1994). The effects of auditory integration training on autism. *American Journal of Speech–Language Pathology*, **3**, 16–24.

Rimland, B. and Edelson, S. M. (1995). Auditory integration training in autism: a pilot study. *Journal of Autism and Developmental Disorders*, **25**, 61–70.

Sallows, G. O. and Graupner, T. D. (2005). Intensive behavioral treatment for children with autism: four-year outcome and predictors. *American Journal on Mental Retardation*, **110**, 417–38.

Sasso, G. M. and Rude, H. A. (1987). Unprogrammed effects of training high-status peers to interact with severely handicapped children. *Journal of Applied Behavior Analysis*, **20**, 35–44.

Schopler, E. and Reichler, R. J. (1971). Parents as cotherapists in the treatment of psychotic children. *Journal of Autism and Childhood Schizophrenia*, **1**, 87–102.

Shabani, D. B., Katz, R. C., Wilder, D. A. *et al.* (2002). Increasing social initiations in children with autism: effects of a tactile prompt. *Journal of Applied Behavior Analysis*, **35**, 79–83.

Skinner, B. F. (1957). *Verbal Behavior*. Englewood Cliff, NJ: Prentice-Hall.

Smith, T. (1996). Are other treatments effective? In C. Maurice, G. Green, and S. C. Luce, eds., *Behavioral Intervention for Young Children with Autism*. Austin, TX: Pro-Ed, pp. 45–59.

Smith, T., Groen, A. D., and Wynn, J. W. (2000). Randomized trial of intensive early intervention for children with pervasive developmental disorder. *American Journal on Mental Retardation*, **105**, 269–85.

Stahmer, A. C. (1995). Teaching symbolic play skills to children with autism using pivotal response training. *Journal of Autism and Developmental Disorders*, **25**, 123–41.

Stehli, A. (1991). *The Sound of a Miracle: A Child's Triumph over Autism*. New York: Doubleday.

Strain, P. S. and Timm, M. A. (1974). An experimental analysis of social interaction between a behaviorally disordered preschool child and her classroom peers. *Journal of Applied Behavior Analysis*, **7**, 583–590.

Strain, P. S., Shores, R. E., and Kerr, M. M. (1976). An experimental analysis of "spill over" effects on the social interaction of behaviorally handicapped preschool children. *Journal of Applied Behavior Analysis*, **9**, 31–40.

Sundberg, M. L. and Partington, J. W. (1998). *Teaching Language to Children with Autism or Other Developmental Disabilities*. Pleasant Hill, CA: Behavior Analysts, Inc.

Tang, J. C., Kennedy, C. H., Koppekin, A., and Caruso, M. (2002). Functional analysis of stereotypical ear covering in a child with autism. *Journal of Applied Behavior Analysis*, **35**, 95–8.

Thiemann, K. S. and Goldstein, H. (2001). Social stories, written text cues, and video feedback: effects on social communication of children with autism. *Journal of Applied Behavior Analysis*, **34**, 425–46.

Thorp, D. M., Stahmer, A. C., and Schreibman, L. (1995). Effects of sociodramatic play training on children with autism. *Journal of Autism and Developmental Disorders*, **25**, 265–82.

Tustin, R. D. (1995). The effects of advance notice of activity transition on stereotypic behavior. *Journal of Applied Behavior Analysis*, **28**, 91–2.

Twardosz, S. and Baer, D. M. (1973). Training two severely retarded adolescents to ask questions. *Journal of Applied Behavior Analysis*, **6**, 655–61.

Van Houten, R. V., Axelrod, S., Bailey, J. S. *et al.* (1988). The right to effective behavioral treatment. *Journal of Applied Behavior Analysis*, **21**, 381–4.

Wacker, D. P., Harding, J., Cooper, L. J. *et al.* (1996). The effects of meal schedule and quantity on problematic behavior. *Journal of Applied Behavior Analysis*, **29**, 79–87.

Zanolli, K., Daggett, J., and Adams, T. (1996). Teaching preschool age autistic children to make spontaneous initiations to peers using priming. *Journal of Autism and Developmental Disorders*, **26**, 407–22.

Zarcone, J. R., Fisher, W. W., and Piazza, C. C. (1996). Analysis of free-time contingencies as positive versus negative reinforcement. *Journal of Applied Behavior Analysis*, **29**, 247–50.

9

The outcome in adult life for people with ASD

Patricia Howlin

Department of Psychology, Institute of Psychiatry

Accounts of adults with autism spectrum disorders (ASD)

Despite the ever-increasing number of publications on the topic of autism, rela-tively little has been written about outcome in adulthood. Moreover, the accounts that are available can present a very confusing picture to families seeking to know what may become of their son or daughter as they grow older. On the one hand, the problems shown by adults with ASD often feature prominently in books or papers dealing with "challenging behaviors" (Clements & Zarkowska, 2000). Lurid accounts of crimes committed by individuals with Asperger's syn-drome also appear from time to time in daily newspapers. In contrast, there are impressive personal narratives by people with autism spectrum disorders (ASDs) who have managed to cope admirably with many of the problems they have encountered throughout their lives (see for example autobiographical accounts by Gerland, 1997; Grandin, 1995; Holliday Willey, 1999, Lawson, 2002; Williams, 1992, 1994). There are individual case reports, too, of individuals who, although impaired in many aspects of their functioning, show remarkable skill in certain specific areas, such as art, music, or numerical calculations (Hermelin, 2001).

In fact, most people with ASD fall into none of these categories, but families are provided with very little guidance or information on what the future is likely to hold. Many come to dread the onset of adolescence, in particular, fearing that this is certain to bring increased difficulties and almost all parents have serious concerns about the ability of their son or daughter to cope when they are no longer there to care for them.

Long-term research is costly and fraught with a host of problems but over the past few decades there has been a number of studies that have followed up individuals with ASD as they reach adolescence or adulthood. Drawing firm conclusions from this research is not easy because of the limited numbers of

Autism and Pervasive Developmental Disorders, 2nd edn, ed. Fred R. Volkmar.
Published by Cambridge University Press. © Cambridge University Press 2007.

studies involved, the small sample size and heterogeneity of subjects, and the variability of outcome measures. Nevertheless, the findings provide important information for individuals with autism and their families.

The first descriptive studies

In the mid to late 1950s there began to appear a number of studies on outcomes in children diagnosed as suffering from "childhood psychosis," "early childhood schizophrenia," or "infantile autism." It is apparent from the descriptions in these reports that many of the cases involved showed the characteristic symptoms of autism. However, the heterogeneity of the groups, in terms of age, intellectual level, diagnosis, and etiology, made the interpretation of outcome data extremely difficult. Thus, Victor Lotter (1978), reviewing a total of 25 follow-up studies of "psychotic children" concluded that the majority suffered from such serious flaws in research design (including inadequate diagnostic criteria, subjective reporting, or very mixed subject groups) that "very little could be concluded about prognosis."

One of the earliest reports focusing on children who clearly met diagnostic criteria for autism was that of Leon Eisenberg, a child psychiatrist at Johns Hopkins Medical School, in 1956. Although the account is largely anecdotal, with many cases still in their early teens when assessed, Eisenberg, like many subsequent authors, documented the wide variety of possible outcomes. Many of the individuals described remained very dependent but about one-third were found to have made "at least a moderate social adjustment," despite the lack of any specialist provision or treatment available at that time. A minority had managed to achieve good independence, although even among this group social impairments remained apparent. As an illustration of this Eisenberg cited the case of one young man who, called upon to speak as a student leader at a soccer rally, announced (with undeniable accuracy) that his team was going to lose.

In a slightly later report from Britain, Mildred Creak (1963) described a hundred cases of "childhood psychosis." Again the information is very anecdotal and because the figures do not distinguish clearly between adult and child cases the longer-term outcome remains unclear. Out of the total sample, 43 were living in institutional care, 40 remained at home, attending school or day centers, and 17 were coping with mainstream schooling or employment.

By far the most fascinating and detailed accounts of this period are those of Kanner, who like Eisenberg was a psychiatrist at Johns Hopkins. Kanner kept meticulous records of what happened to the children under his care and followed up many into their twenties and beyond (Kanner, 1973). He, too, noted the great variability in outcome, and stressed the importance of well-developed communication skills and intellectual ability for a good prognosis. Individuals who remained mute had the least favorable outcome. The majority of this group remained highly dependent as they grew older, living either with their parents, in sheltered communities, in state institutions for people with learning disabilities, or in psychiatric hospitals. Among cases with better communication skills outcome was rather more positive. Just over half of this group were functioning relatively well, at home or in the community, although with varying degrees of support (Kanner & Eisenberg, 1956).

Of special interest is Kanner's account of 96 individuals, first seen before 1953, and in their twenties and thirties when followed up (Kanner, 1973; Kanner & Eisenberg, 1956). Twelve cases were reported to have done remarkably well as they grew older, and as "mingling, working and maintaining themselves in society."* Kanner also notes that in the majority of these cases "a remarkable change took place" around their mid teens. "Unlike most other autistic children they became uneasily aware of their peculiarities and began to make a conscious effort to do something about them." In particular, they tried to improve their interactions with their peers, often using their obsessional preoccupations or special skills "to open a door for contact."

Among these more successful individuals, 11 had jobs (ranging from an accountant, a lab technician, and a meteorologist in the navy, to dish-washing and shelf-stacking) and one was still at college. However, jobs were often at a lower level than the individuals' qualifications might have predicted. One young woman, who was training to be a nurse, failed because she would stick rigidly to the rules. Thus, having been told that 20 minutes was the usual time it took for breast-feeding, she would remove babies from their mothers' breasts if they exceeded this. She later succeeded as a hospital lab technician. Another individual, with a postgraduate degree in economics, was working as an accounts clerk because he could not cope with the managerial demands of a higher-level job. Yet another, with a degree in history, had a "blue-collar job" in a horticultural research station, and was much disappointed at his failure to work with "educated people."

Seven of the group had their own homes and one individual (who was also a successful music composer) was married with a child. The remainder lived with their parents. Although many belonged to social groups or clubs (involving singing, hiking, sport, transport, bridge, or the church) few had any close sexual relationships. Several explained this on grounds such as "women cost too much

---

* Two other cases are also noted. One, formerly attending college, could no longer be traced, and a "gifted student of mathematics" had been killed in an accident.

money" or that it would not be worthwhile to "waste money on a girl who isn't serious."

Asperger's accounts

Hans Asperger, a Viennese psychiatrist, also noted the very variable outcomes among the individuals he studied. The least favorable outcome was for those with learning disabilities in addition to their autism and Asperger commented that "the fate of the latter cases is often very sad." For those more able individuals who did make progress, it was, again, often their special skills or interests that eventually led to social integration. Asperger described many individuals who had done remarkably well in later life, including a professor of astronomy, mathematicians, technologists, chemists, high-ranking civil servants, and an expert in heraldry. Indeed, he went so far as to suggest that

able autistic individuals can rise to eminent positions and perform with such outstanding success that one may even conclude that *only* such people are capable of certain achievements. It is as if they had compensatory abilities to counterbalance their deficiencies. Their unswerving determination and penetrating intellectual powers . . . their narrowness and single mindedness . . . can be immensely valuable and lead to outstanding achievements in their chosen areas.

(For an annotated translation of Asperger's initial paper, see Frith, 1991.)

Autobiographical writings

Personal accounts, too, illustrate the mixture of success and difficulties encountered by individuals with ASD. Donna Williams, who now makes an independent living as an author, was one of the first to write of the experience of having autism (1992, 1994) but her autobiography has since been followed by many others. Temple Grandin, who also has autism, is an animal psychologist, with an international reputation in the design of livestock handling facilities for farms, abattoirs, and zoos. Many of her designs have been developed from the "squeeze machines" that she first began to construct while she was at school (Grandin, 1995; Sacks, 1993). Although she continues to have difficulties in understanding ordinary social relationships and feelings, describing herself, in many ways, like "an anthropologist on Mars" (Sacks, 1993), she has clearly come a long way from her confused, withdrawn, noncommunicating early childhood. Wendy Lawson was 42 years of age, and the mother of four children (some of whom also have an ASD) before she was diagnosed as having Asperger syndrome. Prior to this she had been diagnosed as "intellectually disabled" and then as schizophrenic, a diagnosis that persisted for over 25 years. Her books tell of how the correct diagnosis finally brought some understanding of, and help for her condition.

She went on to gain graduate and postgraduate degrees, and is now a successful writer and lecturer on autism. (cf. Lawson, 1998, 2002). A somewhat similar account of the isolation and difficulties that confront individuals with ASD if they are not correctly diagnosed has been published by Lianne Holliday Willey (1999, 2001). She has an academic career, specializing in psycholinguistics, but it was not until her youngest daughter was diagnosed as having Asperger' syndrome that she realized that she, too, had the same characteristics. Another well-known autobiographical account is that of Gunilla Gerland (1997) while Clare Sainsbury, an Oxford graduate with a First in Philosophy and Politics (2000) has published an anthology of her own experiences, and those of other children with Asperger's syndrome as they attempt to cope with the many demands of school life. Although written by very different individuals, the common theme running through these books is the confusion and frustration, fear and anxiety they experienced in having to mix and fit in with their peers in school, college, and workplace, and their problems in coping with the demands of family life. The titles themselves tell their own story: *Martian in the Playground*; *Life on the Outside*; *Life Behind Glass*; *Pretending to be Normal*.

There are numerous other accounts of personal experiences of autism that can now be accessed via internet sites. Newsletters, such as those produced by self-help or support groups, also contain many first-hand accounts of the difficulties, tribulations, and achievements experienced by people with autism and Asperger syndrome. These include newsletters produced by Asperger United in the UK and Autism Network International.

Autobiographical writings by people with ASD are, of course, fascinating because of what they reveal about the ways in which people with autism think and feel and understand. Nevertheless, although providing us with a rich source of information, these accounts give little indication of what happens to most individuals as they grow older. In order to investigate this, larger-scale and long-term follow-up studies are required.

Early follow-up reports

Initial studies of the outcome for children with autism were, as noted above, largely anecdotal and unsystematic. However, towards the end of the 1960s Michael Rutter and colleagues carried out a detailed follow-up study of 63 individuals, initially diagnosed as autistic at the Maudsley Hospital in London in the 1950s and early 1960s. Thirty-eight of the group were aged 16 years or over. Of these two were still at school, but of the remainder only three had paid jobs. Over half were placed in long-stay hospitals, seven were still living with their parents, with no outside occupation, three were living in special communities, and four attended day centers. Rutter notes that several individuals living at home or in a special community could have been capable of employment "at least in a sheltered setting, had adequate training facilities been available." General outcome for the adult cases in this study is not differentiated from that for the under 16s, but overall only 14% of the group was said to have made a good social adjustment. Nevertheless, most individuals tended to improve with age, and although there was a number of cases who showed a worsening in certain aspects of behavior over time "it was rare to see marked remissions and relapses as in adult psychotic illnesses." No significant sex differences were found, although girls were somewhat less likely to fall either within the good or very poor groups. (For details, see Lockyer & Rutter, 1969, 1970; Rutter & Lockyer, 1967; Rutter et al., 1967).

Although a number of other follow-up studies appeared around this time (Mittler et al., 1966; DeMyer et al., 1973) most of the individuals involved were still in their early teens, so that they contain little information on later outcome and progress. The first study to look specifically at outcome in an older age group was that of Victor Lotter (Lotter, 1974a, b). Twenty-nine young people between the ages of 16 and 18 years, who had been diagnosed as autistic when younger were assessed. In general, the findings were similar to those of Rutter and colleagues although many more children (24%) were still at school, reflecting improvements in educational provision over the previous decade (less than half of the children seen by Rutter had received as much as two years' schooling and many had never attended school at all). Nevertheless, among the 22 individuals who had left school only one had a job. Almost half the sample were in long-stay hospital provision, two individuals were living at home, and five were attending day training centers. In terms of overall social adjustment, 14% were described as having done well, although the majority was described as having a "poor" or "very poor" outcome. Overall, girls did less well, with none being rated as attaining either a good or fair outcome.

Later follow-up studies

Throughout the 1980s and 1990s there has been a number of follow-up studies or reports of adults with autism. However, because many of these have involved subjects who were still relatively young, or have focused more specifically on high-functioning individuals, the implications for older people within the *wider* autistic spectrum are somewhat limited.

Chung et al. (1990), for example, followed up 66 children attending a psychiatric clinic in Hong Kong, in the decade from 1976. As in other studies, the best outcome was found for cases who had developed speech before the age of five, and who scored more highly on tests of intellectual and social functioning. However, as only nine cases were above 12 years old, the report provides no information about longer-term outcomes.

There have been a number of follow-up studies conducted in Scandinavia, where social and psychiatric databases tend to be particularly well maintained. Gillberg's Swedish group (Billstedt *et al.*, 2004) have followed up 83 individuals aged 17 or over (mean age 25 years), with a childhood diagnosis of autistic disorder. Only three people were found to be fully self-supporting as adults. Of the remainder, around a quarter was described as functioning fairly well, but the majority (76%) had a "poor" or "very poor" outcome. Three individuals had died (one, possibly two, of status epilepticus, and one in a fire accident). IQ at initial diagnosis was one of the most important prognostic indicators. In some, but not all cases, the development of epilepsy around puberty seemed to result in a worse outcome. There was no difference in the outcomes for males and females. Another Swedish study, this time in the north of the country (von Knorring & Hägglöf, 1993) examined functioning in 34 cases, with a mean age of around 19 years. Although details of social outcome are limited, one individual was described as having lost all autistic symptoms, 3 had only a few remaining symptoms, and 30 remained clearly autistic. In Denmark, Larsen and Mouridsen (1997) completed a 30-year follow-up of 18 individuals, 9 with autism and 9 with Asperger syndrome, all in their 30s or 40s. Cognitive levels ranged from below 50 to 85+. All had been admitted at some stage to adult psychiatric hospitals and two had died. Nevertheless, over 40% lived more or less independently and four were, or had been, married. However, only three were in paid, independent employment, three attended sheltered workshops, five were on disability pensions, and the remainder attended day programs at their local psychiatric hospitals.

In the United States, a telephone survey by Ballaban-Gil *et al.* (1996) found that among 45 adults, initially diagnosed as children, over half (53%) were in residential placements and only one was living independently. Eleven percent were in regular employment (all in menial jobs) and a further 16% were in sheltered placements. Rates of behavioral difficulties were high and only three adults were rated as having no social deficits.

A much larger study of young adults with autism (170 male, 31 female), aged between 18 and 33, was conducted by Kobayashi and colleagues (1992) in Japan. Outcome was assessed by means of postal questionnaires to parents. The average follow-up period was 15 years, during which time four cases, all male, had died (from encephalopathy, age 6; head injury from severe self-injury, age 16; nephritic syndrome, age 20; and asthma, age 22). Almost half the group were reported as having good or very good communication skills, and over a quarter were described as having a good or very good outcome (i.e. able to live independently or semi-independently and succeeding at work or college). Women tended to have better language outcomes than men but there were no significant differences in social functioning between the sexes.

Forty-three individuals were employed, with a further 11 still attending school or college. Jobs were mostly in the food and service industries, but several individuals were described as having realized their "childhood dreams" of being a bus-conductor, car mechanic, or cook. The highest level of jobs obtained were by a physiotherapist, a civil servant, a printer and two office workers. All but three of those with jobs still lived with their parents, one was in a group home, and two had their own apartments; none was married.

Approximately one-fifth of the sample had developed epilepsy (usually in their early teens) but this was well controlled in all but three cases. Generally the outcome for females was worse than for males. Although outcome in males was significantly correlated with early language abilities and intellectual functioning, these relationships were much weaker in females. Although, by virtue of its size, this remains a very informative study, reliance on questionnaire data, with little or no direct contact with the autistic individuals themselves, clearly raises problems. Parents' ratings of how well their children are functioning may not always accurately reflect their true status. Moreover, diagnostic assessment of autism in the past has not always been entirely satisfactory, and hence some current confirmation of diagnosis is also required.

In a more recent study carried out at the Maudsley Hospital in London (Howlin et al., 2004) parents and individuals were all interviewed independently, diagnostic criteria were reconfirmed, and detailed assessments were carried out of language, cognitive, social, and academic functioning. Only individuals with a childhood IQ of at least 50 were included since it is now well established that below this level outcome is almost certain to be limited. Sixty-eight people (61 male and 7 female) were followed up between the ages of 21 and 48 years. As adults their average performance IQ was 75 (range 33–122). By follow-up seven individuals were living independently, or semi-independently, but a third were still with their parents, and half the group lived in sheltered communities, mostly specifically for people with autism; eight individuals were in long-stay hospital care. Despite the fact that one-fifth had obtained some formal qualifications before leaving school (five had attended college or university) employment levels were generally disappointing. Only eight were in regular, paid employment and one was self-employed; 12 others worked on a supported/sheltered or voluntary basis. The remainder attended day or residential centers, where there was little scope for the development of competitive work skills. In terms of social functioning, around a quarter of the group were described as having some friends, with 13 individuals having relationships that involved shared enjoyment or closer intimacy. One individual was married, although he later divorced, and two have married more recently. However, almost two-thirds had no friends at all.

A composite rating of outcome, based on social interactions, level of independence, and occupational status, indicated that 15 individuals could be described as having a "good" or "very good" outcome. Most of these had some friends and either had a job or were undergoing training. Even if they still lived at home they had a relatively high level of independence, being largely responsible for their own finances, buying their own clothes, or taking independent holidays. Thirteen remained moderately dependent on their families or other carers for support, and few in this group had any close friendships. Thirty-one people were in special residential units, which, by their very nature (most were geographically very isolated), severely limited individual independence; outcome in all these individuals was considered "poor." The eight individuals in long-term hospital care were all rated as having a "very poor" outcome.

Follow-up studies of high-functioning people with autism and Asperger's syndrome

In addition to these more general follow-up studies, some have focused more specifically on individuals with autism or Asperger's syndrome who have normal or near-normal intellectual ability.

Rumsey and colleagues (Rumsey et al., 1985), in a very detailed study involving a five-day inpatient assessment, followed up 14 young men aged between 18 and 39 years of age, all of whom fulfilled DSM-III criteria for autism (American Psychiatric Association, 1980). Several cases had initially been diagnosed by Kanner himself and as adults nine were described as "high-functioning," with verbal IQs well within the normal range. In the "lower-functioning" group, three were of normal nonverbal IQ but had continuing language impairments; two were also mildly intellectually impaired. Socially, all the group continued to have marked difficulties. Most were described as "loners." None was married or was thought to have contemplated this; only one had friends, mostly through his church (although he was described as "underinhibited" (not at all inhibited)) and a number, even amongst the intellectually more able group, were said still to show socially inappropriate behaviors. Half the group, including those who were high functioning, showed peculiar use of language, such as stereotyped and repetitive speech or talking to themselves.

Academically, those in the lower-functioning group had needed specialist education into late adolescence, but all had developed basic reading, writing, and mathematical skills commensurate with their intellectual levels. In the higher-ability group, only one had remained in specialist educational provision, five had completed high school, and two had attended junior college; several showed good ability in math and two in foreign languages. Nevertheless, assessment of social outcomes, as measured by the Vineland Social Maturity Scale, indicated that their scores here were often "strikingly" low in relation to IQ. Problems among the more able group were generally related to deficits in the areas of self-direction, socialization, and occupational achievements. Similar difficulties were found among those who were less able but they also had additional impairments in communication and independence of travel.

In terms of independent living, six individuals in the more able group still lived with their parents and two were in supervised apartments; only one lived entirely alone. In the less able group nobody was living independently, three lived with their families, one was in a group home, and one in a state hospital. With the exception of one person who was unemployed, all the lower-ability group attended a sheltered workshop or special job program. Among the others, four were in employment (a janitor, a cab driver, a library assistant, and a key-punch operator); of the remainder, three were in special training or college courses, one was in a sheltered workshop, and one was unemployed. Even among those who had jobs, only two had found these independently – generally "parents played a major role in finding employers willing to give their sons a chance."

Szatmari and colleagues (1989a), working in Toronto, studied a group of 12 males and 5 females aged 17 or over, with an average IQ of above 90. Educationally, half the group had received special schooling but the other half had attended college or university, with six obtaining a degree or equivalent qualification. Two were unemployed and four were in sheltered workshop schemes, three were still studying, one worked in the family business, and six were in regular, full-time employment. Of the latter, one was a librarian, another a physics tutor, two were salesmen with semi-managerial positions, one worked in a factory, and one was a library technician. Ten of the 16 cases still lived at home and one was in a group home, but five lived independently and a further three living at home were said by their parents to be completely independent. Only one individual was felt to need constant supervision at home, one required moderate care, and six required some minimal supervision. Socially, nine individuals had never had a sexual relationship with anyone of the opposite sex but a quarter of the group had dated regularly or had long-term relationships; one was married. In contrast with some other studies, little or no relationship was found between early measures of language or social behavior and later functioning (early IQ data were not available). However, there was a high and significant correlation between current IQ and social functioning as measured by the Vineland.

The authors are open about the problems related to the study, including the small sample size (compounded by a high refusal rate), and, because of the group's high IQ, a lack of representativeness for autistic individuals as a whole. Nevertheless they note that outcome is not necessarily as gloomy as many earlier studies had indicated. They conclude: "A small percentage of non-retarded autistic children . . . can be expected to recover to a substantial degree. It may take years to occur, and the recovery may not always be complete, but substantial improvement does occur."

Another Canadian-based study (Venter et al., 1992) has also assessed later functioning in more able children. Fifty-eight children (35 males and 23 females) with an average full-scale IQ of 79 were given a detailed battery of tests and assessments and the results focus predominantly on intellectual and academic attainments rather than overall functioning. The authors note a marked improvement in children's academic attainments compared with the earlier follow-up studies carried out by Rutter and Bartak in the mid 1970s (Rutter & Bartak, 1973; Bartak & Rutter, 1973). Thus, even among the lower-functioning group, over half could read and do simple arithmetic, compared to about one-fifth in the studies conducted 20 years ago.

Twenty-two individuals in the study were aged 18 or over; of these 6 were competitively employed and 13 were in sheltered employment or special training programs; only 3 had no occupation. Nevertheless, again, all those who were employed were in relatively low-level jobs and all but one had required special assistance in finding employment. Of the three individuals not involved in any adult program two were female, and all of the competitively employed people were male. No individual was married, and only two lived alone, one of these with considerable support from his mother. Four people lived in apartments with minimal supervision.

In a further study based at the Maudsley Hospital (Mawhood et al., 2000) the outcome for 19 young men was studied in great detail, as part of a comparative follow-up study of individuals with autism and developmental language disorders. Individuals had initially been seen between the ages of 4 and 9 years and all had a nonverbal IQ within the normal range. At follow-up the average performance IQ of the group remained well within the normal range and five individuals had attended college or university. Despite this they showed continuing problems in social relationships, and most remained very dependent. Only three individuals were living independently, one of these in sheltered

Table 9.1 Independence and social outcomes in follow-up studies of adolescents and adults[a]

Study (total n)	Age	IQ	Semi/independent (%)	With parents (%)	Residential provision (%)	Hospital care (%)	Married (%)	Some friends (%)	Outcome summary (%)		
									Good	Fair	Poor
Eisenberg, 1956 (50)	12–35		0						6	28	67
Lockyer & Rutler, 1970 (38)	16+	X = 62	0	18	19	53			14	25	61
Kanner, 1973 (96)	22–29		8				1 (1 child)	2	11		
Lotter, 1978 (29)	16–18	55–90	0	28	16	48			14	24	62
Newson et al., 1982 (93)	X = 23		7	71	16		1	15	7	77	16
Rumsey et al., 1985 (14)	18–39	55–129	21	64	7	7			35	35	28
Szatmari et al., 1989 (16)	17–34	68–110	33	63	12	0	29	21	38	31	31
Tantam, 1991 (46)	X = 24		3	41	53	2	2	1			
Kobayashi et al., 1992 (201)	18–33	23% > 70	1	97		2	0		27	27	46
Venter et al., 1992 (22)	18+	X = 90	21			0	0				
Knorring & Hägglöf, 1993 (34)	X = 19								3	9	88
Ballaban-Gil et al., 1996(45)	18+	31 > 70	2	45	53				6	?	?
Larsen & Mouridsen 1997 (18)	32–43	78% > 50	44	17	12	17	22 (2 with children)		28	28	44
Mawhood et al., 2000 (19)	21–26	70–117	16	32	47	5	5	21	26		74
Billstedt et al., 2004 (83)	25.5	53% < 50	4				1		0	24	76
Howlin et al., 2004 (68)	21+	51–137	10	38	38	12	4	19	22	19	57

[a] Summary ratings based on authors' own classifications where provided. Otherwise "Good" = moderate to high levels of independence in living and/or job; some friends/acquaintances. "Fair" = needing support in work and/or daily living but some limited autonomy. "Poor" = living in residential care or hospital provision (or parental home but with close supervision in most activities). Blank cells indicate insufficient information to rate.

accommodation, three had jobs (two of these under special arrangements), none had married, and only three were described as having close friendships. Almost half the group were said never to have had any friends, and about one-third had "acquaintances" only. Fifteen subjects had never had either a close friendship or a sexual relationship. Thirteen were still described as having moderate to severe behavioral difficulties, associated with obsessional or ritualistic tendencies. A composite rating of outcome, based on communication skills, friendships, levels of independence, and behavioral difficulties indicated that, overall, only 3 subjects were considered to have a good outcome, 2 remained moderately impaired, and 14 continued to show substantial impairments.

There are also a number of cross-sectional studies, which, although lacking the advantage of data on functioning in childhood, do provide a detailed description of status in adult life. Tantam (1991), for example, has described outcome in 46 individuals with Asperger syndrome, with an average age of 24 years. Despite being of normal intellectual ability, only two had had any education after school, and only four were in jobs. One individual was married but most continued to live with their parents or in residential care. A somewhat similar group of 93 young adults was described by Newson and her colleagues in 1982. Diagnostic and IQ data on the sample are lacking, but overall more subjects than in Tantam's study had received further education, 22% were in jobs and 7% lived independently. Of this group, 15% were said to have had heterosexual relationships, although only one was married. Nevertheless, at an average age of 23, almost three-quarters still lived with their parents.

What can studies of outcome in adult life tell us?

A summary of studies that have examined outcome in adults with ASD is presented in Table 9.1. Comparisons between them must, of course, be treated with caution for a number of reasons. First, the data from the later studies are much more systematic and objective than those from earlier ones. Second, several of the more recent reports have concentrated on individuals of higher ability, and therefore a more favorable outcome would be expected. Nevertheless, there were many individuals in the earlier reports who were of relatively high intellectual ability, and indeed the average nonverbal IQ of subjects in the Rutter and Lotter studies fell just within the normal range (i.e. above 70). Similarly there were many subjects in the later investigations who were well below average intelligence. Third, overall judgments of whether outcome is "Good," "Fair," or "Poor" tend to be somewhat subjective, even if attempts are made to quantify what is meant by these terms. Finally, no doubt because of factors related to

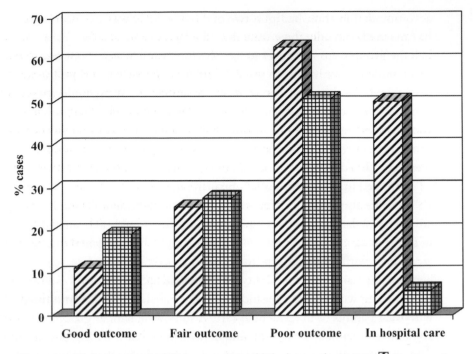

Figure 9.1 Adult outcomes in follow-up studies published pre and post 1980. ▨ Average rating pre-1980, ▦ Average rating post-1980.

the variability in subject selection and assessment, there continue to be quite marked differences between studies in outcome results. Thus "Good" ratings, for example, range from 0% to 38% and "Poor" ratings from 16% to over 80%.

The proportions living independently also remain very variable. The best outcome was reported in the Canadian study of Szatmari and his co-workers, and although this may be partly understood because of the high ability of the subjects involved, it does not explain why the findings should be considerably better than for the British subjects in the Mawhood study, who were of very similar intellectual levels. It may well be that cultural factors play an important role here, since schemes involving supported employment or semi-sheltered living are generally much better established in Canada and the USA than in Britain. The very small number of subjects living independently in the Japanese study is also likely to be related to cultural factors.

Despite these qualifications, improvements do appear to be taking place. Figure 9.1 summarizes the results of studies conducted over the last two decades (1980–2001) with those appearing in the 1950s to 1970s, in terms of general outcome. Whereas the mean percentage of those rated as having a "Good" outcome in follow-up studies conducted before 1980 was around 11%, over the following two decades the proportion had risen to almost 20%. "Poor" outcome ratings declined from an average of 65% to around 50% over the same period. "Fair" ratings remained around 25% to 30%. However, the proportions still living with their families, or in specialist residential provision, remains high, often around 30% or more. One particularly noticeable change has been in the frequency of admissions to long-stay hospital care. Around 40% to 50% of individuals in the earlier studies moved into such placements as adults, but there was a marked decline from the 1980s onwards, with the mean being around 6% (and in many cases far less). Nevertheless, despite the general trend toward the closure of large residential institutions, for some individuals it has proved extremely difficult to find an alternative to hospital care. This is because their behavioral problems, and especially their lack of social understanding, greatly limit their ability to settle into community-based provision.

Over the years there have been increases in the proportion of individuals with ASD finding employment, but numbers are still relatively low, with the average percent in work in studies post-1980 being only around 20%. Even among reports with a focus on higher-functioning individuals the highest proportion reported in work is 47% (Szatmari et al., 1989a) and few studies report employment rates above 30%. Moreover, the majority of job placements reported were menial and poorly paid, in positions such as kitchen hands, unskilled factory workers, or backroom supermarket staff. In addition, jobs had often been procured through the efforts or personal contacts of families rather than through the normal channels (Howlin et al., 2004). Employment stability, too, was poor, with many individuals experiencing lengthy periods without paid work. In the group studied by Howlin et al. (2004), for example, the average IQ in adulthood was 75, with one third having performance IQs of 80 or above. Although around 20% had obtained formal qualifications (several had degrees or diplomas) only 8 were working independently, one was a self-employed fabric printer, 12 worked on a supported/sheltered or voluntary basis, 2 worked for the family business, and 1 worked in a shop run by his residential center. One other man, previously employed in a factory, had been unemployed for some years. Even among those in higher-level jobs involving computing or accountancy, the level at which they functioned was often lower than their educational attainments would have predicted. Only three or four individuals (a cartographer, a scientific analyst for an oil company, and two computer programers) were employed at a level fully appropriate to their qualifications. Those who were not employed attended general work/leisure programs within their day or residential units. If anything, employment prospects tended to worsen with

age and in a subsequent follow-up of the same group, some time after the initial data had been collected Hutton (2004) found no increase in the numbers in
independent work and three previously employed individuals were no longer
working.

Figures for independent living are also disappointing, although again there
have been some improvements over time. Apart from the individuals described
by Kanner in his follow-up, none of the studies conducted prior to 1980 mention
subjects living independently. In the post-1980 studies an average of around 12%
had their own homes.

The quality of interpersonal relationships, although a crucial aspect of adult
life, has not been considered in detail in most follow-up studies. Few describe
individuals who have married or who have children of their own although Howlin
et al. (2004) and Mawhood *et al.* (2000) found that around 15–20% of their participants were described as having friendships that involved both selectivity and
shared enjoyment. A quarter of the individuals studied by Szatmari had close
friendships and over 40% had had some relationships with members of the opposite sex; heterosexual relationships were also reported by 15% of subjects studied
by Newson and her colleagues. Moreover, it is important to remember that as
autism is largely a genetic disorder, many parents of children with autism and
Asperger's syndrome are likely themselves to be undiagnosed individuals within
the spectrum, who have clearly succeeded in maintaining close relationships and
in bringing up families of their own. There are also now many personal accounts
by or about married people with autism or Asperger's syndrome, some involving
several individuals within the same family (see for example Holliday Willey, 1999,
2001; Lawson, 1998; Paradiž, 2002; Pyles, 2002; Slater Walker & Slater-Walker,
2002).

Factors related to outcome

The variability in outcome among individuals with ASD has been noted since
the very earliest follow-up studies of Eisenberg and Kanner (Eisenberg, 1956;
Kanner & Eisenberg, 1956) and there have been many attempts to try to isolate
the variables that best predict later functioning.

Kanner, in his follow-up (1973), noted that lack of appropriate education was
highly damaging and that admission into hospital care, rather than a school
placement, was "tantamount to a death sentence." Subsequent studies (e.g.
Lockyer & Rutter, 1969, 1970; Lotter, 1974a, b) also noted the association between
years of schooling and later outcome. The most positive outcomes are generally
reported for individuals who have attended mainstream schools, but since this

is directly affected by pupils' linguistic and cognitive levels, the influence of schooling per se on long-term functioning remains obscure.

The relationship between the severity of autistic symptomatology in early childhood and later outcome is also unclear. Rutter and colleagues (Lockyer & Rutter, 1969, 1970; Rutter & Lockyer, 1967) found no significant correlation between individual symptoms in childhood (other than lack of speech) and adult outcome, although there was a significant relationship with the total number of major symptoms rated. DeMyer *et al.* (1973) also reported a relationship between overall severity of autistic symptoms and later progress. In contrast, Lord and Venter (1992) found no association between prognosis and total number of early symptoms as rated on the Autism Diagnostic Interview (ADI). Of greater predictive value were the degree of language *abnormality* and the level of disruption caused by stereotyped and repetitive behaviors.

The possible impact of many other variables remains uncertain. In almost every follow-up study in which women have been involved outcome has been poorer for females than males. However, the number of women participants has generally been very small (many studies are exclusively male) and the differences found rarely reach significance; the tendency for females to be of lower IQ also complicates the issue (Lord & Schopler, 1985). In some studies, the presence of epilepsy has been associated with a poorer outcome but, again, epilepsy is more likely to occur in individuals with more severe cognitive impairments. Socioeconomic factors and ratings of family adequacy were correlated with prognosis in some early studies, (DeMyer *et al.*, 1973; Lotter, 1974a, b), but there is little evidence of a direct causal relationship between an impoverished or disruptive family background and later outcome, although, as with any other condition, disruption at home may well result in an increase in problems generally.

The two factors that have been consistently associated with later prognosis are early language development and IQ. Very few children who have not developed some useful speech by the age of 5–6 years are reported to have a positive long-term outcome, although occasionally older children may develop relatively good communication skills. The relationship between adult outcome and cognitive ability in childhood has been noted in many follow-up studies (Gillberg & Steffenberg, 1987; Lockyer & Rutter, 1969, 1970; Lotter, 1974a, b). Thus, individuals who were either untestable as children, or who had nonverbal IQ scores below 50 were almost invariably reported as remaining highly dependent. However, more recent studies suggest that a minimum childhood IQ of 70 is necessary for a positive outcome in adulthood. Howlin *et al.* (2004) found that on virtually every adult measure (academic attainments, communication skills, reading and spelling, employment status, social independence) individuals with a childhood

IQ below 70 were significantly more impaired than those with an initial IQ of 70+. Only one individual with an IQ between 50 and 69 obtained a "Good" outcome rating in adulthood. Nevertheless, even amongst the 45 individuals in this study with an initial IQ above 70, outcome was very mixed. Thus, although almost one third of this subgroup was rated as having a "good" or "very good" outcome, 22% were rated as only "Fair" and 44% obtained ratings of "poor" or "very poor". Moreover, those individuals with an IQ above 100 did no better as a group than those with an IQ in the 70–99 range. Indeed several individuals in this lower range achieved considerably more highly as adults than many with a childhood IQ of above 100.

It is clear that childhood performance on nonverbal tests of intelligence, whilst being a *relatively* good predictor of outcome, is by no means perfect, and Lord and Bailey (2002) have proposed that childhood *verbal* IQ is a far more reliable indicator of later functioning. However, in the Howlin *et al.* study, although correlations between child and adult verbal IQ were highly significant there was a sizeable subgroup of individuals who, despite being unable to score at all on verbal tests when younger, subsequently made considerable improvements in this area. Over a third of individuals who were "untestable" on verbal measures initially, obtained a verbal IQ equivalent of at least 70 at follow-up and several of these children were subsequently rated as having a "Good" or "Very good" outcome as adults. In the case of other children, who *were* able to obtain a verbal IQ score when first assessed, the relationship with adult outcome was very variable. While a third of those who scored above 50 on verbal IQ tests as children obtained an outcome ratings of "Good" or "Very good" in adulthood; one third were rated as "Fair" and a further third as having a "Poor" or "Very poor" outcome. Even among the few children who scored above 70 on a verbal IQ test initially, less than half were rated as having a "Good"/"Very good" outcome as adults. Thus, again, although statistically there is a positive correlation between early verbal IQ and later prognosis, from an individual, clinical perspective, this variable has only limited predictive value.

Lord and Bailey (2002) also suggest that the presence of useful speech by the age of 5 years is highly predictive of later outcome. Certainly, for many young children it is much easier to obtain information of this kind than to obtain a verbal IQ score, although there may be some problems of recall if interviewing parents of older individuals. However, in the Howlin *et al.* study even this variable was only weakly associated with adult outcome. Over 40% of children who had little or no language when first diagnosed had subsequently developed useful language and the higher their linguistic levels as adults the more likely were they to do well on a range of other outcome measures. Other research has pointed to the impact that improvements in language may have on the developmental trajectory of children with autism (Szatmari, 2000) but as yet we have little information on what is associated with such improvement.

To some extent it may prove easier to identify correlates of "Poor" outcome than the variables predictive of good prognosis. In the Howlin *et al.* study, as already noted, most individuals with an initial performance IQ below 70 remained highly dependent as adults. Moreover, *no one* with a childhood performance IQ below 70 *and* a verbal IQ below 30 achieved even a "Fair" rating in adulthood and only one individual with a performance IQ below 70 coupled with a verbal IQ below 50 did so.

Identifying the reasons why some individuals make significant improvements in their general levels of functioning over time, while others show little or no change has major implications for our understanding of autism and of the factors influencing the trajectory from child to adulthood. There is evidence that the ability to function adequately in adulthood life may depend as much on the degree of support offered (by families, educational, employment, and social services) as much as basic intelligence (Lord & Venter, 1992; Mawhood & Howlin, 1999). It may also be, as Kanner postulated, that the presence of *additional* skills or interests (such as specialized knowledge in particular areas, or competence in mathematics, music, or computing), which allow individuals to find their own niche in life, and thus enable them to be more easily integrated into society, is of great importance. Certainly, eccentric or unusual behaviors are more readily acceptable in individuals who demonstrate exceptional skills in certain areas, than they are in those who have no such redeeming features. Thus, as Kanner, Eisenberg, and Rutter all proposed many years ago, adequate educational opportunities, and encouragement to develop skills that may lead to later acceptance, are crucial. Moreover, particularly for those who are more able, it would seem more profitable in the long term for educational programs to concentrate on those areas in which the person with autism already demonstrates potential competence, rather than focusing on areas of deficit.

Are there differences in outcome between individuals with autism and Asperger's syndrome?

The issue of whether autism and Asperger's syndrome are different conditions (albeit part of the same spectrum of disorders) has been a source of continuing debate over recent years (cf. Klin *et al.*, 2000; Schopler *et al.*, 1998). There is also considerable disagreement about the validity of the diagnostic criteria used in DSM-IV and ICD-10 to distinguish between the two conditions (Kim *et al.*, 2000;

Kugler, 1998; Leekam *et al.*, 2000; Manjiviona & Prior, 1999). However, overall, there appears to be no *consistent* evidence that there are any major differences in rates of social, emotional, and psychiatric problems, current symptomatology, motor clumsiness or neuropsychological profiles between the two groups. There are also indications that any differences found in early childhood decrease with age (Gilchrist *et al.*, 2001; Ozonoff *et al.*, 2002; Szatmari *et al.*, 1995). Howlin (2003), for example, compared a group of 34 adults with autism of normal IQ who had shown early delays in language with 42 IQ-, age-, and gender-matched individuals who were reported to have had no such delays. Although, according to parental reports, there were some group differences in early symptomatology up to the age of 3 years no significant differences were reported on ADI algorithm scores, which are mostly based on behavior at 4 to 5 years. Current ADI scores were almost identical in the two groups, as were social outcome ratings and scores on tests of language comprehension and expression. Moreover, in both groups language abilities were well below chronological age level, despite the fact that language development in Asperger's syndrome is postulated as being essentially normal (DSM-IV).

How great is the risk of deterioration in adulthood?

The transition to adulthood can be a time of upheaval and difficulties for many young people and their families and in a number of long-term studies there have been accounts of an increase in disruptive behaviors in adolescence. Rutter *et al.* (1970), for example, noted that five young people (out of the sample of 64) had shown significant deterioration in their communication in adolescence, together with progressive inertia, and general cognitive decline. Three of these cases had also developed epilepsy. Gillberg and his colleagues (Billstedt *et al.*, 2004) also found that 18% of individuals in their follow-up study exhibited marked deterioration in puberty and the majority of these never really recovered. The typical symptoms noted were increases in hyperactivity, aggressiveness, destructiveness and ritualistic behaviors, inertia, loss of language skills, and "slow intellectual decline." Ballaban-Gil *et al.* (1996) noted that ratings of problem behaviors had increased in almost 50% of their adult sample, although the nature of these is not defined. Kobayashi *et al.* (1992) found that 31% of their group of 201 adults showed a worsening of symptoms, mainly after the age of 10 years, and Larsen and Mouridsen, (1997) reported that 5 of 18 high-IQ individuals with ASD had shown deterioration, mostly in late puberty. In both these latter studies the pattern of deterioration described was very similar to that outlined by Rutter *et al.* (1970) and Gillberg and Steffenberg (1987).

In one of the very few systematic investigations of deterioration over time, Hutton (1998) examined data on the emergence of problems in adulthood for 125 individuals with autism and Asperger's syndrome. Over a third were reported to have developed new behavioral or psychiatric difficulties including psychosis, obsessive–compulsive disorder, anxiety, depression, tics, social withdrawal, phobias, and aggression. Most people developed additional symptoms prior to the age of 30 and episodes of periodic disturbance, occurring at fairly regular and frequent intervals, was noted in eight individuals. The increase in problems of this nature was not associated with epilepsy, cognitive decline, or residential placement. Factors associated with a greater risk of deterioration were low verbal IQ in childhood and long-stay hospital placement; women were also more likely to show an increase in problems than men.

Although it is clear that some individuals with ASD do show an increase in problems as they grow older it is also important to note that, in many studies tracing progress from child- to adulthood, the overriding picture is one of *improvement* over time. This was reported in the early follow-up studies of Rutter and his group, and by Kanner, who noted that for some individuals, particularly those who become more aware of their difficulties, mid adolescence was often a period of "remarkable improvement and change" (Kanner, 1973). Over 40% of the individuals in the Kobayashi *et al.* (1992) study were rated as showing marked improvement, and Billstedt *et al.* (2004) noted that 38% of their sample had a remarkably problem-free adolescent period. Mawhood and her colleagues (2000) in their follow-up of young men with autism into their mid-to-late twenties found that verbal ability on formal IQ tests had increased significantly since childhood, and in terms of general social competence almost one third of the group had moved from a rating of "Poor" functioning as children to a "Good" rating as adults. Even in the Ballaban-Gil study (1996) where increases in ratings of behavioral disturbance were higher than in other groups, 16% had improved, and 35% showed no evidence of deterioration. Many other studies, both retrospective and prospective, suggest that change over time is more likely to be positive, rather than negative with scores on standardized assessments such as the ADI and Autism Diagnostic Observation Schedule indicating a decline in the severity and frequency of autistic symptoms with age (Gilchrist *et al.*, 2001; Howlin, 2003; Piven *et al.*, 1996; Seltzer *et al.*, 2003). Improvements have also been reported in groups of individuals with severe learning disabilities in addition to their autism (Beadle-Brown *et al.*, 2000)

In summary, while it is evident that skills may be lost or problem behaviors increase in adolescence or early adulthood, it is also essential to get the picture into perspective. Conclusions about "improvement" or "deterioration" may depend on the particular measures used, and whereas individuals may fail to make progress in certain areas (for example, in the ability to form close friendships), other skills, notably those related to communication, may show positive and significant change. The number of adults who show marked deterioration in all aspects of their functioning is, fortunately, relatively small and significant regression appears to be the exception, not the rule

Psychiatric disturbances in adulthood

It is hardly surprising, given the many difficulties that they have to deal with in their daily lives, that many individuals with autistic disorders experience mental health problems as they grow older. However, the nature of the association between autism and other disorders, particularly schizophrenia, is often misunderstood.

Autism and schizophrenia

Kanner himself initially considered that autism was an early manifestation of schizophrenia, writing in 1949: "I do not believe that there is any likelihood that early infantile autism will at any future time have to be separated from the schizophrenias." His view was supported by many other psychiatrists at the time, and indeed the suggestion that there is a link between autism and schizophrenia or schizoid-type disorders has persisted for many decades (cf. Wolff, 1991; Wolff & Chick, 1980; Wolff & McGuire, 1995). However, work by Rutter (1972) and Wing (1981) has documented the many crucial differences between the two conditions and there is no evidence to suggest that individuals with ASD have an increased risk of developing schizophrenia in adult life.

Although there have been a number of individual case reports of schizophrenic illness in individuals with ASD (Clarke et al. 1989; Petty et al., 1984; Sverd et al., 1993; Szatmari et al., 1989b; Wolff & McGuire; 1995) Larger-scale studies have failed to find any evidence of increased rates of schizophrenia (Chung et al., 1990; Ghaziuddin et al., 1998). None of the cases followed up by Kanner over a period of 40 years was reported as showing positive psychotic symptoms (i.e. delusions or hallucinations) and Volkmar and Cohen (1991) found only one individual with an unequivocal diagnosis of schizophrenia in a sample of 163 cases. Similarly, Gillberg and colleagues (Billstedt et al., 2004) report on one case with a diagnosis of schizophrenia in their follow-up of 83 people diagnosed with autistic disorder. Schizophrenia also appears to be relatively uncommon among more able individuals or those with Asperger's syndrome. Asperger (1944) noted that only 1 out of his 200 cases developed schizophrenia and Wing (1981), in a study of 18 individuals with Asperger's syndrome, describes one with an unconfirmed diagnosis of schizophrenia. Rumsey *et al.* (1985), in their detailed psychiatric study, found no evidence of schizophrenia. None of the relatively able subjects in the studies of Mawhood *et al.* (2000) or Howlin *et al.* (2004) had developed a schizophrenic illness, and only one individual in a similar group studied by Szatmari *et al.* (1989b) had been treated for chronic schizophrenia. Tantam (1991) diagnosed 3 cases of schizophrenia amongst 83 individuals with Asperger's syndrome, but these were all psychiatric referrals.

Volkmar and Cohen (1991) have suggested that the frequency of schizophrenia in individuals with autism is around 0.6% (roughly comparable to that in the general population) and that: "it does not appear that the two conditions are more commonly observed together than would be expected on a chance basis." Similar conclusions are reached in the more recent overviews by Lainhart (1999) and Howlin *et al.* (2004). Thus, although some studies have suggested that there may be "an excess of schizophrenia in later life," particularly among individuals with Asperger's syndrome (Wolff & McGuire, 1995) there is little evidence for such claims, which Wing (1981) has criticized as being "distressing without being constructive."

Affective disorders

In contrast to the relatively small number of cases with a formal diagnosis of schizophrenia, there are very many more case reports of individuals with affective disorders. As early as 1970, Rutter noted the risk of depressive episodes occurring in adolescents or older individuals with autism and subsequent reviews have reported a high frequency of affective disorders both among individuals with autism (Lainhart & Folstein, 1994) and within their families (Bolton *et al.*, 1998; Smalley *et al.*, 1995). Abramson and colleagues (1992) suggest that around one third of people with autism suffer from affective disorders, and high rates of depression are found among high-functioning individuals, as well as those of lower ability. Tantam (1991), in his study of 85 adults with Asperger's syndrome, noted that 2% had a depressive psychosis and 5% had a bipolar disorder. A further 13% suffered from nonpsychotic depression and/or anxiety. In the study by Rumsey *et al.* (1985) of 14 relatively high-functioning individuals, generalized anxiety problems were found in half the sample. Similar figures were reported by Wing (1981) who found that around a quarter of her group of 18 individuals with Asperger's syndrome showed signs of an affective disorder. Bipolar affective disorders, or mania without depression tend to be reported less frequently than depression alone, although Wozniak *et al.* (1997) found that up to 21% of their autism/PDD sample had been diagnosed as having mania.

Other psychotic conditions

Although the occurrence of first-rank schizophrenic symptoms is relatively unusual, there are reports of individuals who show isolated psychotic symptoms, including delusional thoughts. Tantam (1991) suggests that the delusional content is often linked with autistic-type preoccupations. For example, one young man described by Lorna Wing (1981) could not be deterred from his conviction that some day Batman was going to come and take him away as his assistant. Ghaziuddin and colleagues (1992) describe another who was unduly concerned about the ozone layer and believed the air in Michigan was not pure enough to breathe. One patient of the author's was threatening to take revenge on the US President and the UK Prime Minister because he believed the American and British air control authorities had conspired to prevent him from qualifying as an airline pilot. Another young man had, since childhood, had "voices" to whom he could talk when he was particularly angry or upset. He believed firmly that the voices were real but they did not provoke any distress or make him do things that he did not wish to do. Instead they appeared to offer him a means of working through difficult situations, and if he became particularly agitated his parents would send him off to "talk to his voices."

A number of other authors have described cases of delusional disorder, various unspecified psychoses (occasionally associated with epilepsy), paranoid ideation, catatonia, and hallucinations (Clarke *et al.*, 1989; Ghaziuddin *et al.*, 1992; Tantam, 1991, 2000; Rumsey *et al.*, 1985; Szatmari *et al.*, 1989b; Wing & Shah, 2000). Obsessive–compulsive disorders have also been reported although it can often prove very difficult to distinguish between these and the ritualistic and stereotyped behaviors that are characteristic of autism. Thus, in their study of more able individuals, Szatmari *et al.* (1989b) caution: "We found it very difficult . . . to distinguish between obsessive ideation and the bizarre preoccupations so commonly seen in autistic individuals."

Case studies of psychiatric disorder among individuals with autistic spectrum disorders

Because data on mental health problems in autism are based on clinical case reports or small group studies there are no systematic studies of incidence and estimates of the frequency of comorbid psychiatric disorders vary from 4% to 58% (Lainhart, 1999). A systematic search for case reports of psychiatric disorder in individuals with autism resulted in 35 different studies involving 200 patients aged 16 years and older. Eighty-six cases were diagnosed with autism or PDD; 114 were described as having Asperger's syndrome or were within the

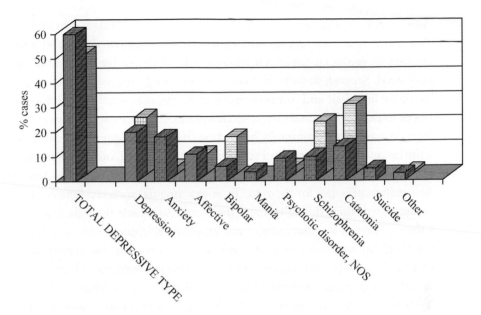

Figure 9.2 Psychiatric diagnoses reported in individuals with autism and those with Asperger syndrome or high functioning autism. ■ HF A/Asp ($n = 114$), ▨ Aut/PDD ($n = 86$).

high-functioning range of the autistic spectrum. As is apparent from Figure 9.2, by far the most frequent psychiatric diagnoses given (in 55% of cases) related to depression or anxiety disorders (including major and minor depression, mood disorders or bipolar affective disorder, depression + anxiety, severe social withdrawal, and attempted suicide). Mania alone occurred much less frequently, in only 2% of the total. The relatively high number of cases of catatonia reported largely reflects the special interest in this disorder of Lorna Wing and her colleagues. This also illustrates how case reports cannot be used to determine the prevalence of psychiatric illness since the researchers' particular areas of expertise or interest will lead to systematic bias in the types of cases seen. However, the figure does provide a *rough* guide to the relative frequency of different disorders, and data from this and other reviews consistently suggest that schizophrenia is relatively infrequent. The development of symptoms related to depressive and anxiety disorders, on the other hand, appears to be a significant risk for people with autism as they grow older.

Are higher-functioning individuals at greater risk of psychiatric disturbance?

It is often suggested that the risk of psychiatric disturbance, especially related to depression and anxiety, is particularly high among more able individuals with autism or those with Asperger's syndrome. There are several reasons for this view. First, because of these individuals' relatively good cognitive ability and *apparently* competent use of language, they frequently fail to receive the level of support they need. Second, despite their superficially good expressive skills, many have extensive linguistic and comprehension difficulties (especially involving abstract or complex concepts) and their understanding of the more subtle aspects of social interaction is often profoundly limited. Such deficits frequently prove an almost insurmountable barrier to full social integration. Third, others' expectations of their social and academic potentials are often unrealistically high and there may be constant pressure for them to "fit in" to "normal society." Finally, their own awareness of their difficulties and the extent to which they are isolated from others can result in great sadness and very low self-esteem. All these factors can place enormous pressures on the individuals concerned, and sometimes result in intolerable levels of anxiety and stress. Nevertheless, there is little evidence of differential rates of mental health problems among subgroups within the autistic spectrum. On the whole, the findings from the case studies summarized in Figure 9.2 did not indicate a higher-incidence of such problems in higher-functioning compared to less-able individuals; and, although the former group were somewhat more likely to be diagnosed as having mania or anxiety disorders, this may be because it is much more difficult to diagnose these conditions in individuals who have little ability to describe their moods and feelings effectively (Sturmey, 1998). In their cases the problems may simply be labeled as unspecified "mood disorders." However, many of the clinical case studies reviewed did not distinguish clearly between high-functioning and low-functioning individuals, or between those with autism or Asperger's syndrome. Even if separate categories were used, diagnostic criteria were rarely specified, and very few reports provided information on the IQ levels of the individuals concerned. Szatmari *et al.* (1989b), in one of the few well-controlled studies in this area, failed to find any marked differences in rates of psychiatric disturbance between adults with a diagnosis of Asperger's syndrome and those with high-functioning autism although the autism group tended to show more bizarre preoccupations.

In summary, crucial data on the prevalence and nature of mental health problems across the autistic spectrum are still lacking and there is a particular need for epidemiological studies in this area. None of the studies reported above are based on representative samples, and the resulting estimates of the prevalence of psychiatric disturbance must be treated with caution. The difficulties inherent in making a valid diagnosis of psychosis in people with autism are also considerable. Impoverished language (Howlin, 1996), literal interpretation of questions (Wing, 1981), concrete thinking (Dykens *et al.*, 1991), and obsessionality

(Volkmar & Cohen, 1991) can all give rise to misunderstandings, leading to possible misdiagnosis, even in the cases of relatively able individuals. For those with little or no speech, the risks of an incorrect diagnosis (or failure to diagnose when problems do exist) are even higher.

Other disorders

Tourette's syndrome is another disorder that has been linked with autism (Baron-Cohen et al., 1999a,b; Ringman & Jankovic, 2000). However, there can be great difficulty in reliably distinguishing the involuntary movements associated with tic disorders with the stereotyped motor movements that characterize autism; comorbidity findings vary markedly. In the follow-up study of Howlin et al. (2004), for example, no one was diagnosed as having a tic disorder, whereas 23% of the individuals followed up by Billstedt et al. (2004) were reported to suffer from motor tics, and one woman had a severe case of Tourette's syndrome.

Epilepsy

As noted in the earliest descriptions of autism (Kanner, 1971; Lotter, 1966; Rutter, 1970) epilepsy is a further complicating factor and occurs in around 25–30% of cases (Lord & Bailey, 2002). The risk of developing fits appears to be higher among those who are profoundly retarded, but there does not seem to be a marked difference between groups of normal IQ and those with mild–moderate retardation. Eleven (16%) of the adults with an IQ of 50 or above assessed by Howlin et al. (2004) had had at least one fit. In four of these cases IQ was between 50 and 69; in seven IQ was in the normal range. Occasionally the onset of epilepsy is associated with marked behavioral changes and regression in adolescence (see below) although this is by no means always the case.

Suicide and other causes of death

Recent research suggests that death rates may be higher in individuals with ASDs than in the population as a whole. Isager and colleagues (1999) followed 207 cases with autism or autism-like conditions over a 24-year period and found that seven individuals had died, giving a crude mortality rate of 3.4%, approximately double the expected rate. Mortality was highest in those with severe–profound learning disabilities, or those of higher intelligence. In the former group ($n = 4$), all of whom were in residential institutions, two deaths were attributed to choking while unsupervised, one to pneumonia and one to meningitis. In the more able group ($n = 3$), who lived either independently or with parents, one death followed an epileptic attack and two were due to drug overdoses (one deliberate, the other *probably* accidental). The largest single study of mortality rates (Shavelle *et al.*, 2001), based on over 13 000 individuals with autism registered on the California Department of Developmental Services database, concluded that, "on average . . . mortality was more than double that of the general population." In individuals with mild mental retardation or those of normal IQ, deaths from seizures, nervous system dysfunction, drowning, and suffocation were three times more common than in nondisabled controls. Among individuals with more severe mental retardation there was a threefold increase in deaths from all causes (other than cancer). Occasional deaths, due to a range of different causes, have been reported, too, in long-term follow-up studies (Lotter, 1978). Causes of death include car accidents (Kanner, 1973; Larsen & Mouridsen, 1997), encephalopathy, self-injury, nephritic syndrome and asthma (Kobayashi *et al.*, 1992), unrecognized volvulus (in a woman in a long-term psychiatric institution; Larsen & Mouridsen, 1997), status epilepticus (Howlin *et al.*, 2004), and cases of drowning, pneumonia, and complications arising from long-term psychotropic medication (Ballaban-Gil *et al.*, 1996).

Suicide as a cause of death has also been noted in a number of follow-up studies. Among the "schizoid" individuals (several of whom appeared to meet criteria for Asperger's syndrome) studied by Wolff and McGuire (1995), 10 out of 17 women and 17 out of 32 men had attempted suicide. Tantam (1991) described the case of one man who threw himself into the river Thames because the Government refused to abolish British Summer Time and he believed that watches were damaged by the necessity of being altered twice a year. In Wing's group of 18 individuals with Asperger's syndrome, 3 had attempted suicide although, fortunately, their attempts had not been successful. One young man, who had become very distressed by minor changes in his work routine, tried to drown himself but failed because he was a good swimmer. When he tried to strangle himself the attempt also failed because, as he said, "I am not a very practical person."

Nordin and Gillberg (1998) have suggested that higher death rates of individuals with ASDs may be due to the association of autism with severe mental retardation and epilepsy. However, the examples cited above indicate that many other causes are also operating. Although the number of deaths related to the inadequate medical and physical care of individuals living in institutions is a particular cause of concern, it is evident that better understanding of the difficulties that lead some young people to attempt suicide could also avoid unnecessary loss of life.

Is there a link between autism and criminality?

Although there is little evidence of any significant association between autism and criminal offending, occasional and sometimes lurid publicity has led to suggestions that there may be an excess of violent crimes among more able people with autism, particularly those diagnosed as having Asperger's syndrome. Certainly tragic events do sometimes occur. In 2001, for example, a London newspaper reported the case of a 7-year-old boy with Asperger's syndrome who had killed his 6-month-old brother, stabbing him 17 times and cutting off his left hand. He had then gone to the police to inform them of what he had done. The first his mother (who had been at home all the while) knew was when the police arrived at the house.

A number of reports of criminal offending has also appeared in the academic literature from time to time. In her original account of 34 people with Asperger's syndrome, Lorna Wing describes the case of one individual who had injured another boy, apparently because of his obsession with chemical experiments (Wing, 1981). Mawson and colleagues (1985) report on a 44-year-old man with Asperger's syndrome who was committed to Broadmoor Special Hospital after attacking a baby. This followed a series of other attacks, including stabbing, on young women or children, which had begun in his teens. The attacks seemed to be related to his obsession with getting a girlfriend, his dislike of certain styles of dress, and his dislike of the noise of crying. He also had a fascination with poisons. Simon Baron-Cohen (1988) describes the strange case of a 21-year-old man who had, over a period of several years, violently assaulted his 71-year-old "girlfriend." Chesterman and Rutter (1994) describe a young man with Asperger's syndrome who had been charged with a number of sexual offenses. However, these seemed to relate mainly to his obsession with washing machines and women's nightdresses. The case was complicated by the fact that he struck the interviewing police officer when it was suggested that he might also have been contemplating burglary; as far as he was concerned "he was merely intending to make use of the occupant's washing machine."

Everall and Le Couteur (1990) describe a case of fire-setting in an adolescent boy with Asperger's syndrome, and Tantam (1991) notes five cases of fire-setting, four of which occurred when other people were in the building. Tantam also cites another case in which someone had killed his schoolmate "probably as an experiment." Nevertheless, he also adds that violence, in a fight, in an explosion of rage, or in sexual excitement is rare. Among the men with Asperger's syndrome he studied, sexual offending, too, was unusual, although some got into trouble for indecent exposure. Property offenses were also rare except as the "side-effects of the pursuit of a special interest."

There is a number of other, largely anecdotal reports of offending by people with autism or Asperger's syndrome. Inappropriate social responses, especially to strangers, may result in police involvement, and crimes may also be linked to obsessional interests. Because of this, offending may well be of an unusual or even bizarre nature, such as attempting to drive away an unattended railway engine because of an obsession with trains, or causing explosions and fires because of an obsessional interest in chemical reactions (Wing, 1986).

Estimates of offending by people with autism or Asperger's syndrome

On the basis of their single-case report, Mawson and colleagues suggest that many people who come to the attention of secure units because of violent offenses may have Asperger's syndrome. In fact, evidence in support of such a statement is extremely limited. Scragg and Shah (1994) assessed the entire male population of Broadmoor Special Hospital, using case notes to identify possible autistic cases. They identified three cases with autism (using personal interviews and the Handicap, Behavior, and Skills schedule of Wing and Gould, 1978) and six with Asperger's syndrome. From a total of 392 patients this represented a prevalence rate of just over 2%, clearly a much higher figure than the rates for autism or Asperger's syndrome in the general population. The offenses committed included violence or threats of violence (five cases), unlawful killing (three cases, including one of matricide), and fire-setting (one case). Solitariness or lack of empathy was noted in each case. Six of the cases had a fascination for topics such as poisons, weapons, murder books, or combat. Because the prevalence of Asperger's syndrome in this special hospital setting was higher than predicted. Scragg and Shah also conclude that there is an association between Asperger's syndrome and violence. Nevertheless, as Ghaziuddin and his colleagues point out, the number of reports of violence or offenses by people with autism or Asperger's syndrome is actually very small. In their review of offending by people with Asperger's syndrome (Ghaziuddin et al., 1992) only 3 out of a total of 132 cases had a clear history of violent behavior (these are the cases described by Wing, 1981; Baron-Cohen, 1988, and Mawson et al., 1985 as noted above). The low incidence of violence found by Ghaziuddin is compared with a rate of 7% of violent crimes (rape, robbery, and assault) in the 20 to 44-year age group in the USA (US Bureau of Justice Statistics, 1987).

As Scragg and Shah (1994) suggest, there may well be more people with autism in prisons or secure accommodation than is realized, and it is clearly important that such individuals are correctly identified and treated. However, estimates of the prevalence of violence in this group can only be made on the basis of community studies. Until then, speculation on the alleged links between violence and autism or Asperger's syndrome is only likely to increase the stigma and distress of people with ASD and their families. Currently there is no reason to suppose that people with autism are more prone to committing offenses than anyone else; indeed, because of the very rigid way in which many tend to keep to rules and regulations, they may well be more law-abiding than the general population.

Causes of offending

Although it has been suggested that lack of empathy may be a significant factor in violent attacks by people with autism or Asperger's syndrome, other significant variables include their lack of social understanding, the pursuit of obsessional interests, and a failure to recognize the implications of their behavior, either for themselves or others. Rigid adherence to rules may also give rise to problems. Occasionally, too, crimes may be unwittingly, or unwillingly, committed at the instigation of others. Very often, of course, a combination of these factors is involved, but only rarely does there appear to be deliberate intention to hurt or harm others

How far can early interventions affect outcome in adult life?

Parents of young children with autism are faced by bewildering and often conflicting claims about the merits of different interventions. Among the treatments said to have a dramatic impact on outcome are Holding Therapy (Welch, 1988), scotopic sensitivity training (Irlen, 1995), sensory integration (Ayres, 1979), auditory integration (Stehli, 1992), drug and vitamin treatments (Rimland, 1994a,b), music therapy (Alvin & Warwick, 1991), facilitated communication (Biklen, 1990), and intensive behavioral programs (Lovaas, 1987; McEachin et al., 1993).

Unfortunately, on the whole, the more extravagant the promises the more limited are the data on which they are based. Moreover, even when there is evidence of short-term gains, reliable information on the impact on adult outcome is generally non-existent. So far there is no evidence of any cures for autism, any more than there is for other chromosomal or genetically determined conditions, such as fragile X or Down's syndromes. The fact that many individuals now attend mainstream schools, find jobs, get married, or have children of their own does not mean that they are cured, nor that the treatment advocated has been responsible for their progress. Many individuals of high IQ do well despite totally inadequate provision, and to a great extent eventual outcome is dependent on innate cognitive, linguistic, and social abilities. Nevertheless, although there is little evidence to suggest that *long-term outcome* can be dramatically improved following the implementation of any particular therapy (Howlin, 2004), this does not mean that appropriate intervention and education in the earliest years have no positive effects. Appropriate intervention in childhood can make all the difference in helping to minimize or avoid secondary behavioral problems, and can have a significant impact on ensuring that children develop their innate abilities to the fullest extent possible. However, autism is a lifelong condition and there are many more adults with autism in this world than there are children. Current attempts to improve access to high-quality preschool programs should not be at the expense of interventions for older children, adolescents, and adults.

Conclusion

Follow-up studies of adults with ASD suggest that although intrinsic factors such as high IQ and good language abilities are important for outcome, these alone are not enough to ensure a positive outcome. External factors, including appropriate junior and secondary school provision, improved transitional programs for entry into college and supported employment schemes are also crucial. A recent study by Alcock and Howlin (2004), for example, has shown how employment success rates can be significantly improved and maintained in the long-term by means of specialist employment services; the success of such programs has also been reported by Keel *et al.*, (1997) and Smith *et al.* (1995). Much greater financial, practical, and social support is also required in order to extend the current very limited facilities for individuals requiring independent or semi-independent residential provision.

It is clear that many individuals with ASD, although continuing to be affected by their condition, autism, can find work, live independently, and maintain close relationships with others. However, such achievements do not come easily. While some individuals have access to specialist support schemes, in many cases jobs are often found only with the support of families; and opportunities to live independently depend heavily on local provision, and often, too, on parental determination and persistence. A common fear among so many adults, even those who on the surface seem to be very high functioning, is "What am I going to do when my parents are no longer around?" Many parents, too, express deep distress at not knowing what will happen to their sons or daughters when they die or become too ill to offer practical help. Although there can be no doubt that the future for most people with ASD now appears far less bleak than was once assumed, ultimately the extent to which they can succeed will be heavily dependent on the support systems to which they have access. Improving access to such provision is the major challenge for the decade to come.

REFERENCES

Abramson, R., Wright, H. H., Cuccara, M. L. *et al.* (1992). Biological liability in families with autism. *Journal of the American Academy of Child and Adolescent Psychiatry*, **31**, 370–1.

Alvin, J. and Warwick, A. (1991) *Music Therapy for the Autistic Child*, 2nd edn. New York: Oxford University Press.

Asperger, H. (1944). Autistic psychopathy in childhood. Translated and annotated by U. Frith, ed., in *Autism and Asperger Syndrome* (1991). Cambridge: Cambridge University Press, pp. 37–92.

Ayres, J. A. (1979). *Sensory Integration and the Child*. Los Angeles: Western Psychology Service.

Ballaban-Gil, K., Rapin, I., Tuchman, R., and Shinnar, S. (1996). Longitudinal examination of the behavioral, language, and social changes in a population of adolescents and young adults with autistic disorder. *Pediatric Neurology*, **15**, 217–23.

Baron-Cohen, S. (1988). Assessment of violence in a young man with Asperger's syndrome. *Journal of Child Psychology and Psychiatry*, **29**, 351–60.

Baron-Cohen, S., Mortimore, C., Moriarty, J., Izaguirre, J., and Robertson, M. (1999a). The prevalence of Gilles de la Tourette's syndrome in children and adolescents with autism. *Journal of Child Psychology and Psychiatry*, **40**, 213–18.

Baron-Cohen, S., Scahill, V. L., Izaguirre, J., and Robertson, M. M. (1999b). The prevalence of Gilles de la Tourette syndrome in children and adolescents with autism: a large scale study. *Psychological Medicine*, **29**, 1151–9.

Bartak, L. and Rutter, M. (1973). Special educational treatment of autistic children: a comparative study. I. Design of study and characteristics of units. *Journal of Child Psychology and Psychiatry*, **14**, 161–79.

Beadle-Brown, J., Murphy, G., Wing, L., Shah, A., and Holmes, N. (2000). Changes in skills for people with intellectual disability: a follow-up of the Camberwell Cohort. *Journal of Intellectual Disability Research*, **44**, 12–24.

Biklen, D. (1990). Communication unbound: autism and praxis. *Harvard Educational Review*, **60**, 291–315.

Billstedt, A., Gillberg, C., and Gillberg, C. I. (2005). Autism after adolescence: population-based 13 to 22-year follow-up study of 120 individuals with autism diagnosed in childhood. *Journal of Autism and Developmental Disorders*, **35**, 351–60.

Bolton, P., Pickles, A., Murphy, M., and Rutter, M. (1998). Autism, affective and other psychiatric disorders: patterns of familial aggregation. *Psychological Medicine*, **28**, 385–95.

Chesterman, P. and Rutter, S. C. (1994). A case report: Asperger's syndrome and sexual offending. *Journal of Forensic Psychiatry*, **4**, 555–62.

Chung, S. Y., Luk, F. L., and Lee, E. W. H. (1990). A follow-up study of infantile autism in Hong Kong. *Journal of Autism and Developmental Disorders*, **20**, 221–32.

Clarke, D. J., Littlejohns, C. S., Corbett, J. A., and Joseph, S. (1989). Pervasive developmental disorders and psychoses in adult life. *British Journal of Psychiatry*, **155**, 692–9.

Clements, J. and Zarkowska, E. (2000). *Behavioural Concerns and Autistic Spectrum Disorders*. London: Jessica Kingsley Publishers.

Creak, M. (1963). Childhood psychosis: a review of 100 cases. *British Journal of Psychiatry*, **109**, 84–9.

DeMyer, M. K., Barton, S., DeMyer, W. E. *et al.* (1973). Prognosis in autism: a follow-up study. *Journal of Autism and Childhood Schizophrenia*, **3**, 199–246.

Dykens, E., Volkmar, F., and Glick, M. (1991). Thought disorder in high-functioning autistic adults. *Journal of Autism and Developmental Disorders*, **21**, 303–14.

Eisenberg, L. (1956). The autistic child in adolescence. *American Journal of Psychiatry*, **112**, 607–12.

Everall, I. P. and Le Couteur, A. (1990). Fire-setting in an adolescent boy with Asperger's syndrome. *British Journal of Psychiatry*, **157**, 284–7.

Frith, U. (1991). *Autism and Asperger Syndrome*. Cambridge: Cambridge University Press.

Gerland, G. (1997). *A Real Person: Life on the Outside*. London: Souvenir Press.

Ghaziuddin, M., Tsai, L. Y., and Ghaziuddin, N. (1992). Co-morbidity of autistic disorder in children and adolescents. *European Journal of Child and Adolescent Psychiatry*, **1**, 209–13.

Ghaziuddin, M., Weidmer-Mikhail, E., and Ghaziuddin, N. (1998). Comorbidity in Asperger syndrome: a preliminary report. *Journal of Intellectual Disability Research*, **42**, 279–83.

Gilchrist, A., Green, J., Cox, A., Rutter, M., and Le Couteur A. (2001). Development and current functioning in adolescents with Asperger syndrome: a comparative study. *Journal of Child Psychology and Psychiatry*, **42**, 227–40.

Gillberg, C. and Steffenberg, S. (1987). Outcome and prognostic factors in infantile autism and similar conditions: a population-based study of 46 cases followed through puberty. *Journal of Autism and Developmental Disorders*, **17**, 272–88.

Grandin, T. (1995). The learning style of people with autism: an autobiography. In K. A. Quill, ed., *Teaching Children with Autism: Strategies to Enhance Communication and Socialization*. New York: Delmar, pp. 33–52.

Hermelin, B. (2001). *Bright Splinters of the Mind. A Personal Story of Research with Autistic Savants*. London: Jessica Kingsley Publishers.

Holliday Willey, L. (1999). *Pretending to be Normal*. London: Jessica Kingsley Publishers.

Holliday Willey, L. (2001). *Asperger Syndrome in the Family*. London: Jessica Kingsley Publishers.

Howlin, P. (1996). Asperger Syndrome: differential diagnosis and current treatment strategies. *Directions in Psychiatry*, **16**(20), 1–12.

Howlin, P. (2003). Outcome in high-functioning adults with autism with and without early language delays: implications for the differentiation between autism and Asperger syndrome. *Journal of Autism and Developmental Disorders*, **33**, 3–13.

Howlin, P., Alcock, J., and Burkin, C. (2005). As eight year follow-up of a supported employment service for high ability adults with autism or Asperger Syndrome. *Autism*, **9**, 533–49.

Howlin, P., Goode, S., Hutton, J., and Rutter, M. (2004). Adult outcomes for children with autism. *Journal A Child Psychology and Psychiatry*, **45**, 212–29.

Hutton, J. (1998). *Cognitive Decline and New Problems Arising in Association with Autism*. Doctor of Clinical Psychology Thesis, Institute of Psychiatry, University of London.

Irlen, H. (1995). Viewing the world through rose-tinted glasses. *Communication*, **29**, 8–9.

Isager, T., Mouridsen, S. E., and Rich, B. (1999). Mortality and causes of death in pervasive developmental disorders. *Autism: International Journal of Research and Practice*, **3**, 7–16.

Kanner, L. (1971). Follow-up study of eleven autistic children originally reported in 1943. *Journal of Autism and Childhood Schizophrenia*, **1**, 119–45.

Kanner, L. (1973). *Childhood Psychosis: Initial Studies and New Insights*. New York: Winston/Wiley.

Kanner, L. and Eisenberg, L. (1956). Early infantile autism 1943–55. *American Journal of Orthopsychiatry*, **26**, 556–66.

Keel, J. H., Mesibov, G., and Woods, A. V. (1997). TEACCH-supported employment programme. *Journal of Autism and Developmental Disorders*, **27**, 3–10.

Kim, J. A., Szatmari, P., Bryson, S., Streiner, D. L., and Wilson, F. (2000). The prevalence of anxiety and mood problems among children with autism and Asperger syndrome. *Autism: International Journal of Research and Practice*, **4**, 117–32.

Klin, A., Volkmar, F. R., and Sparrow, S. S., eds. (2000). *Asperger Syndrome*. New York: Guildford Press.

Kobayashi, R., Murata, T., and Yashinaga, K. (1992). A follow-up study of 201 children with autism in Kyushu and Yamaguchi, Japan. *Journal of Autism and Developmental Disorders*, **22**, 395–411.

Kugler, B. (1998). The differentiation between autism and Asperger syndrome. *Autism: International Journal of Research and Practice*, **2**, 11–32.

Lainhart, J. E. (1999). Psychiatric problems in individuals with autism, their parents and siblings. *International Review of Psychiatry*, **11**, 278–98.

Lainhart, J. E. and Folstein, S. E. (1994). Affective disorders in people with autism: a review of published cases. *Journal of Autism and Developmental Disorders*, **24**, 587–601.

Larsen, F. W. and Mouridsen, S. E. (1997). The outcome in children with childhood autism and Asperger syndrome originally diagnosed as psychotic. A 30-year follow-up study of subjects hospitalized as children. *European Child and Adolescent Psychiatry*, **6**, 181–90.

Lawson, W. (1998). *Life Behind Glass: A Personal Account of Autistic Spectrum Disorder.* Lismore, Australia: Southern Cross University Press.

Lawson, W. (2002). *Understanding and Working with the Spectrum of Autism: An Insider's View.* London: Jessica Kingsley Publishers.

Leekam, S., Libby, S., Wing, L., Gould, J., and Gillberg, C. (2000). Comparison of ICD-10 and Gillberg's criteria for Asperger syndrome. *Autism: International Journal of Research and Practice*, **4**, 11–28.

Lockyer, L. and Rutter, M. (1969). A five to fifteen year follow-up study of infantile psychosis. III. Psychological aspects. *British Journal of Psychiatry*, **115**, 865–82.

Lockyer, L. and Rutter, M. (1970). A five to fifteen year follow-up study of infantile psychosis. IV. Patterns of cognitive ability. *British Journal of Social and Clinical Psychology*, **9**, 152–63.

Lord, C. and Bailey, A. (2002). Autism spectrum disorders. In M. Rutter and E. Taylor, eds., *Child and Adolescent Psychiatry*, 4th edn. Oxford: Blackwell, pp. 636–63.

Lord, C. and Schopler, E. (1985). Differences in sex ratios in autism as a function of measured intelligence. *Journal of Autism and Development Disorders*, **15**, 185–93.

Lord, C. and Venter, A. (1992). Outcome and follow-up studies of high functioning autistic individuals. In E. Schopler and G. B. Mesibov eds., *High Functioning Individuals with Autism*. New York: Plenum Press, pp. 187–200.

Lotter, B. (1974a). Factors related to outcome in autistic children. *Journal of Autism and Childhood Schizophrenia*, **4**, 263–77.

Lotter, B. (1974b). Social adjustment and placement of autistic children in Middlesex: a follow-up study. *Journal of Autism and Childhood Schizophrenia*, **4**, 11–32.

Lotter, B. (1978). Follow-up studies. In M. Rutter and E. Schopler, eds., *Autism: A Reappraisal of Concepts and Treatment.* New York: Plenum Press, pp. 475–96.

Lotter, V. (1966) Epidemiology of autistic conditions in young children. 1. Prevalence. *Social Psychiatry*, **1**, 124–37.

Lovaas, O. I. (1987). Behavioral treatment and normal educational and intellectual functioning in young autistic children. *Journal of Consulting and Clinical Psychology*, **55**, 3–9.

Manjiviona, J. and Prior, M. (1999). Neuropsychological profiles of children with Asperger syndrome and autism. *Autism: International Journal of Research and Practice*, **3**, 327–54.

Mawhood, L. M. and Howlin, P. (1999). The outcome of a supported employment scheme for high functioning adults with autism or Asperger syndrome. *Autism: International Journal of Research and Practice*, **3**, 229–53.

Mawhood, L., Howlin, P., and Rutter, M. (2000). Autism and developmental receptive language disorder: a follow-up comparison in early adult life. I. Cognitive and language outcomes *Journal of Child Psychology and Psychiatry*, **41**, 547–59.

Mawson, D., Grounds, A., and Tantam, D. (1985). Violence in Asperger's syndrome: a case study. *British Journal of Psychiatry*, **147**, 566–9.

McEachin, J. J., Smith, T., and Lovaas, O. I. (1993) Long-term outcome for children with autism who received early intensive behavioral treatment. *American Journal of Mental Retardation*, **97**, 359–72.

Mittler, P., Gillies, S., and Jukes, E. (1966). Prognosis in psychotic children: report of a follow-up study. *Journal of Mental Deficiency Research*, **10**, 73–83.

Newson, E., Dawson, M., and Everard, T. (1982). The natural history of able autistic people: their management and functioning in a social context. Unpublished report to the Department of Health and Social Security, London. Summary published in four parts in *Communication*, **19–21** (1984–85).

Nordin, V. and Gillberg, C. (1998). The long-term course of autistic disorders: update on follow-up studies. *Acta Psychiatrica Scandinavica*, **97**, 99–108.

Ozonoff, S., South, M., and Miller, J. N. (2002). DSM-IV defined Asperger syndrome: cognitive, behavioural and early history differentiation from high-functioning autism. *Autism Journal of Research and Practice*, **4**, 29–46.

Paradiž, V. (2002). *Elijah's Cup: A Family's Journey into the Community and Culture of High-Functioning Autism and Asperger's Syndrome.* New York: The Free Press.

Petty, L. K., Omitz, E. M., Michelman, J. D., and Zimmerman, E. G. (1984). Autistic children who become schizophrenic. *Archives of General Psychiatry*, **41**, 129–35.

Piven, J., Arndt, S., Bailey, J., and Andreasen, N. (1996). Regional brain enlargement in autism: a magnetic resonance imaging study. *Journal of the American Academy of Child and Adolescent Psychiatry*, **35**, 530–6.

Pyles, L. (2002). *Hitchhiking Through Asperger Syndrome.* London: Jessica Kingsley Publishers.

Rimland, B. (1994a). Comparative effects of treatment on child's behavior (drugs, therapies, schooling, and several non-treatment events). *Autism Research Review International*, publication 34b.

Rimland, B. (1994b). Information pack on drug treatments for autism. *Autism Research Review International*, Information Pack P6.

Ringman, J. M. and Jankovic, J. (2000). Occurrence of tics in Asperger's syndrome and autistic disorder. *Journal of Child Neurology*, **15**, 394–400.

Rumsey, J. M., Rapoport, J. L., and Sceery, W. R. (1985). Autistic children as adults: psychiatric social and behavioural outcomes. *Journal of the American Academy of Child Psychiatry*, **24**, 465–73.

Rutter, M. (1970). Autistic children: infancy to adulthood. *Seminars in Psychiatry*, **2**, 435–50.

Rutter, M. (1972). Childhood schizophrenia reconsidered. *Journal of Autism and Childhood Schizophrenia*, **2**, 315–37.

Rutter, M. and Bartak, L. (1973). Special educational treatment of autistic children: a comparative study. II. Follow-up findings and implications for services. *Journal of Child Psychology and Psychiatry*, **14**, 241–70.

Rutter, M. and Lockyer, L. (1967). A five to fifteen year follow-up study of infantile psychosis. I. Description of sample. *British Journal of Psychiatry*, **113**, 1169–82.

Rutter, M., Greenfield, D., and Lockyer, L. (1967). A five to fifteen year follow-up study of infantile psychosis. II. Social and behavioural outcome. *British Journal of Psychiatry*, **113**, 1183–99.

Sacks, O. (1993). A neurologist's notebook: an anthropologist on Mars. *New Yorker*, December 27, 106–25.

Sainsbury, C. (2000). *Martian in the Playground: Understanding the School Child with Asperger's Syndrome*. Bristol: Lucky Duck Publishing.

Schopler, E., Mesibov, G. B., and Kunce, L. J. (1998). *Asperger Syndrome or High Functioning Autism?* New York: Plenum.

Scragg, P. and Shah, A. (1994). Prevalence of Asperger's syndrome in a secure hospital. *British Journal of Psychiatry*, **161**, 679–82.

Seltzer, M. M., Krauss, M. W., Shattuck, P. T. *et al.* (2003). The symptoms of autism spectrum disorders in adolescence and adulthood. *Journal of Autism and Developmental Disorder*, **33**, 565–81.

Shavelle, R. M., Strauss, D. J., and Pickett, J. (2001). Causes of death in autism. *Journal of Autism and Developmental Disorder*, **31**, 569–76.

Slater-Walker, G. and Slater-Walker, C. (2002). *An Asperger Marriage*. London: Jessica Kingsley Publishers.

Smalley, S., McCracken, J., and Tanguay, P. (1995). Autism, affective disorders, and social phobia. *American Journal of Medical Genetics (Neuropsychiatric Genetics)*, **60**, 19–26.

Smith, M. D., Belcher, R. G., and Juhrs, P. D. (1995). *A Guide to Successful Employment for Individuals with Autism*. Baltimore: Paul H. Brookes.

Stehli, A. (1992). *The Sound of a Miracle: A Child's Triumph over Autism*. New York, USA: Doubleday.

Sturmey, P. (1998). Classification and diagnosis of psychiatric disorders in persons with developmental disabilities. *Journal of Developmental and Physical Disabilities*, **10**, 317–30.

Sverd, J., Montero, G., and Gurevich, N. (1993). Brief report: case for an association between Tourette's syndrome, autistic disorder and schizophrenia-like disorder. *Journal of Autism and Developmental Disorders*, **23**, 407–14.

Szatmari, P. (2000). Perspectives on the classification of Asperger syndrome. In A. Klin, F. R. Volkmar, and S. S. Sparrow, eds., *Asperger Syndrome*. New York: Guilford Press, pp. 403–17.

Szatmari, P., Bartolucci, G., Bremner, R. S., Bond, S., and Rich, S. (1989a). A follow-up study of high-functioning autistic children. *Journal of Autism and Developmental Disorders*, **19**, 213–26.

Szatmari, P., Bartolucci, G., and Bremner, R. S. (1989b). Asperger's syndrome and autism: A comparison of early history and outcome. *Developmental Medicine and Child Neurology*, **31**, 709–20.

Szatmari, P., Archer, L., Fisman, S., Streiner, D. L., and Wilson, F. (1995). Asperger's syndrome and autism: Differences in behaviour, cognition, and adaptive functioning. *Journal of the American Academy of Child and Adolescent Psychiatry*, **34**, 1662–71.

Tantam, D. (1991). Asperger's syndrome in adulthood. In U. Frith, ed., *Autism and Asperger Syndrome*. Cambridge: Cambridge University Press, pp. 147–83.

Tantam, D. (2000). Psychological disorder in adolescents and adults with Asperger Syndrome. *Autism*, **4**, 47–62.

US Bureau of Justice Statistics (1987). *Adolescents* (Fall 1989). Princeton, NJ: The Robert Wood Johnson Foundation.

Venter, A., Lord, C., and Schopler, E. (1992). A follow-up study of high-functioning autistic children. *Journal of Child Psychology and Psychiatry*, **33**, 489–507.

Volkmar, F. R. and Cohen, D. J. (1991). Comorbid association of autism and schizophrenia. *American Journal of Psychiatry*, **148**, 1705–7.

Von Knorring, A.-L. and Hägglöf, B. (1993). Autism in northern Sweden: a population-based follow-up study: psychopathology. *European Child and Adolescent Psychiatry*, **2**, 91–7.

Welch, M. (1988). *Holding Time*. London: Century Hutchinson.

Williams, D. (1992). *Nobody Nowhere*. London: Corgi Books.

Williams, D. (1994). *Somebody Somewhere*. London: Corgi Books.

Wing, L. (1981). Asperger's syndrome: a clinical account. *Psychological Medicine*, **11**, 115–29.

Wing, L. and Gould, J. (1978). Systematic recording of behaviors and skills of retarded and psychotic children. *Journal of Autism and Childhood Schizophrenia*, **8**, 79–97.

Wing, L. and Shah, A. (2000). Catatonia in autistic spectrum disorders. *British Journal of Psychiatry*, **176**, 357–62.

Wolff, S. (1991). Schizoid personality in childhood and adult life. 1. The vagaries of diagnostic labelling. *British Journal of Psychiatry*, **159**, 615–20.

Wolff, S. and Chick, J. (1980). Schizoid personality in childhood: a controlled follow-up study. *Psychological Medicine*, **10**, 85–100.

Wolff, S. and McGuire, R. J. (1995). Schizoid personality in girls: a follow-up study. What are the links with Asperger's syndrome? *Journal of Child Psychology and Psychiatry*, **36**, 793–818.

Wozniak, J., Biederman, J., Faraone, S. V. *et al.* (1997). Mania in children with pervasive developmental disorder revisited. *Journal of the American Academy of Child and Adolescent Psychiatry*, **36**, 1552–9.

10

Autism, social neuroscience, and endophenotypes

Lynn Waterhouse
The College of New Jersey

Deborah Fein
The College of New Jersey

Emily G. W. Nichols
Georgetown University School of Medicine

Introduction

There are two current impediments for genetic and neuroscience research in autism. First, there is no standard comprehensive model of the brain circuits and neurochemistry regulating human social behaviors (Beer & Ochsner, 2006). Second, there is as yet no mapping of gene to brain function to phenotypic expression for component skills of human social behavior (Insel & Fernald, 2004; Panksepp, 2006). Although a complete neural framework for the range of human social skills does not yet exist, research in social neuroscience has led researchers and theorists to construct models of the brain bases of social skills (Adolphs, 2002; Allman et al., 2002; Brothers, 2002; Davidson & Irwin, 2002; Erikson & Shulkin, 2003; Harmon-Jones, 2003; LaBar & Cabeza, 2006; Matthews et al., 2002; Meltzoff & Prinz, 2002; Panksepp, 2006; Porges, 2003; Posamentier & Abdi, 2003; Raichle, 2003; Rapcsak, 2003; Reich et al., 2003; Rolls, 1999; Royzman et al., 2003; Singer et al., 2004). Moreover, although there is no gene–brain–phenotype map for social behaviors, social neuroscience research models do suggest possible links between brain circuits and endophenotype component skills for complex social behavior.

This chapter constructs a component model of the brain bases of social skill from current social neuroscience findings. Three questions are addressed:

(1) To what extent are human social behaviors innately determined?

Autism and Pervasive Developmental Disorders, 2nd edn, ed. Fred R. Volkmar.
Published by Cambridge University Press. © Cambridge University Press 2007.

(2)   What brain circuits and component skills for complex social behavior have been proposed?

(3)   What do these proposed brain circuits and component skills for complex social behavior tell us about the components of the diagnostic phenotype of autism?

In addressing these questions we argue for two claims. First, we claim that social neuroscience research suggests a component model of six neurally distinct evolved domains of human social behaviors:

(1)   mammalian social bonding governed by steroid–peptide interactions in the HPA axis;

(2)   imitative social motor learning regulated in part by prefrontal cortex mirror neurons;

(3)   experience, expression, and comprehension of emotions arising in a complex circuitry including left and right hemisphere, amygdala, ventral striatum, anterior cingulate cortex, and insular cortex;

(4)   face recognition and identification of, and attention to, facial expressions of emotion and social gaze dependent upon fusiform face areas, right occipital face area, amygdala, and a posterior-to-anterior ventral circuit;

(5)   ongoing assessment of the behavior and knowledge of others based in complex circuits including regions of prefrontal cortex and the amygdala;

(6)   syntactic language skill governed by left and right temporal and frontal lobe cortex and basal ganglia circuits.

Second, we claim that the first five of these six neurally distinct groups of human social behaviors should be identified as subskills within the social diagnostic behaviors for autism in order to provide more meaningful and testable endophenotypes of autistic impairment. At present the standard diagnostic criteria for autism (APA, 1994; WHO, 1993) include autistic individuals with widely varying unrelated brain and social skill impairments. This inclusiveness is commonly justified by defining autism as a behavioral diagnosis, but it has become a critical problem for genetic and brain research in autism (Bauman & Kemper, 2005; Coon, 2006; Jamain *et al.*, 2003; Klauck, 2006; Nicolson & Szatmari, 2003; Shao *et al.*, 2003; Volkmar & Pauls, 2003; Yonan *et al.*, 2003).

The social neuroscience studies reviewed in this chapter suggest that bonding, imitation, emotional expression, face and gaze attention and recognition, and ascertaining the dispositional state of others are based in distinct brain circuits, and research in autism suggests that these specific social skills contribute to the diagnostic behaviors of autism (e.g. lack of friends, lack of social reciprocity, lack of imaginative play). Thus impairment in these social subskills may be genetically significant endophenotypes of the autism phenotype. We therefore propose that the social diagnostic criteria in autism should be revised to include the specific additional identification of impairment in bonding, imitation, emotional expression, face and gaze recognition, and ascertaining dispositional state.

It has been argued that finding genes that make an individual susceptible to autism will depend on establishing a broader phenotype of autism generally (Volkmar & Pauls, 2003) or on creating dimensional measures that span a broader phenotype of autism (Dawson *et al.*, 2002). Dawson and colleagues (2002) reviewed autism and developmental research and identified six domains to define a broader phenotype of autism: face processing; sensitivity to social reward; imitation of body actions; memory; executive function; and phonology. We agree with Volkmar and Pauls (2003), and with Dawson *et al.* (2002), that the autism phenotype requires serious revision. However, we propose that the behavioral syndrome of autism may represent an aggregate of many subdisorders, most of which arise from genetically significant distinct endophenotypes. We agree with Dawson *et al.* (2002) that clearly specified domains should be recognized in the revision of the autism phenotype, and our review uncovered two of the same domains to be specified: face recognition and imitation. Our focus in this chapter, however, has been to identify "units" of human sociability for which distinct brain circuits have already been identified in social neuroscience research. We believe that forming research-based social endophenotypes within the autism diagnostic criteria will better serve genetic and brain research.

QUESTION 1: TO WHAT EXTENT ARE HUMAN SOCIAL BEHAVIORS INNATELY DETERMINED?

Humans are social animals. Until the spread of agriculture 8000 years ago we lived in small social groups of 30 to 50 hunter–gatherers. Small groups of humans still hunt and gather in South America, Africa, Indonesia, the Philippines, and the South Pacific, but the majority of us live in or near towns and cities that range from a few hundred to 25 million people. We seek social contact and group cohesion (Richerson & Boyd, 2004), and the size of the human neocortex has increased in parallel with increasing social group size (Dunbar, 2002, 2003).

With the exception of the orang-utan, all large primates are social. De Waal (1996) has argued that all social primates share 14 prosocial behaviors: (1) mother–child and male–female attachment and pair-bonding; (2) succorance or active care for another individual; (3) emotional contagion; (4) social mimicry; (5) long-term bonds of friendship; (6) reciprocity in support and aggression; (7) peace-making; (8) conflict avoidance; (9) adjustment of behavior toward, and special care of disabled individuals and helpless infants; (10) active maintenance of social bonds; (11) play and teasing; (12) monitoring of the social interactions of others; (13) social teaching; and (14) the accommodation of differing needs through active negotiation.

Both humans and nonhuman social primates use these interaction behaviors to establish and maintain elaborate social group relationships of dominance hierarchies, subgroup cliques, and shifting alliances (de Waal & Tyack, 2003). Nonhuman primates conduct social interaction by means of a set of innate communicative displays that combine vocalization, gesture, facial expression, and body postures (Corballis, 2003; Crockford & Boesch, 2003; Slocombe & Zuberbühler, 2005). Research suggests that these displays are governed both by thalamic circuits and by temporal and frontal cortex regions (Corballis, 2003; Sherwood et al., 2003).

Humans, of course, also use facial expressions, gestures, and body postures to communicate, but only a small basic subset of our expressive facial displays – joy, fear, disgust, rage, surprise, and sadness – appear to be identical across all cultures (Ekman, 2003). Moreover, our communicative displays depend most heavily on formal language, which allows for an infinitely varying array of statements that express and explain multitudes of emotional states, plans, ideas, and which can be used to create an infinite variety of commands, complaints, requests, and questions as well as other forms of utterance in order to weave complex conversations and group social interactions.

Reasoning from the evidence of complex social behaviors in nonhuman primates, theorists have proposed that human social skills must have evolved before the emergence of formal language (Brinck & Gardenfors, 2003; Corballis, 2003). As is true for apes and chimpanzees, early human prelanguage social behaviors would have offered the adaptive advantages of enhanced social care for infants and children, enhanced group cohesion for protection from threat, and a hierarchy of social food-sharing that would have allowed for more individuals in the group to survive.

Adaptive human skills have been argued to have emerged from a variety of mechanisms including generative complexity (Kauffman, 1993), spandrelism (Gould & Lewontin, 1979), phylogenetic construction of brain circuits, tissue regions and neurochemistry, phylogenetic inflection, ontogenetic construction, and ontogenetic inflection (Heyes, 2003).

Kauffman (1993) proposed that organisms and their constitutive internal systems (e.g. the brain and the immune system) will self-generate greater and greater systemic complexity through the biophysical replicating forces of the genome. He called his model "generative complexity plus Darwinian selection" (1993). In Kauffman's view individuals and their internal systems are kept from mutating into chaotic disorganized complexity precisely by means of environmental selection pressures. Darwin proposed that natural selection caused changes within a species and created new species by selecting for the reproductive success of beneficent variants. While Kauffman has supported the modern synthesis – that all variation and speciation are a spontaneous and continuous function of DNA itself – Kauffman has proposed that even beneficent and benign variations are normally overproduced by the genome and it is only through selection that an organism maintains a stable structure and set of traits: "selection must hold (an organism and its internal) networks in this poised ensemble (so that adaptive) features may be expected to shine through across the aeons and across phyla" (1993, p. 535).

Gould and Lewontin (1979) proposed the term "spandrel" to identify an adaptation that is the unintended byproduct of selection for another trait. A spandrel is an architectural term describing the space left between the outer curve of an arch and the rectangular frame around the arch. The arch is intended, the rectangular framework is intended, but the two triangular spaces between the left and right sides of the arch and frame, the spandrels, are unintended byproducts. Gould and Lewontin (1979) suggested that much of human social behavior could be the result of a "spandrel" of the increase in human brain size. Calvin (1994) argued that our brains increased in size because we needed more brain tissue to support memory of where we found raw materials for tools, and memory of the sequence of actions required to make and effectively use tools (Calvin, 1994).

Conversely, Ingold (1994) and Dunbar (2002) have argued that brain adaptations for social behavior are not the result of a "spandrel byproduct" of the brain's increase in size for tool-making, but rather that human brain size increased in direct response to the need to manage increasingly complex social interactions among humans. Dunbar (2002) has found a positive association between primate group size and the size of the brain's neocortex, and has proposed that primate group size is limited by the individuals' abilities to manipulate information about social relationships (2002, p. 77). For Dunbar, increased neocortical tissue evolved in primates because increased working memory and increased associative memory was necessary to support the social interaction and social cognition skills required to maintain complex social systems.

Heyes (2003) has outlined a differentiated framework of four mechanisms of human cognitive evolution that is applicable to human social behaviors and social cognition. In Heyes' model both gene-based natural selection and developmental selection in individual ontogeny operate on three controls for behavior:

(1)   the formation of brain circuits, regions, and chemistry;
(2)   how a circuit solves a cognitive problem;
(3)   what information is the focus of mental computation.

Heyes defines phylogenetic construction as natural selection operating on the brain to adaptively alter its tissue, circuits, and chemistry. In Dunbar's claim that the neocortex increased in size in order to better manage social relationships, the neocortical increase is an example of phylogenetic construction. Heyes defines phylogenetic inflection as the way in which natural selection biases the brain's automatic attention to the environment for computation. In de Waal's 14 primate social behaviors, the automatic monitoring of the behavior of others would be a specific phylogenetic inflection of brain attention capacities.

Ontogenetic construction, in Heyes' model, is a process of developmental selection through experiences that alter the way in which a pre-existing brain mechanism operates. The primate social skill of face recognition is an example of ontogenetic construction because although infants do recognize faces (de Haan et al., 2003) humans improve in face discrimination over the course of infancy and toddlerhood (Pellicano & Rhodes, 2003).

Heyes' fourth proposed cognitive evolution mechanism is ontogenetic inflection, which she defines as an adaptation whose source is information from the social copying of behaviors "selected" over the course of an individual's development. Heyes has proposed that social copying is distinct from any imitative learning fostered by the presence of mirror neurons in the frontal lobe (Rizzolatti & Craighero, 2004). Heyes has argued that when one individual watches and copies the motor behaviors of another individual, this copying is not governed by mirror neurons but by the reconfiguration of motor representations in the observer's brain by means of general brain circuits for motor learning. Many of the 14 universal primate social behaviors, such as play, negotiation, and social teaching, depend on social copying.

All six evolutionary mechanisms outlined above – generative complexity, spandrelism, phylogenetic construction, phylogenetic inflection, ontogenetic construction, and ontogenetic inflection – go beyond Darwinian selection to explain how complex traits such as human social behaviors and social cognition may have evolved to be innately determined. Ascertaining the relative validity of these mechanisms remains speculative. For example, Dunbar's reported association between primate neocortex size and primate social group size (2002) may be (1) the result of generative complexity of the genes for the central nervous system constrained by the environmental selection of birth canal size; or (2) the result of spandrel brain growth for tool use where increased tool use was necessary to support greater group size; or (3) the result of phylogenetic construction of increased brain size to manage the adaptive complexity of human social behavior.

Despite their differing mechanisms all models argue that many simple and complex component human social behaviors are the product of evolution, and that these behaviors depend on innate brain structures and functions. As social primates some of our most adaptive behaviors are those that enable us to interact with others. The recent emergence of the field of social neuroscience has led to research working to identify specific brain regions and circuits associated with human sociability and social cognition.

QUESTION 2: WHAT HAS SOCIAL NEUROSCIENCE RESEARCH DISCOVERED ABOUT HUMAN SOCIAL BEHAVIOR AND COGNITION?

A review of current social neuroscience research suggests that human social skills are likely to depend on six distinct groups of evolved brain adaptations.

One: hormones in brain–body circuits have been found to regulate mammalian social attachment (Carter, 2002; Insel & Fernald, 2004; Porges, 2003).

Two: prefrontal cortex mirror neurons guiding motor imitative learning programs have been found in monkeys and humans (Corballis, 2003; Meltzoff & Prinz, 2002; Rizzolatti & Craighero, 2004; Wohlschlager & Bekkering, 2002).

Three: evidence for neurochemical circuits and brain loci that determine the ability to experience and express one's own emotions, and understand and empathically experience the emotions of others has been found in humans (Adolphs *et al.*, 2003; Davidson & Irwin, 2002; Lang *et al.*, 2002; LeDoux, 2002; Panksepp, 2006; Rolls, 1999; Sander *et al.*, 2003; Singer *et al.*, 2004).

Four: neocortical and subcortical tissues which become specialized to distinguish faces, facial expressions, and social gaze have been found in humans (Adams & Kleck, 2003; Batty & Taylor, 2003, 2006; Deaner & Platt, 2003; Gauthier *et al.*, 2002; Hooker *et al.*, 2003; Kanwisher *et al.*, 2002; Pageler *et al.*, 2003; Pizzagalli *et al.*, 2002; Posamentier & Abdi, 2003; Yovel & Duchaine, 2006).

Five: evidence for brain systems that support forms of complex social cognition in humans has been reported (Allman *et al.*, 2002; Beer & Ochsner, 2006; Kringelbach & Rolls, 2003; Paller *et al.*, 2003; Royzman *et al.*, 2003; Ziv & Frye, 2003).

Six: evidence for many human brain regions involved with syntactic language processing, most notably left hemisphere neocortex and basal ganglia tissues, has been found (Josse & Tzourio-Mazoyer, 2004; Kotz *et al.*, 2003; Lieberman, 2006).

Each of these six groups of proposed brain adaptations for social behavior has a large body of associated research. The present review of each, however, is necessarily brief and selective.

1   Hormones in brain–body circuits that regulate social attachment

Based on studies of the social behaviors of the prairie vole, Carter (2002) has proposed that the hormone peptides oxytocin and vasopressin are crucial to a network in which "steroid–peptide interactions involving hormones of the HPA axis (hypothalamus, pituitary, adrenal cortices) . . . provide neuroendocrine substrates for species-typical social behaviors and emotions" (2002, p. 875). Carter's model identifies this circuit and these hormones as the basis for the pair-bonding between male and female prairie voles, and between mother and offspring. Carter also proposed that this circuit reduces neophobia (fear of the new or different) and increases learning and memory of each other for the individuals in the pair-bond.

Insel and Fernald's work with prairie voles (2004) led them to conclude that vasopressin in the hippocampus increases active and passive avoidance learning, and that vasopressin the lateral septum of the amygdala is crucial to learning to identify the other individual in the pair-bond, and to identify individuals in the social group. Insel and Fernald (2004) also reported that oxytocin activity in females and vasopressin activity in males is crucial for the achievement of the pair-bond and that the activity of both oxytocin and vasopressin in the cingulate is crucial for the production of the voles' distress calls.

Bielsky *et al.* (2004) found that vasopressin a-type receptor knockout mice exhibited normal skill on spatial and nonsocial olfactory learning and memory tasks, but showed a profound impairment in social recognition.

Porges (2003) has proposed a different model of attachment but it too involves vasopressin and oxytocin. Porges has argued that mammals have two vagal pathways as part of their autonomic systems. The older vagal pathway directs consummatory behaviors and lies in the dorsal motor nucleus of the vagus, which contains oxytocin receptors. The newer vagal pathway, in Porges' model, directs our viscerally felt need to be near and interact with others. The newer vagal pathway lies in the nucleus ambiguus of the vagus and contains both oxytocin and vasopressin receptors. Porges (2003) has claimed that in the newer vagal pathway vasopressin triggers actions leading to social interactions, and that the newer vagal pathway's interconnections with the sympathetic nervous system direct mammals to seek one another when stressed or excited.

Kurup and Kurup (2003) have outlined the level of cortical serotonin as another possible neural system supporting bonding in humans. They found a significant association between the degree of family cohesiveness reported by individual family members and the presence of left-hemisphere dominance and increased serotonin levels in the family members. Individuals in extended families with more members having left-hemisphere dominance and higher serotonin levels reported a greater degree of family closeness.

Although human relationships depend on complex interactions governed by conversations, cultural etiquette, institutional policies, and legal rules, it is nonetheless likely that hormone mechanisms for mammalian pair-bonding and group cohesion remain as adaptive forces for human sexual reproduction, care for infants, and social group formation.

2 Prefrontal cortex mirror neurons that guide motor imitative learning

Mirror neurons have been identified in area F5 of the macaque's brain (Rizzolatti & Craighero, 2004). Mirror neurons do not discharge when the macaque sees objects, but do discharge when the macaque observes another monkey using its hand to grasp, tear, manipulate, or place objects. Most importantly mirror neurons discharge to trigger the observer macaque's hand action when it moves its own hand in exactly the way it has seen the other macaque move its hand. Rizzolatti and Craighero (2004) have concluded that mirror neurons link action recognition to action production.

Area F5 in the macaque is the ventral premotor cortex homologous to humans' Brodmann's area 44 and consistent with Broca's area. For this reason, and because Broca's area may be active during human hand movements, Rizzolatti and Craighero (2004) have argued that a gestural communication system based on mirror neurons was the first form of early human language that moved beyond the limits of the fixed communicative displays of our nonhuman primate cousins. As a consequence they have further concluded that formal spoken syntactic language emerged from manual gestural communication based in the mirror neuron system.

Mirror neurons are also argued to be the basis for primate imitative behavior in general (Meltzoff & Prinz, 2002). Wohlschlager and Bekkering (2002) reported evidence for mirror neurons in humans, and Tai *et al.* (2004) reported that human study participants observing another person grasping an object exhibited a significant neural response in the left premotor cortex. Hauk and Pulvermuller (2004) reported that the processing of action words referring to leg, arm, and face movements was associated with distinct neural activity; reading leg-related words activated dorsal frontoparietal areas more strongly, while reading face-words produced more activity at left inferior-frontal sites. Corballis (2003) has reviewed theories of language evolution and reviewed the research on mirror neurons, and has concluded that the evidence for the lateralization of mirror neurons in the human left prefrontal cortex – as opposed to mirror neurons bilaterally in the macaque F5 – suggest that handedness must have been part of the evolution of human language skills.

Mimicry has also been linked to increased sociability (van Baaren *et al.*, 2004). Van Baaren and colleagues reported that individuals whose behaviors were mimicked (by an experimental confederate) significantly increased their social interactions with others.

Whether social mimicry is governed by mirror neurons is not yet known. However, evidence is accruing to support the existence of mirror neurons. Mirror neurons may contribute to the acquisition of social interaction skills through nonconscious mimicry of social displays, may contribute to language acquisition, and motor skills acquisition. Furthermore nonconscious mimicry may contribute to emotional reciprocity in social interactions, as well as increased sociability.

3   Neurochemical circuits and brain loci that determine the ability to experience and express one's own emotions, and understand and empathically experience the emotions of others

Many researchers have offered evidence for the brain basis of emotion processing. We consider here the ideas and findings of Adolphs *et al.* (2003), Davidson and Irwin (2002), Lang *et al.* (2002), LeDoux (2002), Panksepp (2006), Rolls (1999), Sander *et al.* (2003), and Singer *et al.* (2004).

Davidson and Irwin (2002) constructed a comprehensive account of the many sources of human affects. Based on their own work, and the research of others, they have proposed that there are eight distinct affect circuits:

(1)   approach, related to positive affect and moving toward others and objects, is associated with increased left prefrontal cortex metabolism;

(2)   withdrawal, related to fear, disgust, and other negative affects and moving away from others and objects, is associated with increased right prefrontal cortex metabolism;

(3)   anticipating future negative or positive outcomes are affect states that depend on working memory, which, in turn, depend on bilateral ventromedial prefrontal cortex;

(4)   perception, experience, and expression of negative emotions stem from amygdala activity;

(5)   computing the meaning of the emotional expressions of others takes place in the posterior region of the right hemisphere of the cortex;

(6)   experiencing reward states depends on the ventral striatum;

(7)   attention to the emotional states of others depends on anterior cingulate cortex;

(8)   body state visceral feedback to the brain depends on the insular cortex.

Panksepp (2006) has proposed that specific emotions signal a particular adaptive challenge, and that arousal, reward, and fear originate in the brainstem, hypothalamus, hippocampus, amygdala, and basal ganglia in order to regulate our responses to the environment. Panksepp further argued that cognition is a separate brain function from emotion based on the evidence of a difference between the two in subjective experience, a difference in patterns of the cortical–subcortical locus of control, and differences in development, expression states, and in cerebral laterality. Harmon-Jones (2003) reviewed research on the emotion of anger. He reported that although anger has often been associated with approach motivation and with increased left prefrontal cortex metabolism, the asymmetrical frontal cortical activity found for anger is due to motivational direction and not affective valence.

In contrast to Davidson and Irwin (2002), Panksepp (2006), and Harmon-Jones (2003), Lang *et al.* (2002) have argued that it is unlikely that emotions operate in discrete modules. They have suggested that it would not be adaptive to have isolable tactical emotions. They have proposed instead that emotions exist in a "motivation–emotion circumplex" in which positive and negative affect components combine synergistically to create complex motivating states of emotion.

LeDoux (2002) has concluded that many mammalian amygdala-based defense responses are not operants – motor skills learned through a series of repeated actions – but are actually respondents, that is, fixed motor programs reacting to a specific pattern in the environment. Based on his research LeDoux has claimed that hardwired respondents in the amygdala include reactive freezing, fighting, and fleeing, as well as facial grimaces. He has outlined that such respondents are governed by the amygdala and its circuits with the ventral striatum of the forebrain and the brainstem motor system. Sander *et al.* (2003), however, have proposed a broader role for amygdala function in primates. They have argued that research to date has not proven that the amygdala's sole function is the generation of fear. They have claimed that it is likely that the amygdala in primates computes a wide range of interpretations of emotional stimuli, especially socially relevant stimuli.

Rolls (1999) has further argued that both cortical and subcortical activations are necessary for the experience of emotion. His argument is based on the evidence that primates require view-invariant representations of objects and individuals in order to learn to make and use tools, and also require view-invariant representations of objects in order to collect food. From this Rolls has concluded that these cortical representations must be activated by primate emotions because emotions "drive" adaptive behaviors such as food-gathering and tool-making.

Adolphs *et al.* (2003) reported a case of an individual with extensive bilateral brain lesions who could not recognize static representations of emotions but could recognize emotions in dynamic displays. They argued that this individual's brain damage and behavioral deficits suggest that bilateral inferior and anterior temporal lobe and medial frontal cortices are critical for linking perception of static stimuli to recognition of emotions.

Singer and colleagues (2004) reported that fMRI of individuals witnessing their partner experiencing painful hand stimulation showed brain activation of a subset of their own pain reaction pattern. An individual experiencing his or her own pain activated the entire neural pain matrix including the secondary somatosensory cortex, primary somatosensory cortex, thalamus, bilateral anterior insula, rostral anterior cingulate cortex, brainstem, and cerebellum. Witnessing their partner experiencing the same hand pain activated only the bilateral anterior insula, rostral anterior cingulate cortex, brainstem, and cerebellum. The researchers argued that anterior insula and rostral anterior cingulate cortex comprise the core of an autonomic-affective system that provides our experience of pain and our experience of empathy for the feelings of others (2004, p. 1160).

In sum, social neuroscience research is generating increasing evidence for a variety of innate brain circuits that reflect the evolution of our ability to experience and distinguish and be motivated by our own emotions, and to comprehend and empathize with the emotions of others.

4   Neocortical and subcortical tissues that become specialized to distinguish faces, facial expressions, and social gaze

Face recognition and face expression interpretation

There are two ongoing debates in the studies of face recognition and facial expression. The first debate is whether or not "face-recognition" brain regions are solely dedicated to face recognition or serve to recognize and discriminate other complex visual images as well (Yovel & Duchaine, 2006). The second debate is whether recognition of people's emotional expressions is dependent on face-recognition brain regions or operates separately.

Posamentier and Abdi (2003) reviewed research exploring brain regions for face form identification and facial expression recognition. They concluded that data from neuroimaging studies suggest an overlap of brain activation regions for face form recognition and facial expression recognition. Kanwisher *et al.* (2002) reported that only one brain area is uniquely active in response to human faces: the fusiform gyrus. They further noted greater activity in the right fusiform gyrus than the left.

Contrary to Kanwisher and colleagues, Gauthier *et al.* (2002) reported finding that people who have special expertise in object recognition (birdwatchers and car model experts) activate the fusiform face areas and the right occipital face area both when they identify human faces and also when they identify bird species or specific car models. Gauthier and colleagues have concluded that all humans become face-identification experts because we have seen so many human faces over the course of development. They have also concluded that because the extensiveness of expertise possessed by bird and car experts is significantly correlated with the amount of activation recorded in their right fusiform face-recognition areas that the "face" recognition areas of all of us are better understood as tissue dedicated to increasingly complex figural analysis, which is not unique to human faces.

In an earlier related study, Swithenby *et al.* (1998) also found early automatic stimulus-bound stages of configural feature extraction of facial expressions of emotion. Batty and Taylor (2003, 2006), too, reported data that support the notion that recognition of facial expression of emotions is a rapid, automatic process. Batty and Taylor's localization analyzes indicated that both positive and negative face expression of emotions are registered by the N170 ERP from the superior and middle-temporal regions for early processing of facial expressions. However, in later processing at 300–400 ms differentiable patterns for processing positive and negative face expression of emotions appeared in frontal lobe activation.

Face expression and face-feature processing both appear to be organized along a back-to-front ventral stream of activation running from the occipital cortex to the temporal cortex. This stream may also be altered by the reactions of the individual doing the processing. Pizzagalli *et al.* (2002) found that study participants with positive attitudes showed a different pattern of activation along this ventral stream to both liked and disliked faces than did participants with negative attitudes.

Recognition of social gaze

Adams and Kleck (2003) reported that study participants combined information about gaze direction with information about facial expression in the processing of emotionally relevant facial information. Deaner and Platt (2003) have demonstrated that both rhesus macaques and humans automatically orient their visual attention in the same direction as they observe a rhesus macaque to be looking. Hooker *et al.* (2003) found increases in neural activity in the amygdala when individuals were actively monitoring human gaze cues for emotional events, but found increased activity in the superior temporal sulcus when individuals were attempting to discern social spatial information. However, Hooker and colleagues' distinction is in conflict with Batty and Taylor's (2003, 2006) findings of increased activity in superior temporal regions for early processing of facial expressions of emotion.

Supporting Batty and Taylor (2003, 2006), Pageler *et al.* (2003) reported finding that the fusiform gyrus and the superior temporal sulcus both showed increased activity to gaze processing. They reported that the fusiform gyrus responded with the greatest activation to face and gaze forward (directly at the observer), and that both the fusiform gyrus and superior temporal sulcus showed increased activity when subjects looked at a direct face compared to an angled face, regardless of gaze direction. Calder *et al.* (2002) found that theory of mind (ToM) tasks and eye-gaze processing engage a similar region of the posterior–superior temporal sulcus as well as a similar region of medial prefrontal cortex. These studies, and other such studies, suggest that social gaze attention circuits do exist and are likely to be integrated in processing with recognition of faces and facial expression of emotion, and with the interpretation of the possible mental state of another as well.

5   Possible brain systems that support forms of complex social cognition

Willingham and Dunn (2003) proposed that social cognition skills are second-order processes that depend on necessary first-order processes such as memory and attention. They also argued that few brain constructs are uniquely dedicated to social cognition or social behavior, basing their claim on evidence that both early prefrontal brain damage and bilateral amygdala damage yield a wide range of impaired social behaviors and impaired social cognition skills. Supporting Willingham and Dunn's claims, Pessoa and Ungerleider (2004) reported finding that all regions of the brain that are normally activated to faces with emotional content (fusiform face areas, right occipital face area, and the amygdala) are activated only when the individual has sufficient attentional resources to do so, suggesting that the social cognition of understanding facial expressions may be a second-order mental process relying on the first-order process of attention.

Opposed to Willingham and Dunn's thesis (2003) and Pessoa and Ungerleider's (2004) data, Sander *et al.* (2003) have argued that the wide range of types of social impairment that result from amygdala damage is evidence that the amygdala has adapted its function in primates to be a general processing device for all socially relevant stimuli. In their view, amygdala processing would be primary not secondary and will be activated by a wide range of primate (human) social situations. At present, however, there are insufficient data to determine the relationship between complex social cognition skills and attention.

A review of current research in the neuroscience of social cognition suggests that there are an increasing number of claims for distinct social cognitive skills (Beer & Ochsner, 2006). Research exploring five theorized social cognitive skills will be briefly reviewed here:

(1)   epistemic egocentrism and ToM (Royzman *et al.*, 2003);
(2)   rapid cue reversal learning for interaction (Allman *et al.*, 2002; Kringelbach & Rolls, 2003);
(3)   detection of the dispositional state of another (Adolphs, 2002; Brothers, 2002);

(4)   social evaluation (Cunningham *et al.*, 2003);

(5)   global emotional intelligence (Goleman, 1995, Matthews *et al.*, 2002).

Epistemic egocentrism and theory of mind

Royzman *et al.* (2003) reviewed research on ToM, and research on perspective-taking skills in children and adults. They proposed a functional interconnection between three concepts:

(1)   theory of mind, defined as having an idea that other people have different mental contents from one's own (Ziv & Frye, 2003);

(2)   the illusion of transparency, defined as overestimating what other people know about our own unexpressed mental states and knowledge (Savitsky & Gilovich, 2003);

(3)   the failure to preserve privileged knowledge about the mental states of others, defined as being unable to inhibit one's own state of knowledge from interfering with privileged knowledge of another person's mental contents (Nickerson, 1999).

Royzman *et al.* (2003) argued that ToM, the illusion of transparency, and the failure to separate one's own knowledge from privileged information about the mental knowledge of another are three versions of the same social cognitive human limitation, which they have defined as "epistemic egocentrism." For Royzman *et al.*, epistemic egocentrism is our difficulty in maintaining all privileged information separately. In tasks that test for theory of mind, very young children cannot maintain the privileged information they are given about a doll's lack of knowledge of a hiding place, and studies of the illusion of transparency have indicated that adults often fail to recognize that their own mental contents are privileged information that others do not have (Savitsky & Gilovich, 2003).

Royzman and colleagues concluded from their research review that the ability to maintain mental content information as "privileged" (whether it is our own mental contents that are privileged to us but not others, or it is the mental contents of others "privileged" to us because we know their mental contents) improves over the course of our lifetime of social interactions, and that even most competent adults still have trouble setting aside privileged information. Royzman *et al.* have argued that what improves over our lifetime of interactions is the ability to inhibit the salience of any privileged information, and they have argued that this particular form of inhibitory control improves with the development of prefrontal cortex.

Supporting Royzman *et al.* (2003), Sabbagh and Taylor (2002) reported event-related potential data that they suggested indicates that brain processing of information about mental contents is not an automatic process. However, in contrast to Royzman and colleagues, Sabbagh and Taylor have argued that effortful processing of the mental contents of others is unlikely to be simply the result of a failure to inhibit privileged information.

Rapid cue reversal learning

Another skill thought to be crucial to social cognition is rapid cue reversal learning. Kringelbach and Rolls (2003) and Allman *et al.* (2002) have argued that rapid cue reversal learning is necessary for successfully following the often-changing emotional cues provided by human facial and vocal expressions in conversation. Both research teams have identified a brain circuit involving the prefrontal cortex and the anterior cingulate as the basis for rapid cue reversal learning. In addition, Allman *et al.* (2002) proposed that our body's reactions to the behavior of others are fed into our ability to learn changing cues by means of spindle cell neurons that convey body (visceral) reaction states information via insular tissue to the cingulate–prefrontal circuit. Allman and colleagues argued that social insight and comprehension depend on visceral reaction-informed cue reversal learning, which improves over our lifetime as we expand our repertoire of interaction experiences.

Detection of dispositional intent

Brothers (2002) argued that comprehending the dispositional intent of another person is likely to reside in a brain social cognition module in which distinct groups of neurons code for four specific pieces of information about another person. These are first, the person's identity, second, the direction of the person's movement, particularly their ongoing hand movements, third, the person's body posture, and fourth, the person's facial expression. Brothers (2002) proposed that additional information outside the module is required to determine another person's dispositional intent: the context of the other persons present must be assessed and knowledge of the relationships of those other people must also be computed.

Adolphs (2002) has also proposed a mixture of innate modules and more global processing as a basis for the comprehension of the dispositional intent and behavior or other people. Adolphs argued that "it is likely that domain-specific processing draws upon innately specified modules, as well as upon self-organized maps that emerge as a consequence of experiences with the world" (2002, p. 316).

Social evaluation

In an fMRI study, Cunningham *et al.* (2003) found that good versus bad evaluations of other people were associated with greater medial and ventrolateral prefrontal cortex activity than in past versus present judgments (of the person's existence). They argued that both automatic processing in medial and ventrolateral prefrontal tissue and controlled processing in associative cortex are involved in the social evaluation of other people.

Emotional intelligence

Goleman (1995) proposed that all social cognition depends on a global skills he labeled "emotional intelligence." Goleman defined emotional intelligence as a unitary skill that computes self and other recognition and self and other regulation. Matthews *et al.* (2002) reviewed research on emotional intelligence and reported that research studies have failed to confirm "self and other recognition" and "self and other regulation" as subgroups of skills. Matthews *et al.* also reported that there is no research evidence to support the belief that emotional intelligence exists as a unitary ability. They concluded that Goleman's emotional intelligence cannot be tested empirically because it is "too open-ended and loosely specified to constitute good scientific theory" (2002, p. 15). Matthews and colleagues research review also led them to conclude that the concept "emotional intelligence" has been applied too widely both by Goleman (1995) and other researchers to include distinct social skills ranging from the ability to experience different emotions, to the ability to evaluate the dispositions of others, to the ability to alter one's own expressions appropriately during the course of a conversation.

While there is no evidence to support the notion of emotional intelligence as a unitary mental process, research does suggest that social cognition requires a wide range of effortful mental processes. Processing information about the mental contents of others and ourselves is a tricky mental task, prone to error and subject to improvement over time in all of us. Similarly, rapid cue reversal learning, deemed a requisite for successfully conducting a conversation, improves with practice. Certainly both social evaluation and ascertaining the dispositional intent of another person, which depends on keeping track of the direction of their movement, their body posture, and their facial expression, remain daily problems to solve even for typical adults living in urban areas, and working within large institutions.

6   Cortical and subcortical tissues that understand and produce syntactic language

Josse and Tzourio-Mazoyer (2004) reviewed research on hemispheric specialization for language and concluded that although there is a great deal of interindividual variability, left temporal and frontal lobe specialization for language is a very consistent finding, and that size of the left but not the right planum temporale is significantly associated with skill in language comprehension. Salustri and Kronberg (2004) conducted an independent component analysis of brain sources of activity during language tasks in unimpaired adults. They found three critical active brain regions associated with language skill – right-frontal, left-parietal, and left-frontal areas – and each showed well-defined dipolar field distributions.

Research has also suggested other brain specializations for language. Kotz *et al.* (2003) reported that patients with left temporoparietal lesions in an imaging language-processing study had a P600 wave but no N400 wave, while, conversely, patients with lesions of the basal ganglia had no P600 wave but did have an odd form of an N400 wave. Similar to prior findings by other research teams, the researchers concluded that the basal ganglia modulate the P600 brain wave which signals syntax processing, and the left temporal and parietal lobes – along with the basal ganglia – modulate the N400, which signals semantic integration processing in sentence comprehension. In a related model, Ullman (2001) argued that word knowledge and grammar knowledge depend on two brain memory systems. For Ullman, word memory depends on declarative memory (fact and event knowledge), which may be specialized for computing and learning arbitrary relations, and is based in temporal lobe structures. In Ullman's model, processing grammar requires procedural memory, which resides in basal ganglia structures linked to frontal structures.

Finally, as outlined in the section above on mimicry and mirror neurons, there may be a role for human frontal mirror neurons in language skill (Lieberman, 2006). Rizzolatti and Craighero (2004) have argued that frontal lobe mirror neurons are likely to provide both sequencing of hand and arm gestures and sequencing of verbal syntax. They also proposed that mirror neurons regulate the learning of gesture and syntactic speech through the process of nonconscious motor imitation.

QUESTION 3: WHAT CAN THESE SIX GROUPS OF BRAIN ADAPTATIONS FOR SOCIAL BEHAVIOR TELL US ABOUT THE DIAGNOSTIC PHENOTYPE OF AUTISM?

Evidence for six groups of proposed brain adaptations for human social behavior was outlined above. These six groups are: (1) steroid–peptide interactions in the HPA axis governing mammalian bonding; (2) prefrontal cortex mirror neurons governing primate and human imitative motor learning; (3) multiple brain circuits and tissue (left and right hemisphere, amygdala, ventral striatum, anterior cingulate cortex, and insular cortex) governing human emotions; (4) fusiform face areas, right occipital face area, amygdala, and a posterior-to-anterior ventral circuit governing human face identification, gaze attention and identification of facial expressions of emotion; (5) regions of prefrontal cortex and the amygdala governing human social cognition of the behavior of other individuals; and (6) left and right temporal and frontal lobe cortex and thalamic circuits governing human language.

Research evidence has indicated that there are autistic individuals who do have brain deficits and dysfunctions in each of these six groups of brain adaptations for sociability and social cognition. Only a few of the most recent of these studies will be mentioned here but relevant current reviews include Brambilla *et al.* (2003) and Ronald *et al.* (2006).

Abnormal levels of plasma oxytocin in autistic individuals were reported by our research group (Modahl *et al.*, 1998). Luna *et al.* (2002) found that autistic subjects demonstrated significantly less task-related activation in dorsolateral prefrontal cortex and posterior cingulate cortex in comparison with healthy subjects during a spatial working memory task. Lower than normal blood oxygen level-dependent signal changes in the fusiform gyrus of autistic individuals during visual processing of faces have been reported (Hubl *et al.* 2003), and Schultz *et al.* (2003) have reported hypoactivation of the fusiform face area in autism which they suggest is a core social cognitive impairment. Howard *et al.* (2000) found that individuals with high-functioning autism who demonstrated impairment in the recognition of facial expressions and perception of eye-gaze direction also had abnormalities of the medial temporal lobe, including bilaterally enlarged amygdala volumes. Bauman and Kemper (2005) systematically analyzed brain tissue in autism and found three regions with consistent abnormalities:

(1)   reduced numbers of Purkinje cells in the cerebellum;
(2)   small, tightly packed neurons in the entorhinal cortex;
(3)   small, tightly packed neurons in the medially placed nuclei of the amygdala.

Herbert *et al.* (2004) found increased white matter enlargement localized to the radiate white matter in all cortical lobes in autism which would alter intrahemispheric and corticocortical connections. In a magnetoencephalographic study of brain activation to speech sounds Tecchio *et al.* (2003) found no evidence for the detection of a change in the physical characteristics of a repetitive sound in autistic subjects, suggesting abnormal function in temporal lobe processing of speech sounds. Turkeltaub *et al.* (2004) reported that autistic hyperlexia was associated with hyperactivation of the left superior temporal cortex. Barnea-Goraly *et al.* (2004) found reduced white matter in the brains of autistic individuals in ventromedial prefrontal cortices, anterior cingulate gyri, temporoparietal junctions, adjacent to the superior temporal sulcus bilaterally, in the temporal lobes approaching the amygdala bilaterally, in occipitotemporal tracts, and in the corpus callosum.

The first five of the six groups of brain adaptations for human social skills reviewed here invite a reconsideration of the social diagnostic criteria for autism. "Impairment in social interaction," including (a) impaired eye gaze, (b) lack of social reciprocity, (c) poor or absent joint attention, and (d) limited or absent peer relationships, is the first subset of criteria for autism. "Qualitative impairments in communication" including (a) no language, (b) impaired language, and (c) lack of appropriate imaginative play is the second subset of diagnostic criteria. ("Restricted patterns of behavior and interest," including (a) abnormal interests, (b) difficulties with change, and (c) stereotyped mannerisms is the third) (APA, 1994; WHO, 1993).

Consider the autism diagnostic criteria "lack of social reciprocity." It is possible that " lack of social reciprocity" in an autistic individual could arise from any of the following:

(1) *impaired bonding* stemming from abnormal oxytocin and / or vasopressin or other abnormality in the HPA axis system function would result in a consequent lack of behavioral drive to interact with others and thus no reciprocal social interest in another person;

(2) *impaired functioning of prefrontal cortex mirror neurons* governing imitative motor learning would result in failed nonconscious mimicry of language, social, and motor behavior of others that would appear as failed social reciprocity;

(3) *impaired experience, expression, and/or understanding of emotions* resulting from impairment in any of the multiple brain circuits and tissue (left and right hemisphere, amygdala, ventral striatum, anterior cingulate cortex, insular cortex) that govern emotional processing could yield absence of social reciprocity;

(4) *impaired ability to recognize or attend to gaze, faces and facial expression of emotions* stemming from impairment of one or more of the regions governing these skills – the fusiform face areas, right occipital face area, amygdala, and a posterior-to-anterior ventral circuit (including superior temporal sulcus) could lead to lack of social reciprocity;

(5) *impaired ability to update changing interaction information* arising from impaired regions of prefrontal cortex or amygdala or any of their reciprocal connections could also give rise to lack of social reciprocity; and, finally,

(6) *absence of language or language impairment* stemming from a dysfunction in neocortical circuits and / or thalamic circuits governing human language could clearly be a basis for lack of social reciprocity.

Similarly, it can be argued that the diagnostic criteria of impaired or absent joint attention, limited or absent peer relationships, and lack of appropriate imaginative play could result from: (1) absent or impaired bonding; and/or (2) impaired imitation; and/or (3) impaired experience and comprehension of emotions; and/or (4) impaired face recognition, gaze attention, or impaired recognition of facial expression of emotions; and/or (5) impaired ability to update changing interaction information; and/or (6) impaired language.

These subskill contributions also point to the problem of the interrelatedness of the existing diagnostic criteria for autism. For example, Dawson *et al.* (2004) studied 72 children with autism spectrum disorder (ASD) reporting that structural equation modeling indicated that *joint attention* was the best predictor of concurrent *language ability*, and that *social orienting* and attention to distress were *indirectly related to language* through their relations with joint attention.

Volkmar and Pauls (2003) argued that twin and family genetic studies suggest that autism is the core syndrome of a broader existing range of milder phenotypes of social and cognitive impairment, and proposed that research in autism must more clearly define discrete behavioral elements of the autism phenotype for use as quantitative traits in genetic association studies. A successful example of this approach is a study by Shao *et al.* (2003). Using principal–component factor analysis they identified a factor representing insistence on sameness (IS) – derived from the Autism Diagnostic Interview-Revised – and found that families sharing high scores on the IS factor increased linkage evidence for the 15q11-q13 region, from a LOD score of 1.45 to a LOD score of 4.71.

However Yonan and colleagues (2003) conducted a genome-wide screen of 345 families, each with at least two siblings with autism. They found 408 markers associated with autism across the entire genome. Like Volkmar and Pauls (2003), Yonan *et al.* (2003, p. 895) concluded that

we must recognize the possibility that even dramatic increases in sample size may fail to detect linkage, or association, if the diagnosis of autism or ASD does not significantly increase the likelihood of carrying any single genetic variant . . . Thus it will be important to identify and characterize autism-related quantitative traits and/or endophenotypes that are more directly correlated with underlying genetic variation.

In a review of genetic research in autism Jamain *et al.* (2003) argued that the multiple markers that have emerged from linkage studies combined with the sharp difference in the concordance rates between monozygotic (identical) and dizygotic (fraternal) twins indicates that autism must be both genetically heterogeneous (different sets of genes cause autism in different families) and polygenic (based on multiple altered genes for each autistic individual).

CONCLUSION: SIX SOCIAL ENDOPHENOTYPES SHOULD BE INCLUDED IN AUTISM DIAGNOSTIC CRITERIA

Nicolson and Szatmari (2003) reviewed genetic research in autism and suggested that autism is likely to be genetically heterogeneous such that "each gene (or set of genes) may be a risk factor for a specific component of the autism phenotype" (2003, p. 529). They concluded that future genetic research may have to "disentangle the autism phenotype" (by) "focusing on the core features of autism" (2003, p. 529). This may not be so easy to do. The six domains of social skills reviewed in this chapter identify the very wide variety of brain dysfunctions and behavioral deficits that could contribute to each of the seven social and communication behavioral impairments diagnostic for autism. Even though a group of autistic individuals may share the same specific diagnostic impairment, nonetheless they may not necessarily share the deficits contributing to that shared diagnostic behavioral impairment. These specific underlying deficits may be endophenotypes of autism. Therefore, conducting a genetic study of autistic individuals who all share one diagnostic impairment such as "failed social reciprocity" will be likely to include multiple subgroups each with a different endophenotype generating the shared diagnostic assessment: "failed social reciprocity." If Nicolson and Szatmari (2003) are correct in their claim that there may be correspondence between a gene and a risk factor for a component of the autism phenotype, even grouping by a single shared diagnostic impairment would be problematic for a genetic study.

Currently when autistic individuals are noted to have impairment in bonding, social imitation, emotional expression and comprehension, face recognition, or inability to follow rapidly changing social cues, these impairments are labeled as nondiagnostic-associated deficits of autism, just as level of cognitive impairment and savant skills are defined as associated deficits of autism, largely because these impairments vary widely across diagnosed individuals (Fombonne, 2003; Lord *et al.*, 2006; Volkmar & Pauls, 2003). Nonetheless, it has been shown that level of cognitive impairment is crucial in defining a subgroup of the autistic spectrum as Asperger's disorder (Volkmar & Pauls, 2003), and our team reported that a follow-up study of 138 autistic children showed that preschool high- and low-cognitive function subgroup membership significantly predicted functioning at school age, whereas school-age functioning was not predicted by preschool autistic symptoms (Stevens *et al.*, 2000). More importantly, a genetic study that isolated autistic siblings with higher scores on a savant skills cluster from the Autism Diagnostic Interview (Nurmi *et al.*, 2003) suggested that there may be a genetic contribution of the 15q locus to autism susceptibility in a subset of affected individuals exhibiting savant skills. The researchers noted that Prader–Willi syndrome, which results from deletions of this chromosomal region, can also yield savant-type skills as well.

Following from this, because the social skills reviewed in this chapter appear to be based in distinct brain circuits, and because impairments in these social skills have been demonstrated in subgroups of autistic individuals, and thus must contribute to the social diagnostic impairments in autism, therefore impairment in these social skills – bonding, imitation, emotional expression, face recognition, changing social cues, ascertaining dispositional state – are likely to be genetically significant endophenotypes of the autism phenotype. Consequently we propose that impairment in these specific social skills should be incorporated into the diagnostic criteria for autism.

Incorporating clearly defined subskill impairments within the current standard social diagnostic criteria of autism will help researchers to select better defined groups of autistic individuals and their family members for genetic and brain dysfunction research. We believe that the addition of these subskill impairment descriptions within the standard diagnostic criteria will permit significant inferences from future studies by reducing the confounding problem of multiple endophenotypes within a study sample.

REFERENCES

Adams, R. B. Jr., and Kleck, R. E. (2003). Perceived gaze direction and the processing of facial displays of emotion. *Psychological Science*, **14**, 644–7.

Adolphs, R. (2002). Social cognition and the human brain. In J. T. Cacioppo, G. G. Berntson, R. Adolphs *et al.*, eds., *Foundations in Social Neuroscience*. Cambridge, MA: MIT Press, pp. 313–32.

Adolphs, R., Tranel, D., and Damasio, A. R. (2003). Dissociable neural systems for recognizing emotions. *Brain Cognition*, **52**, 61–9.

Allman, J., Hakeem, A., and Watson, K. (2002). Two phylogenetic specializations in the human brain. *Neuroscientist*, **8**, 335–46.

American Psychiatric Association (1994). *Diagnostic and Statistical Manual of Mental Disorders*, 4th edn. Washington, DC: APA.

Barnea-Goraly, N., Kwon, H., Menon, V. *et al.* (2004). White matter structure in autism: preliminary evidence from diffusion tensor imaging. *Biological Psychiatry*, **55**, 323–6.

Batty, M. and Taylor, M. J. (2003). Early processing of the six basic facial emotional expressions. *Brain Res Cogn Brain Res.*, **17**, 613–20.

Batty, M. and Taylor, M. J. (2006). The development of emotional face processing during childhood. *Developmental Science*, **9**, 207–20.

Bauman, M. L. and Kemper, T. L. (2005). Neuroanatomic observations of the brain in autism: a review and future directions. *International Journal of Developmental Neuroscience*, **23**, 183–7.

Beer, J. S. and Ochsner, K. N. (2006). Social cognition: a multilevel analysis. *Brain Research*, **1079**, 98–105.

Bielsky, I. F., Hu, S. B., Szegda, K. L., Westphal, H., and Young, L. J. (2004). Profound impairment in social recognition and reduction in anxiety-like behavior in vasopressin v1a receptor knockout mice. *Neuropsychopharmacology*, **3**, 483–93.

Brambilla, P., Hardan, A., di Nemi, S. U. *et al.* (2003). Brain anatomy and development in autism: review of structural MRI studies. *Brain Research Bulletin*, **61**, 557–69.

Brinck, I. and Gardenfors P. (2003). Co-operation and communication in apes and humans. *Mind and Language*, **18**, 484–501.

Brothers, L. (2002). The social brain: a project for integrating primate behavior and neurophysiology in a new domain. In J. T. Cacioppo *et al.*, eds., *Foundations in Social Neuroscience*. Cambridge, MA: MIT Press, pp. 367–86.

Calder, A. J., Lawrence, A. D., Keane, J. *et al.* (2002). Reading the mind from eye gaze. *Neuropsychologia*, **40**, 1129–38.

Calvin, W. H. (1994). The unitary hypothesis: a common neural circuitry for novel manipulations, language, plan-ahead, and throwing. In K. Gibson and T. Ingold, eds., *Tools, Language and Cognition in Human Evolution*. New York: Cambridge University Press, pp. 429–45.

Carter, S. (2002). Neuroscience perspectives on attachment and love. In J. T. Cacioppo *et al.*, eds., *Foundations in Social Neuroscience*. Cambridge, MA: MIT Press, pp. 853–90.

Coon, H. (2006). Current perspectives on the genetic analysis of autism. *American Journal of Medical Genetics. Part C, Seminars in Medical Genetics*, **142**, 24–32.

Corballis, M. C. (2003). From mouth to hand: gesture, speech, and the evolution of right-handedness. *Behavioral and Brain Sciences*, **2**, 199–208.

Crockford, C. and Boesch, C. (2003). Context-specific calls in wild chimpanzees, *Pan troglodytes*, verus analysis of barks. *Animal Behavior*, **66**, 115–25.

Cunningham, W. A., Johnson, M. K., Gatenby, J. C., Gore, J. C., and Banaji, M. R. (2003). Neural components of social evaluation. *Journal of Personal and Social Psychology*, **85**, 639–49.

Davidson, R. J. and Irwin, W. (2002). The functional neuroanatomy of emotion and affective style. In J. T. Cacioppo *et al.*, eds., *Foundations in Social Neuroscience*. Cambridge, MA: MIT Press, pp. 473–90.

Dawson, G., Webb, S., Schellenberg, G. D. *et al.* (2002). Defining the broader phenotype of autism: genetic, brain, and behavioral perspectives. *Developments in Psychopathology*, **14**, 581–611.

Dawson, G., Toth, K., Abbott, R. *et al.* (2004). Early social attention impairments in autism: social orienting, joint attention, and attention to distress. *Developments in Psychology*, **2**, 271–83.

Deaner, R. O. and Platt, M. L. (2003). Reflexive social attention in monkeys and humans. *Current Biology*, **13**, 1609–13.

De Haan, M., Johnson, M., and Halit, H. (2003). Development of face-sensitive event-related potentials during infancy: a review. *International Journal of Psychophysiology*, **51**, 45–58.

De Waal, F. (1996). *Good Natured: The Origins of Right and Wrong in Humans and Other Animals*. Cambridge, MA: Harvard University Press.

De Waal F. and Tyack, P. (2003). *Animal Social Complexity: Intelligence, Culture, and Individualized Societies*. Cambridge, MA: Harvard University Press.

Dunbar, R. (2002). The social brain hypothesis. In J. T. Cacioppo, G. G. Berntsson, R. Adolphs *et al.*, eds., *Foundations in Social Neuroscience*. Cambridge, MA: MIT Press, pp. 69–88.

Dunbar, R. (2003). Evolution of the social brain. *Science*, **302**, 1160–1.

Ekman, P. (2003). *Emotions Revealed: Recognizing Faces and Feelings to Improve Communication and Emotional Life*. New York: Times Books/Henry Holt.

Erikson, K. and Shulkin, J. (2003). Facial expressions of emotion: a cognitive neuroscience perspective. *Brain and Cognition*, **52**, 52–60.

Fombonne, E. (2003). Modern views of autism. *Canadian Journal of Psychiatry*, **48**, 503–6.

Gauthier, I., Skudlarski, P., Gore, J. C., and Anderson, A. W. (2002). Expertise for cars and birds recruits brain areas involved in face perception. In J. T. Cacioppo *et al.*, eds., *Foundations in Social Neuroscience*. Cambridge, MA: MIT Press, pp. 277–92.

Goleman, D. (1995). *Emotional Intelligence*. New York: Bantam Books.

Gould, S. and Lewontin, R. (1979). The spandrels of San Marco and the Panglossian paradigm: a critique of the adaptionist programme. *Proceedings of the Royal Society of London*, **285**, 281–8.

Harmon-Jones, E. (2003). Early career award. Clarifying the emotive functions of asymmetrical frontal cortical activity. *Psychophysiology*, **40**, 838–48.

Hauk, O. and Pulvermuller, F. (2004). Neurophysiological distinction of action words in the fronto-central cortex. *Human Brain Mapping*, **21**, 191–201.

Herbert, M. R., Ziegler, D. A., Makris, N. *et al.* (2004). Localization of white matter volume increase in autism and developmental language disorder. *Annals Neurology*, **55**, 530–40.

Heyes, C. (2003). Four routes of cognitive evolution. *Psychological Review*, **110**, 713–27.

Hooker, C. I., Paller, K. A., Gitelman, D. R. *et al.* (2003). Brain networks for analyzing eye gaze. *Brain Research Cognition Brain Research*, **17**, 406–18.

Howard, M. A., Cowell, P. E., Boucher, J. *et al.* (2000). Convergent neuroanatomical and behavioural evidence of an amygdala hypothesis of autism. *NeuroReport*, **11**, 2931–5.

Hubl, D., Bolte, S., Feineis-Matthews, S. *et al.* (2003). Functional imbalance of visual pathways indicates alternative face processing strategies in autism. *Neurology*, **61**, 1232–7.

Ingold, T. (1994). Tool-use, sociality and intelligence. In K. R. Gibson and T. Ingold, eds., *Tools, Language and Cognition in Human Evolution*. New York: Cambridge University Press, pp. 429–45.

Insel, T. R. and Fernald, R. D. (2004). How the brain processes social information. *Annual Review of Neuroscience*, **27**, 697–722.

Jamain, S., Betancur, C., Giros, B., Leboyer, M., and Bourgeron, T. (2003). Genetics of autism: from genome scans to candidate genes. *Medical Science*, **11**, 1081–190.

Josse, G. and Tzourio-Mazoyer, N. (2004). Hemispheric specialization for language. *Brain Research Brain Research Reviews*, **44**, 1–12.

Kanwisher, N., McDermott, J., and Chun, M. M. (2002). The fusiform face area: a module in human extrastriate cortex specialized for face perception. In J. T. Cacioppo *et al.*, eds., *Foundations in Social Neuroscience*. Cambridge, MA: MIT Press, pp. 259–76.

Kauffman, S. (1993). *The Origins of Order*. New York: Oxford University Press.

Klauck, S. M. (2006). Genetics of autism spectrum disorder. *European Journal of Human Genetics*, **6**, 714–20.

Kotz, S. A., Frisch, S., von Cramon, D. Y., and Friederici, A. D. (2003). Syntactic language processing: ERP lesion data on the role of the basal ganglia. *Journal of the International Neuropsychology Society*, **9**, 1053–60.

Kringelbach, M. L. and Rolls, E. T. (2003). Neural correlates of rapid context-dependent reversal learning in a simple model of human socialinteraction. *NeuroImage*, **20**, 371–83.

Kurup, R. and Kurup, P. (2003). Hypothalamic digoxin, hemispheric dominance, and family bonding behavior. *International Journal of Neuroscience*, **113**, 989–98.

LaBar, K. S. and Cabeza, R. (2006). Cognitive neuroscience of emotional memory. *Nature Reviews. Neuroscience*, **7**, 54–64.

Lang, P. J., Bradley, M. M., and Cuthbert, B. N. (2002). A motivational analysis of emotion and affective style. In J. T. Cacioppo *et al.*, eds., *Foundations in Social Neuroscience*. Cambridge, MA: MIT Press, pp. 462–73.

LeDoux, J. E. (2002). Emotion: clues from the brain. In J. T. Cacioppo *et al.*, eds., *Foundations in Social Neuroscience*. Cambridge, MA: MIT Press, pp. 411–24.

Lieberman, P. (2006). The FOXP2 gene, human cognition and language. *International Congress Series*, **1296**, 115–26.

Lord, C., Risi, S., DiLavore, P. S. *et al.* (2006). Autism from 2 to 9 years of age. *Archives of General Psychiatry*, **63**, 694–701.

Luna, B., Minshew, N. J., Garver, K. E. *et al.* (2002). Neocortical system abnormalities in autism: an fMRI study of spatial working memory. *Neurology*, **59**, 834–40.

Matthews, G., Zeidner, M., and Roberts, R. D. (2002). *Emotional Intelligence: Science and Myth*. Cambridge, MA: MIT Press.

Meltzoff A. N. and Prinz W., eds. (2002). *The Imitative Mind: Development, Evolution and Brain Bases*. Cambridge, UK: Cambridge University Press.

Modahl, C., Green, L., Fein, D. *et al.* (1998). Plasma oxytocin levels in autistic children. *Biological Psychiatry*, **43**, 270–7.

Nickerson, R. S. (1999). How we know – and sometimes misjudge – what others know: imputing one's own knowledge to others. *Psychological Bulletin*, **126**, 747–53.

Nicolson, R. and Szatmari, P. (2003). Genetic and neurodevelopmental influences in autistic disorder. *Canadian Journal of Psychiatry*, **48**, 526.

Nurmi, E. L., Dowd, M., Tadevosyan-Leyfer, O. *et al.* (2003). Exploratory subsetting of autism families based on savant skills improves evidence of genetic linkage to 15q11-q13. *Journal of the American Academy of Child and Adolescent Psychiatry*, **7**, 856–63.

Pageler, N. M., Menon, V., Merin, N. M. *et al.* (2003). Effect of head orientation on gaze processing in fusiform gyrus and superior temporal sulcus. *NeuroImage*, **20**, 318–29.

Paller, K. A., Ranganath, C., Gonsalves B. *et al.* (2003). Neural correlates of person recognition. *Learned Memory*, **10**, 253–60.

Panksepp, J. (2006). Emotional endophenotypes in evolutionary psychiatry. *Progress in Neuropsychopharmacology and Biological Psychiatry*, **30**, 774–84.

Pellicano, E. and Rhodes, G. (2003). Holistic processing of faces in preschool children and adults. *Psychological Science*, **14**, 618–22.

Pessoa, L. and Ungerleider, L. G. (2004). Neuroimaging studies of attention and the processing of emotion-laden stimuli. *Progress in Brain Research*, **144**, 171–82.

Pizzagalli, D., Lehmann, D., Koenig, T., Regard, M., and Pascual-Marqui R. D. (2002). Face-elicited ERPs and affective attitude: brain electric microstate and tomography analyses. In J. T. Cacioppo *et al.*, eds., *Foundations in Social Neuroscience*. Cambridge, MA: MIT Press, pp. 599–614.

Porges, S. W. (2003). The polyvagal theory: phylogenetic contributions to social behavior. *Physiology and Behavior*, **79**, 503–13.

Posamentier, M. and Abdi, H. (2003). Processing faces and facial expressions. *Neuropsychology Reviews*, **13**, 113–43.

Raichle, M. E. (2003). Functional brain imaging and human brain function. *Journal of Neuroscience*, **23**, 3959–62.

Rapcsak, S. (2003). Face memory and its disorders. *Current Neurology and Neuroscience Reports*, **3**, 494–501.

Reich, J. W., Zautra, A., and Davis, M. (2003). Dimensions of affect relationships: models and their integrative implications. *Review of General Psychology*, **7**, 66–83.

Richerson, P. J. and Boyd, R. (2004). *Not by Genes Alone: How Culture Transformed Human Biology*. Chicago: University of Chicago Press.

Rizzolatti, G. and Craighero, L. (2004). The Mirror–neuron system. *Annual Review of Neuroscience*, **27**, 169–82.

Rolls, E. T. (1999). *The Brain and Emotion*. New York: Oxford University Press.

Ronald, A., Happe, F., Bolton, P. *et al.* (2006). Genetic heterogeneity between the three components of the autism spectrum: a twin study. *Journal of the American Academy of Child and Adolescent Psychiatry*, **45**, 691–9.

Royzman, E., Cassidy, K., and Baron, J. (2003). "I know, you know": epistemic egocentrism in children and adults. *Review of General Psychology*, **7**, 38–65.

Sabbagh, M. A. and Taylor, M. (2002). Neural correlates of Theory-of-Mind reasoning: an event-related potential study. In J. T. Cacioppo *et al.*, eds., *Foundations in Social Neuroscience*. Cambridge, MA: MIT Press, pp. 235–44.

Salustri, C. and Kronberg, E. (2004). Language-related brain activity revealed by independent component analysis. *Clinical Neurophysiology*, **115**, 385–95.

Sander, D., Grafman, J., and Zalla, T. (2003). The human amygdala: an evolved system for relevance detection. *Reviews in Neuroscience*, **14**, 303–16.

Savitsky, K. and Gilovich, T. (2003). The illusion of transparency and the alleviation of speech anxiety. *Journal of Experimental Social Psychology*, **39**, 618–25.

Schultz, R. T., Grelotti, D. J., Klin, A. *et al.* (2003). The role of the fusiform face area in social cognition: implications for the pathobiology of autism. *Philosophical Transactions of the Royal Society of London B Biological Science*, **358**, 415–27.

Shao, Y., Cuccaro, M. L., Hauser, E. R. *et al.* (2003). Fine mapping of autistic disorder to chromosome 15q11-q13 by use of phenotypic subtypes. *American Journal of Human Genetics*, **72**, 539–48.

Sherwood, C., Broadfield, D., Holloway, R., Gannon, P., and Hof, P. R. (2003). Variability of Broca's area homologue in African great apes: implications for language evolution. *Anatomy Record*, **27**, 276–85.

Singer, T., Seymour, B., O'Dougherty, J. *et al.* (2004). Empathy for pain involves the affective but no sensory components of pain. *Science*, **303**, 1157–62.

Slocombe, S. and Zuberbühler, K. (2005). Functionally referential communication in a chimpanzee. *Current Biology*, **15**, 1779–84.

Stevens, M. C., Fein, D. A., Dunn, M. *et al.* (2000). Subgroups of children with autism by cluster analysis: a longitudinal examination. *Journal of the American Academy of Child and Adolescent Psychiatry*, **39**(3), 346–52.

Swithenby, S. J., Bailey, A. J., Braeutigam, S., Josephs, O. E., Jousmäki, V., and Tesche, C. D. (1998). Neural processing of human faces: a magnetoencephalographic study. *Experimental Brain Research*, **18**, 501–10.

Tai, Y. F., Scherfler, C., Brooks, D. J., Sawamoto, N., and Castiello, U. (2004). The human premotor cortex is 'mirror' only for biological actions. *Current Biology*, **14**, 117–20.

Tecchio, F., Benassi, F., Zappasodi, F. *et al.* (2003). Auditory sensory processing in autism: a magnetoencephalographic study. *Biological Psychiatry*, **54**, 647–54.

Turkeltaub, P. E., Flowers, D. L., Verbalis, A. *et al.* (2004). The neural basis of hyperlexic reading. An fMRI case study. *Neuron*, **41**, 11–25.

Ullman, M. T. (2001). A neurocognitive perspective on language: the declarative procedural model. *Nature Reviews. Neuroscience*, **2**, 717–26.

Van Baaren, R. B., Holland, R. W., Kawakami, K., and van Knippenberg, A. (2004). Mimicry and prosocial behavior. *Psychological Science*, **15**, 71–4.

Volkmar, F. R. and Pauls, D. (2003). Autism. *The Lancet*, **362**, 1133–41.

Willingham, D. T. and Dunn, E. W. (2003). What neuroimaging and brain localization can do, cannot do and should not do for social psychology. *Journal of Personal and Social Psychology*, **85**, 662–71.

Wohlschlager, A. and Bekkering, H. (2002). Is human imitation based on a mirror-neurone system? Some behavioural evidence. *Experimental Brain Research*, **143**, 335–41.

World Health Organization (1993). *The International Classification of Diseases and Disorders 10* (ICD-10). Classification of Mental and Behavioural Disorders: Diagnostic Criteria for Research. Geneva: WHO.

Yonan, A. L., Alarcón, M., Cheng, R. *et al.* (2003). A genomewide screen of 345 families for autism-susceptibility loci. *American Journal of Human Genetics*, **73**, 886–97.

Yovel, G. and Duchaine, B. (2006). Specialized face perception mechanisms extract both part and spacing information: evidence from developmental prosopagnosia. *Journal of Cognitive Neuroscience*, **18**, 580–93.

Ziv, M. and Frye, D. (2003). The relation between desire and false belief in children's theory of mind: no satisfaction? *Developmental Psychology*, **39**, 859–76.

Index

recency effects 84
recognition memory 84
role of organization and meaning 85
rote memory 83–4
short-term memory 83–4
working memory 85–6
methylphenidate 222–3
mirror neurons and imitative motor learning 313,
    315–16
mirtazapine 233–4
modifier genes, and autism susceptibility 172
mood stabilizing drugs 238–9
mortality rates in adults with autism 295–6
    causes of death 295–6
motor development 73–4
multilocus genetic models 166–8

naltrexone 241–2
neuroanatomy 187–9
    brain imaging studies 189–95
    cerebellar abnormalities in autism 188–90
neurobiology of autism
    brain imaging studies 189–95
    classification schemes and instruments 179–80
    comorbidity 180
    data interpretation challenges 179–80
    neuroanatomy 187–9
    neurochemistry 195–200
    neurology and related conditions 180–7
    neurophysiology 200–5
neurochemistry 195–200
    adrenergic function and stress 199–200
    brain catecholamine dysfunction 199
    dopamine 195, 199
    epinephrine 195, 199–200
    hyperserotonemia 195–8
    maturation effects on monoaminergic systems
        195
    noradrenergic system 195
    norepinephrine 195, 196–7, 199–200
    opioid peptides 199
    purposes of autism research 195
    serotonin 195–8
    tryptophan 195, 197–8
neurofibromatosis, association with autism 42–3
neurological dysfunction 180–2
neurology and related conditions 180–7
    EEG abnormalities in autism 185–7
    epilepsy association with autism 185–7
    neurological dysfunction 180–2
    pre- and perinatal conditions 182–5
    seizure disorders in autism 185–7
neurophysiology 200–5
    brainstem auditory-evoked responses 200
    event-related potentials 200–2
    medical conditions associated with autism 202–5
'nonautistic' pervasive developmental disorders 4–7
nonspeaking children 139, 140
nonspeaking older people 143, 144
noradrenergic system 195

norepinephrine 195, 196–7, 199–200
    drugs affecting function 235–7

olanzapine 225–6
oligogenic multilocus genetic models 166–8
ontogenetic construction 312
ontogenetic inflection 312
opioid peptides 199
outcomes see adult life outcomes
oxytocin 242

paroxetine 230–1
PDD (pervasive developmental disorder)
    prevalence (all types) 47–50
    time trends in incidence rates 35–7, 50–7
PDD-NOS (PDD-not otherwise specified)
    development of diagnostic concepts 7–8
    differential diagnosis 19
    prevalence estimations 43–4, 45
peer modeling 259
perceptual development 70–3
pharmacology see psychopharmacology
phonology and syntax 130, 131
phylogenetic construction 311–12
phylogenetic inflection 312
pictures, use to communicate 139, 143, 144
PKU (phenylketonuria), association with autism
    42–3
pleiotropy 163–4
polygenic multilocus genetic models 166–8
postural abnormalities 180–2
pragmatic problems 95
pragmatics 131
pre- and perinatal conditions 182–5
pregnancy and birth complications 182–5
prevalence estimations
    Asperger syndrome 45–6, 47
    autistic disorder 35–7, 41–2
    childhood disintegrative disorder 45, 47, 48
    PDD (all types) 47–50
    PDD-NOS 43–4, 45
pronoun reversal 136–7
prosodic disorders 137–8
psychiatric disturbances in adulthood 290–5
psychological factors in autism 69–70
    academic function 78–80
    attachment behavior 87–8
    attentional abnormalities 74–5
    autistic savants 80–2
    central coherence theory 106–9
    cognitive flexibility 102–3, 104, 105–6
    communication impairment 94–8
    deviant behaviors 90–1
    echolalia 83–4, 95
    emotion perception 91–3
    executive function theory 102–6
    face perception 91–3
    hyperlexia 78–9, 80–1
    'idiot savant' abilities 80–2
    influence of level of functioning 69–70